Miracle Man of The Western Front
Dr. Varaztad H. Kazanjian

PIONEER PLASTIC SURGEON

BY

HAGOP MARTIN DERANIAN, D.D.S., F.A.C.D., F.I.C.D.

Miracle Man of The Western Front

Dr. Varaztad H. Kazanjian

PIONEER PLASTIC SURGEON

BY

HAGOP MARTIN DERANIAN, D.D.S., F.A.C.D., F.I.C.D.

Foreword by
JOSEPH E. MURRAY, M.D.
Nobel Prize Laureate In Medicine

There were other people too who lived in the quarter and came to the Lilas, and some of them wore Croix de Guerre ribbons in their lapels and others also had the yellow and green of the Médaille Militaire, and I watched how well they were overcoming the handicap of the loss of limbs, and saw the quality of their artificial eyes and the degree of skill with which their faces had been reconstructed. There was always an almost iridescent shiny cast about the considerably reconstructed face, rather like that of a well packed ski run, and we respected these clients more than we did the savants *or the professors, although the latter might well have done their military service too without experiencing mutilation.*

In those days we did not trust anyone who had not been in the war, ...

From Ernest Hemingway's *A Moveable Feast*

Published by Chandler House Press
Worcester, Massachusetts
2007

FIRST EDITION

ISBN-10 1-886284-77-6
ISBN-13 978-1-886284-77-7
Library of Congress Card Number: 2006934878

Library of Congress Cataloging-in –Publication Data

Deranian, Hagop Martin, 1922-
Miracle Man of the Western Front/ Hagop Martin Deranian.-1st ed.
p.cm.
Includes biographical references and index.
ISBN 978-1-886284-77-7
I. Deranian, Hagop Martin, 1922-. Plastic Surgeons-United States-Biography. II. Title

First Printing

PUBLISHED BY
Chandler House Press
PO Box 20100, West Side Station
Worcester, MA 01602 USA
508-753-7419
www.chandlerhousebooks.com

BOOK DESIGN
Kim Cutler Graphic Design, Worcester, MA

For more information about the book: **www.miraclemanofthewesternfront.com**

DEDICATED

To my immediate family
and
To my forebears of another time and place

"The memory of a well-spent life should not be allowed to be forgotten."
Cicero, 106-43 BC, *On Divination*

Contents

Foreword

by Joseph E. Murray, M.D.

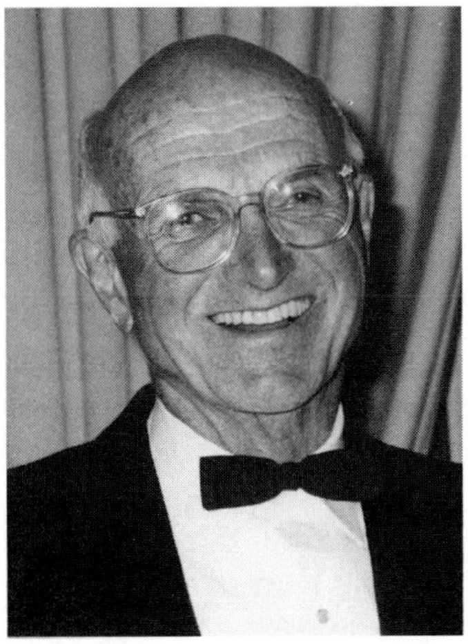

When I started my career in plastic surgery in Boston in 1943, Dr. Kazanjian was already an icon and legend. As a medical student, I had heard the anecdote of a visiting professor from Great Britain speaking to the Harvard medical students after World War I. During the lecture he noticed Dr. Kazanjian's presence and cited his outstanding contributions to the facially injured as a dentist during the war. After the war Dr. Kazanjian had gone on to complete his medical education.

During World War II, assigned as a young general surgeon to Valley Forge General Hospital in Pennsylvania, I learned more about Dr. Kazanjian from Dr. Bradford Cannon. Dr. Cannon was then Chief of Plastic Surgery at VFGH and had worked with Dr. Kazanjian at the Massachusetts Eye and Ear Infirmary.

On my return to Boston after three years of military service, Dr. Cannon asked me to join him as an Associate in the care for the Massachusetts Crippled Children's Program at the Mt. Auburn Hospital in Cambridge. There I first met Dr. K as a professional colleague. He welcomed me warmly.

In my early days, whenever I needed professional consultation, Dr. K was always available. In his recent Kazanjian lecture Dr. Robert Goodwyn recalls that when he was a senior resident at the Brigham on the Surgical Service, a woman in her twenties, a clinic patient, had an ameloblastoma of her lower jaw. Dr. Murray advised resection and immediate iliac bone graft. He suggested, however, that we consult with Dr. Kazanjian. Dr. Goldwyn writes:

Although I had heard of him I had only glimpsed him at a couple of Harvard Medical Alumni reunions. Knowing of my desire to go into plastic surgery, Dr. Murray wanted to give me the opportunity to meet Dr. Kazanjian. He drove the patient and me to Dr. Kazanjian's office in Kenmore Square. Unhurriedly, Dr. Kazanjian talked to us and the patient, making us feel at home and, by his behavior, conveying to the patient the truth: that she was the most important person in the room. After having carefully taken her history and after having examined her, he thoughtfully discussed her with us. He reassured her but not in a cavalier fashion. His reassurance to us also meant a great deal. He agreed with our plan and fortunately, she had the expected outcome.

In the early 1950s, I gave my first talk before the Boston Surgical Society in a Symposium on Surgical Treatment of Cancer. I was assigned treatment of "Head and Neck Cancer With Immediate Reconstruction." I was a bit nervous, a neophyte among the giants of Boston Surgery. Dr. Kazanjian and Dr. Cannon sat together in the audience and I sensed their increasing satisfaction with my presentation. Dr. Kazanjian's support will always remain as an indelible memory.

He was one of the kindest persons I have ever known. Possibly because of his troubled childhood fleeing from the Turks, he developed a special sense of caring. Dr. Deranian has devoted a lifetime in perpetuating the truly outstanding contributions of Dr. Kazanjian. It is a special privilege for me to be part of this superb tribute to one of the world pioneers in plastic surgery.

Author's Note

" . . . in order to understand the life of Kazanjian, one must sit at his feet and look up—rather than lean from an imaginary pedestal. . . . "

—Dr. Moses Strock

The dignified, yet unpretentious, memorial service for Dr. V. H. Kazanjian was held on October 19, 1974, at the Harvard University Memorial Church. My thoughts returned to the first time that I met him. It was during my final year, in 1947, as a student at the University of Pennsylvania School of Dental Medicine, when I heard his name being paged on the loudspeaker. He was in Philadelphia, lecturing to graduate students in oral surgery at the University of Pennsylvania. I ran to meet him and introduced myself. Enthusiastically, yet courteously, he greeted me and seemed genuinely interested in my budding career. Here was the man whose story and exploits I had heard since I was a teenager in Worcester. "I worked next to Dr. Kazanjian in the wire mill," an old man once proudly boasted. "Our families were friends," another remembered. "We lived in the same tenement house on 130 Belmont Street . . . ." These anecdotes and remembrances became a familiar part of my life and a source of inspiration.

His path and that of both my grandfathers must have crossed, as all three of them labored in the Washburn & Moen Manufacturing Company wire mill as immigrants from Ottoman Armenia.

In the years following my student days, during my first years of practice in Boston (1948-1951), we often met, since I practiced a few hundred yards from his office on Commonwealth Avenue. On several occasions, Dr. Kazanjian allowed me to "scrub in" with him on cleft palate operations that he was performing. I also had the rare good fortune to be associated with Dr. Ronald M. King who, as a student at Harvard Dental School, served in General Hospital No. 5 during World War I.

On one particular occasion during the centennial meeting of the American Academy of Dental Science, in October 1967, he took me by the arm and insisted that the photographer capture the moment. Later he autographed the photograph with the inscription:

"To my good friend Dr. Deranian V. H. Kazanjian."

It was fated that I preserve the story of this "Gentle Genius of Plastic Surgery."

H. Martin Deranian

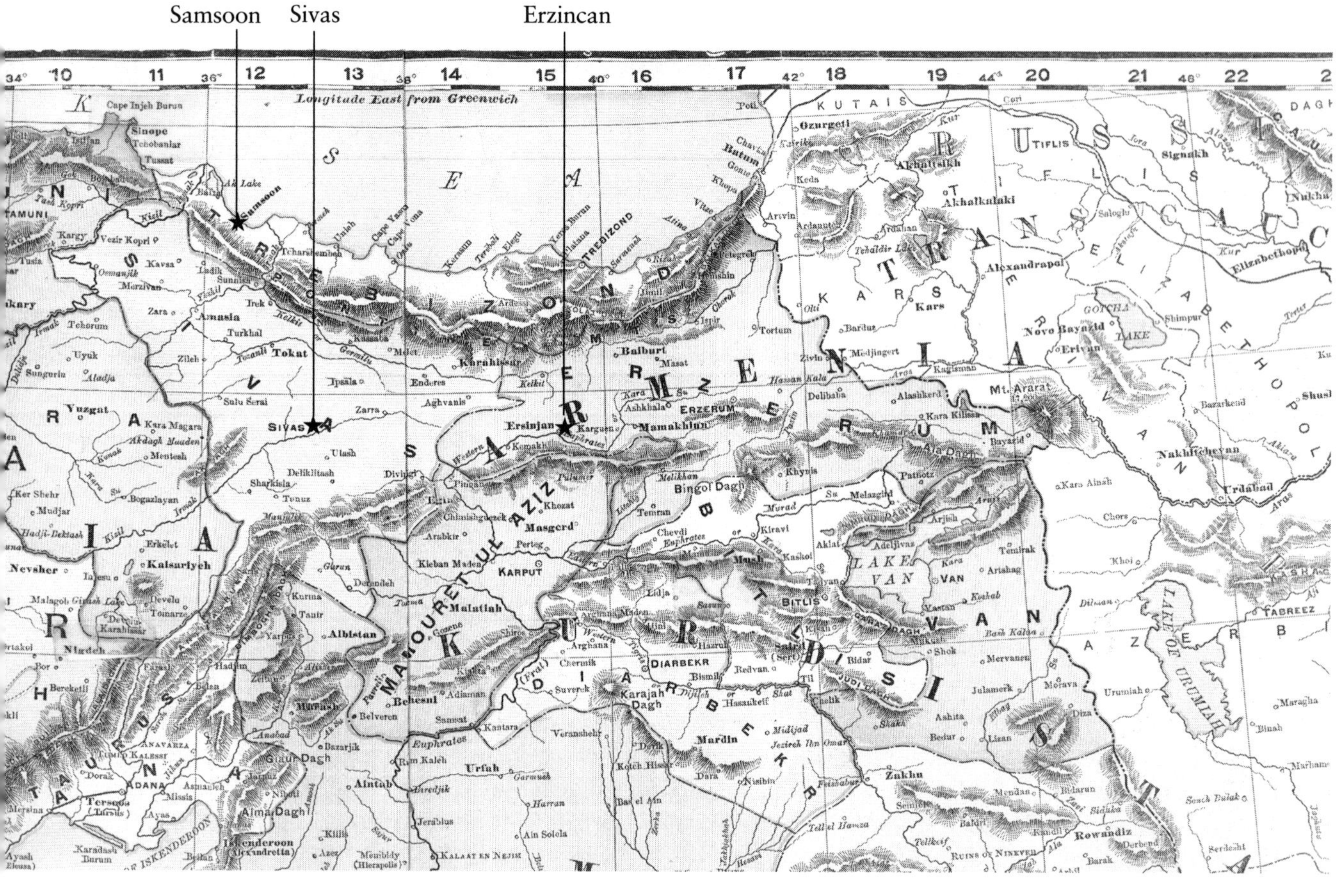

Map of Turkey in Asia in 1895, showing the three towns in which Dr. Kazanjian lived in his youth
Rand McNally Co., 1895, enlarged segment

CHAPTER ONE

Armenia the Homeland

In the regal splendor of Buckingham Palace, Dr. Varaztad Hovhannes Kazanjian, dressed in the uniform of an Honorary Major in the British Royal Army Medical Corps, stood before His Majesty, King George V, on March 15, 1919, for investiture as a Companion of the Most Distinguished Order of Saint Michael and Saint George. It was one of the highest honors that the British Empire could confer upon an individual not a British subject, in this case for outstanding surgical services rendered during World War I. It was an unusual scene; its recipient was until recently an obscure American dentist, who had been born forty years earlier in the declining Ottoman Empire, in a world far away and apart from Buckingham Palace and all that it represented.

For nearly four centuries the ancestral home of the Kazanjian family had been in the city of Erzincan in the province of Erzurum (or Garin) in the heartland of eastern Turkey known as Armenia. At an altitude of 3,900 feet, Erzincan overlooks a rich, well-watered plain through which the western Euphrates River flows. In 1880, a year after Varaztad Kazanjian's birth, its male population was estimated to be 61,109.[1]

The earliest mention of a settlement on the site of Erzincan is in an Urartian inscription from the eighth century B.C. From pagan times, it was an important religious center. A famous temple and gold statue of Anahid, the mother of the Armenians, goddess of fertility and protectress of the nation, were located there. (Anahid is the counterpart of Artemis in Greek mythology, known to the Romans as Diana.) In 35 B.C. the Roman general Mark Antony destroyed the statue of Anahid and distributed the gold among his generals. The shrine was rebuilt but was destroyed forever by Saint Gregory, the Illuminator, who firmly established Christianity in Armenia early in the fourth century (301 A.D.). Armenia became the first nation to adopt Christianity as its state religion; its church is apostolic, claiming succession of spiritual authority from the apostles Thaddeus and Bartholomew.[2]

In the centuries that followed, Erzincan was successively conquered by the Byzantines, Persians, Arabs, and Mongols, by Tamerlane and by Turkoman tribes. In 1473, it was annexed to the Ottoman Empire by Sultan Mohammed II. Surrounded by mountains and somewhat isolated, it was situated on one of the principal seismic faults in Asia Minor. After an earthquake in 1682, the city was moved from the shores of the Euphrates River two kilometers to the north. It continued to suffer from cataclysmic earthquakes and was almost completely destroyed in 1784. The devastating earthquakes and the seemingly endless ingress of conquerors caused the town to lose many inhabitants. After 1600, it never again enjoyed the prosperity of the past.[3]

In their travels through the area, Marco Polo (1254-1324), the Venetian, and Ibn Batuta (1304-1377), the Arab, recorded the fine quality of the textiles and fabrics that were woven in Erzincan.[4] Following weaving, the most widely practiced and highly developed craft in the city was copper-

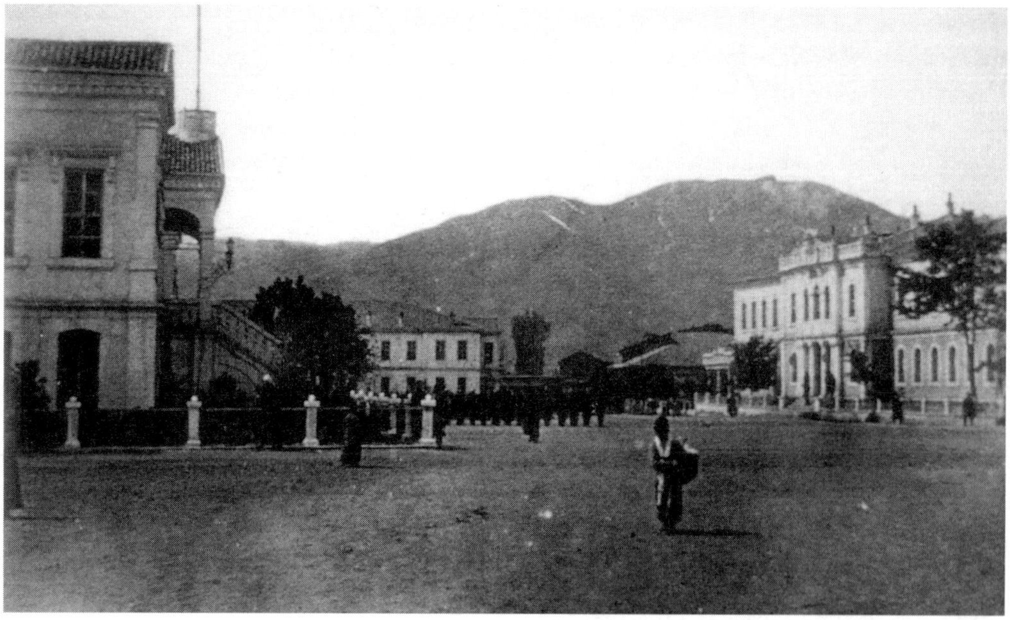

Scene in the center of Erzincan circa 1906
Photograph from Kévorkian and Paboudjian, Les Arméniens: dans l'Empire Ottoman à la Veille du Génocide *(Paris: Les Editions d'Arte et Histoire, 1992) p. 452. Photograph #749*

smithing. The superiority of Erzincan coppersmiths was recognized as far away as Paris, Vienna, and even Philadelphia, where their handiwork was exhibited at the nineteenth century world's fairs. There were two levels of coppersmiths; the products of one were rustic, and, those of the other more refined. The latter were fewer, and the quality and artistry of their production was rivaled only in Constantinople and Tokat, a city in the neighboring province of Sivas.[5]

The original Kazanjian family name was Yerikian, which signified "of noble heritage." Over time, the family name was converted into its Turkish cognomen of Kazanjian, meaning coppersmiths. The family had been kazanjis for generations. They fabricated the huge vats and cauldrons used for cooking and boiling liquids over an open fire. The molding of this brilliant and malleable metal with its peculiar red color was an expert craft that had been practiced in Erzincan from ancient times. "The memory of the bright [copper] metal," a previous Kazanjian biographer observed, "is in the family consciousness like the clash of a cymbal." [6]

True to its tradition as a religious center, Erzincan in 1886 housed a celebrated monastery named for Saint Gregory, as well as eight Armenian schools and five Armenian churches. The Kazanjians belonged to the traditional Armenian Apostolic Church. The family was prominent in the Armenian community; it belonged to the upper middle class and was "fairly well off." Varaztad Kazanjian was born at a time and place where tradition was the guiding principle of life. As Armenians and Christians, the family lived as a minority in an Ottoman Turkish Muslim land. Though subjugated, the Armenians had clung tenaciously to their Christian tradition and had maintained their identity. For centuries they had lived in relative harmony with the Turks. Some of them held high positions of trust in the government. "For although we are a small country and very restricted in numbers, weak in power, and often subject to another's rule," the fifth-cen-

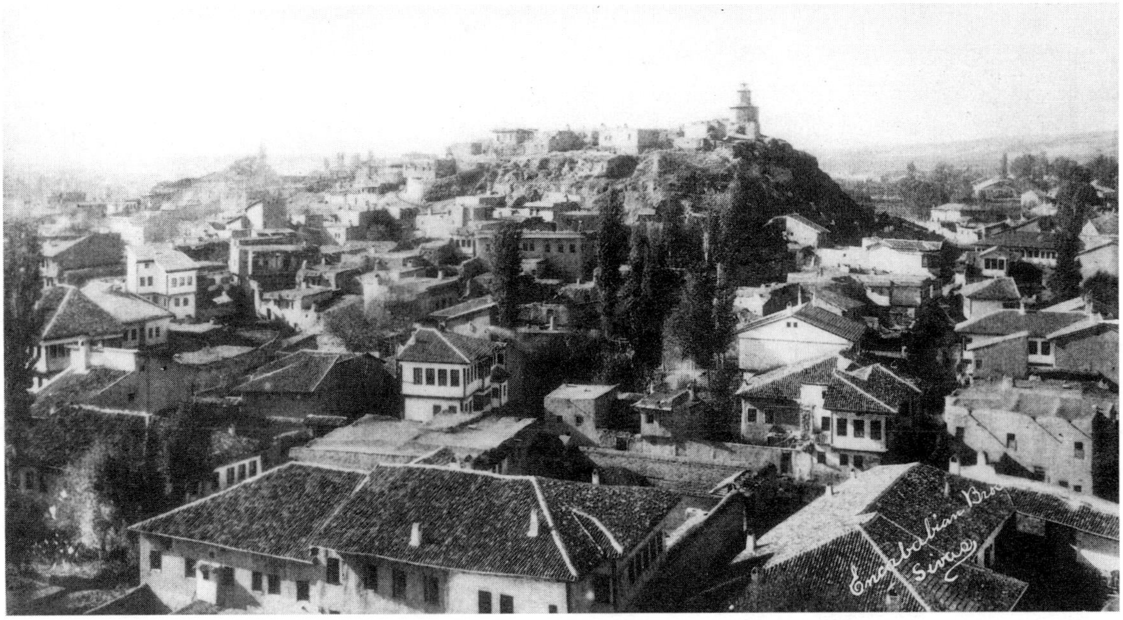

Sivas (Sebastia) circa 1910-12; "View of the clock and the environs of the ancient citadel"
Photographer Encababian Brothers; Courtesy of Yervant Alexanian, Project SAVE Armenian Photograph Archives

tury Armenian historian, Moses Khorenatsi, wrote, "yet many manly deeds have been performed in our land."[7]

Varaztad's father, Hovhannes Kazanjian, like his forebears before him, was a kazanji. His life had tragedy. He had lost his wife after he had fathered five children. He then married Anna Siroonian, a widow with three children. Out of this new union came three more children. The first was Varaztad Hovhannes Kazanjian, born on March 18, 1879, in Erzincan.[8] (Only four days before, on March 14, 1879, Albert Einstein was born in Ulm in the German state of Württemberg.)

The name Varaztad was historically significant. It was the name of a king of Armenia who ruled in the fourth century. He was described as "spirited, personable, strong, full of all deeds of valor and very expert at archery . . . he had killed lions for which he was praised and honored by the contestants of the Olympic games." About 377 A.D. Varaztad was banished to the "'Island of Thule' by which is meant the British Isles."[9]

It was not long before Hovhannes Kazanjian sensed the need for a locale with more financial opportunities and better schools for his children than Erzincan had to offer his growing family. In 1881, when Varaztad was about two-and-a-half years old, his father moved his family and his large copper business from Erzincan to Sivas, 150 miles westward and seven days journey by horse. Sivas, or Sebastia, is the name of both the province and its chief city situated on the broad valley and located on a tributary of the Kizil Irmak (or Halys) River at an altitude of 4,420 feet. Larger and more cosmopolitan than Erzincan, Sivas was considered by Varaztad Kazanjian to be his home-town. Sivas had a large number of coppersmiths. There was a special bazaar with seventy-five shops where coppersmiths and tinsmiths displayed their wares. Varaztad's brother, Roupen (Roopen) Kazanjian, was listed as one of these artisans after his return to Sivas from America in the early 1900s.[10]

Sivas was in existence centuries before there were any Turks in that area. The Romans called it

Sebastia as the Armenians still do. Even then it was an important trade center. Under Diocletian, near the end of the third century, the city of Sivas became the capital of Armenia Minor. For centuries thereafter it was a part of the Byzantine Empire. Under the Seljuk Turks it became one of Anatolia's most important cities and was called "The Pearl of Armenia." Marco Polo, in his travels through Anatolia in 1275, noted that the Armenians in Sivas were weaving "silk fabrics of crimson and other colors of great beauty and richness, and many other kinds of cloth."[11]

Sivas, like Erzincan, had been subjugated by a succession of invaders. One of the most ruthless was Tamerlane (Timur, the Lame, 1336-1405), who invaded Sivas in 1400. The city was defended by 4,000 men, primarily cavalry and archers, and mostly Armenian. After resisting for three weeks, they surrendered upon Tamerlane's promise not to shed blood. However, the conquerors got around their chief's promise by burying all soldiers alive. Thousands of children had met him with garlands of roses. He had both the children and the roses crushed under the hoofs of his horses. The place was called "Black Earth" and became the site of an Armenian church.[12]

From 1880 to 1882 Sivas was the residence of the British military consul-general for Asia Minor. Beginning in 1886, the first American consul to serve in the Turkish interior was sent to Sivas. Until 1915, great emphasis was placed on education among the Armenians. Sivas contained ten Apostolic boys' schools, three Apostolic girls' schools, seven Protestant boys' schools, and one Protestant girls' school. There were six Armenian churches: four Apostolic, one Protestant and one Catholic.[13]

In Sivas was located the Monastery of the Holy Cross, which was built in the ninth century "and ever since [has been] the sanctuary and stronghold of the Christian faith in all the long, bitter years of misfortune and persecution which this oldest of Christian Churches has suffered."[14] It was once the palace of the medieval king of the Armenians. Sivas was the birthplace in 1686 of the abbot, Mekhitar, who established an Armenian religious brotherhood under the patronage of the Roman Catholic Church. He became the founder of the order of the Mekhitarists and of the famous monastery in Venice. The city also had a Jesuit mission as well as a flourishing American mission with churches and schools. In 1880-1881, French Jesuits established a school called the Forty Martyrs (College des Quarante). It taught classes from kindergarten to the twelfth grade and eventually had 300 students, most of whom were Armenian, with the exception of fifteen or twenty Greeks. Instruction was in French. By 1912 there were ten or twelve French fathers and fifteen or twenty nuns located in Sivas.[15]

Sivas also had a strong Protestant presence. The American Board of Commissioners for Foreign Missions established a mission in Sivas in 1851. The missionaries Albert and Emma Hubbard reported that in November 1873 there were five American missionaries in Sivas, including a medical missionary, Dr. West, who "treats all missionaries far and near free of charge." In speaking of their obligations as missionaries in Sivas, Henry Holbrook, one of the later American missionaries, asserted:

> *Our first work here has been . . . with the nominally Christian peoples—Armenians and Greeks. It is very hard to make you realize this . . . for the longing to grapple at once with the Moslem [Muslim] problem dies hard. It seems less heroic . . . to go quietly to work to educate a few hundred Armenian and Greek children.*[16]

Eventually the Protestant missionaries established a circle of twenty elementary schools around the city, enrolling over 700 children, according to Frank A. Stone. In 1880, Dr. Henry T. Perry estab-

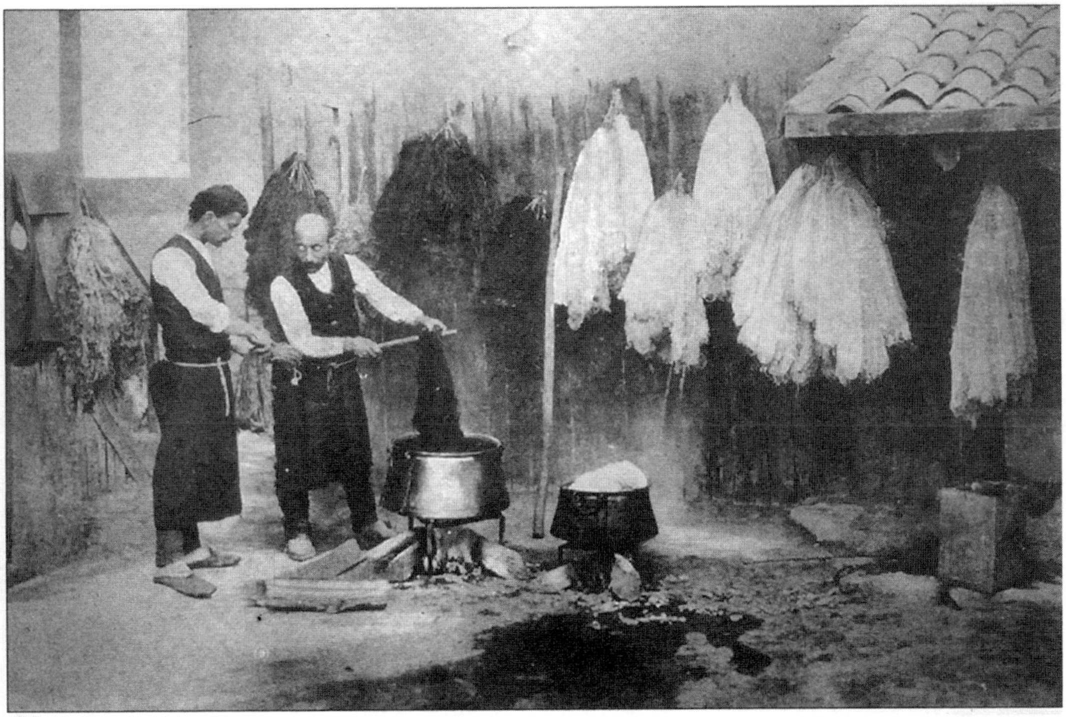

Dyers in Sebastia (Sivas). Pictured are the copper vats or caldrons used for boiling the dye lots
Photograph from Kévorkian and Paboudjian, p. 241, Photograph #393

lished a boys' normal school there in order to prepare the most promising students for teaching careers. "We live right in the heart of a busy city of 75,000 inhabitants," the missionary Henry Holbrook wrote in 1912, "the metropolis of central Asia Minor." In 1912, the normal school became the Sivas Teachers' College, but "sadly 1915 saw all of the Armenians deported from Sivas, snuffing out the life of this first American sponsored program in Turkey on the college level that was completely devoted to preparing teachers."[17]

Varaztad's earliest education was in an American-sponsored Protestant school in Sivas, followed by study with French Jesuits, where he came under their rigid and disciplined schedule, until the age of fourteen. He learned to read and write not only his native Armenian, but French and Turkish as well. He was also taught Armenian and European history, chemistry, physics, and mathematics. Instruction in English was not available. Cholera broke out in Sivas in April 1894, with from thirty to forty deaths daily. The Jesuit fathers went from house to house helping people. Since they were not fluent in Armenian or Turkish, it was young Varaztad who interpreted for them. For the rest of his life he greatly admired the Jesuits, feeling that they were closer to the people than the American missionaries.[18]

Sivas was known for its long and bitter winters. During the three months of summer there was a great deal of mud. "The streets were not built on a plan," one native of Sivas observed. "There was no water system, no sewer or electricity, no central heating or any of the comforts of technology which the western world takes for granted." The railroad did not reach Sivas until

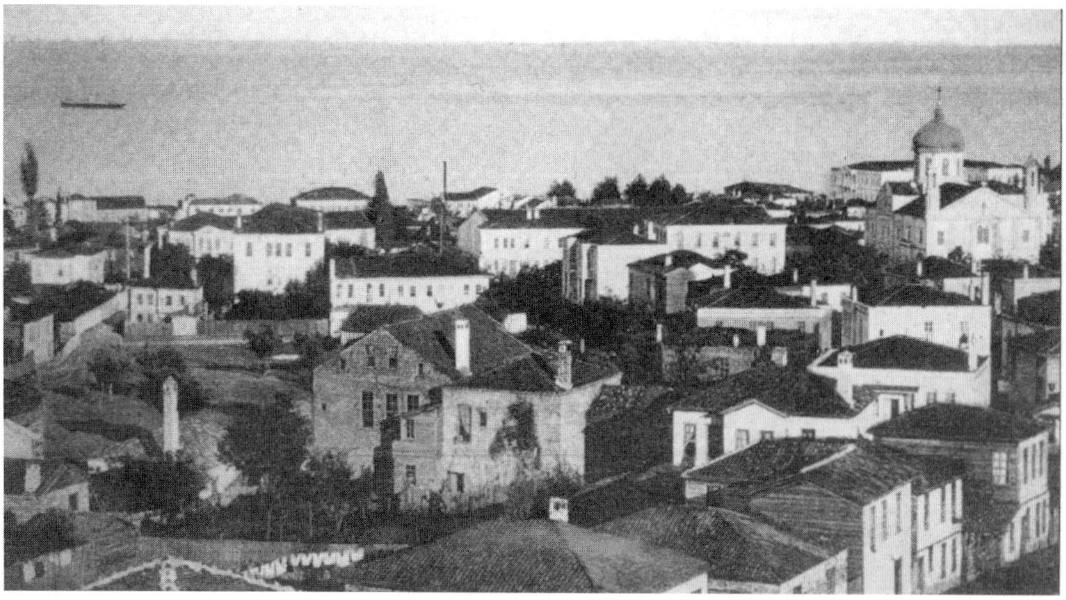

The city of Samsun showing the Greek cathedral
Photograph from Kévorkian and Paboudjian, p. 197, Photograph #324

1930. Holbrook, in commenting of the mud of Sivas, wrote: "Your rubbers, to be of any use at all, must be buttoned. . . . Everybody throws all kinds of refuse into the streets, the sewers often flow in open ditches through the middle of the street, and when covered by an inch of boards, often become clogged and overflow."[19]

Hovhannes Kazanjian, the father, died in 1891, when Varaztad was twelve years old. When he was fourteen years old, the son left Sivas forever. "I wrote a letter to my oldest (half) brother, Hagop [or Jacob]," he later recalled. "He was a commission merchant in Samsun, a port town on the Black Sea, in Turkey [in the Province of Trebizond]. He sent for me and took me into his business." The northerly journey from Sivas to Samsun took ten days by wagon over the mountains. Varaztad did not remain an apprentice commission merchant long, saying, "I wasn't good enough."[20] After working for a few months as a clerk-bookkeeper in his half brother's business, he accepted a position as a clerk in the Austrian post office in Samsun. Being a port city and influenced by European trade and culture, Samsun was somewhat cosmopolitan. At that time, several European countries maintained their own post offices there.

This was also a time of great peril for the Armenians in Turkey. "The increasing Turkish measures of oppression created such an atmosphere of fear," Dr. Carl W. Waldron reported, "that Armenian history books were hidden behind basement foundation stones and were read only in secret." The oppressive and corrupt regime of the Turkish sultans was becoming increasingly unacceptable to the educated segment of the population, which was in contact with western ideas of democracy and nationalism. Faced with growing pressures, the Turkish government issued a series of reform decrees on paper, but in practice became more and more repressive. Conditions were particularly difficult for the Armenians, who were discriminated against in many ways. For example, they were not allowed to own or carry arms, their villages were left unprotected and exposed to neighboring tribes, and their testimony was not accepted in court. In response, Armenians banded together and formed secret societies as a means of seeking justice and protection. The fifteen-year-old Varaztad sympathized with one of these revolutionary societies, known as the Hunchakists. The Hunchak Revolutionary Party was the first socialist party in Turkey and Persia. It was founded in Geneva in August 1887 by seven Russian-Armenian students who were Marxist. "The ideological impact of the times led them to a new view of society . . . To achieve full and real freedom . . . it was imperative to establish a new order based on humanitarian and socialistic principles . . . a new one might be built, based upon `economic truths' and `socialistic justice'." They published a newspaper called *Hunchak* (Bell).[21]

The Armenian patriots in England, France, and Switzerland printed forbidden pamphlets against the Turkish government and against Sultan Abdul Hamid and mailed them to fictitious names in care of the Austrian post office where they were claimed by members of the Armenian patriotic groups. That was the only way leaflets, tracts and all other instruments that the sultan regarded as seditious could enter the country because of the vast system of censorship. "Under a set of rules known as the Capitulations, foreigners living in the empire were exempt from trial in Ottoman courts; they maintained their own postal systems in which Ottoman censorship did not apply. This did not prevent the sultan's spies from maintaining a vigil outside each foreign-operated post office. A careful watch was kept on who entered and left such buildings. Ottoman citizens seen around these post offices were likely to be jailed or banished."[22]

Young Varaztad and four other Armenian youths formed a junior group to work for the cause of freedom. His position in the post office was strategic and frequently in the darkness before dawn he would distribute the pamphlets protesting the massacres of the Armenian people, one source has noted; another has added, "He would throw the pamphlets over the walls of the Turkish homes in the middle of the night. The material he was distributing sought to inform the Turkish people of the persecution of the Armenians."[23] As might be expected, the Turkish authorities began an investigation to discover the source of the forbidden literature. Armenians considered guilty of acts against Turkey were imprisoned, exiled, and sometimes put to death.

After six months, Varaztad's activities came to the attention of the Turkish authorities. Fortunately, his family learned that he was under suspicion. At the crucial moment, he was smuggled by his half-brother Hagop aboard a ship that sailed from Samsun to Marseille. He was accompanied by his twin twenty-six year-old half-brothers, Alexander and Roupen, born of his father's first marriage. Varaztad had to leave or face the repressive measures of the Turkish authorities. Had the Sultan of Turkey carried out the provisions of the 1878 Treaty of Berlin for reform, and had the European Powers "been willing to direct attention to their commitments relative to the Armenians, the continued succession of massacres following 1878 might not have occurred, and Varaztad Kazanjian might well have lived his days in Sivas."[24] "When I left Armenia," he later disclosed to his associate, Dr. John Marquis Converse, "it was not because conditions were bad, but to escape imprisonment." At least one member of his family, his half-brother from his mother's first marriage, Harootiun Siroonian, was in America before 1895 and may have, with others, encouraged his emigration to America.[25]

The Kazanjian brothers arrived in Marseille in the summer of 1895, just before the catastrophic storm of massacres erupted in Turkey that were to seal the fate of the oppressed Armenians. They joined a group of other Armenian expatriates who were en route north to Cherbourg. Among them

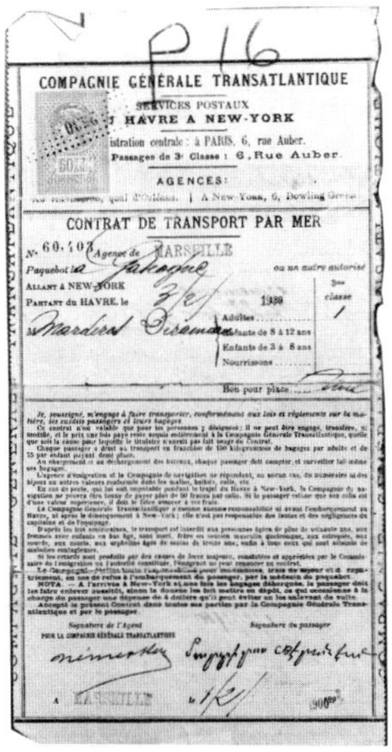
COMPAGNIE GÉNÉRALE TRANSATLANTIQUE

SERVICES POSTAUX

HAVRE A NEW-YORK

istration centrale : à PARIS, 6, rue Auber.

Passages de 3e Classe : 6, Rue Auber.

AGENCES:

A New-York, 6, Bowling Green

CONTRAT DE TRANSPORT PAR MER

No 60,403 Agence de MARSEILLE

Paquebot la ... ou un autre autorisé

ALLANT A NEW-YORK

PARTANT du HAVRE, le ... 1899 ... 3me classe

Adultes ... Enfants de 8 à 12 ans ... Enfants de 3 à 8 ans ... Nourrissons ...

Bon pour place ...

Above:
An example of a third class transatlantic steamship ticket from LeHavre to New York, 1900, used by the author's father

Below:
Sicilia, *Hamburg Amerika Line Courtesy Peabody Essex Museum, Salem, Mass.*

was a friend from Sivas, Boghos Der Bedrosian, who came to the United States later. In LeHavre the Kazanjian brothers boarded a ship bound for New York. In a misadventure typical of the period, the exploiters who arranged their passage forced them to share a cabin with sixty others in virtual steerage and under intolerable conditions. "I was very sick," Varaztad remembered.[26] The crossing was harsh and brutal.

To Varaztad Kazanjian fleeing oppression, the Statue of Liberty, sheathed in copper, must have seemed like the "Mother of Exiles" who welcomed him as one who was "yearning to breathe free." "I arrived at Ellis Island with a bundle on my back and nothing else," he recalled. "You didn't even need a passport in those days." The year was 1895, but the exact date of his arrival had been open to question. He had no visible means of support. The archival evidence points to November 11, 1895, as the date of his arrival aboard the *Sicilia,* a ship of the Hamburg Amerika line.[27]

At Ellis Island, the lad of sixteen years was held for some days before being admitted, as the immigration officials were concerned that he would become a public charge. It was a difficult situation, because he had little or no knowledge of English and no references other than a slip of paper with the name of an Armenian friend of the family who lived in New York. (Another source reports that "his only contact was an Armenian in Worcester," Massachusetts.) Providentially he was admitted to the United States, but little could the immigration official at Ellis Island imagine that standing before him was a sixteen-year-old boy who would become one of the most famous surgeons in the nation and in the world.[28]

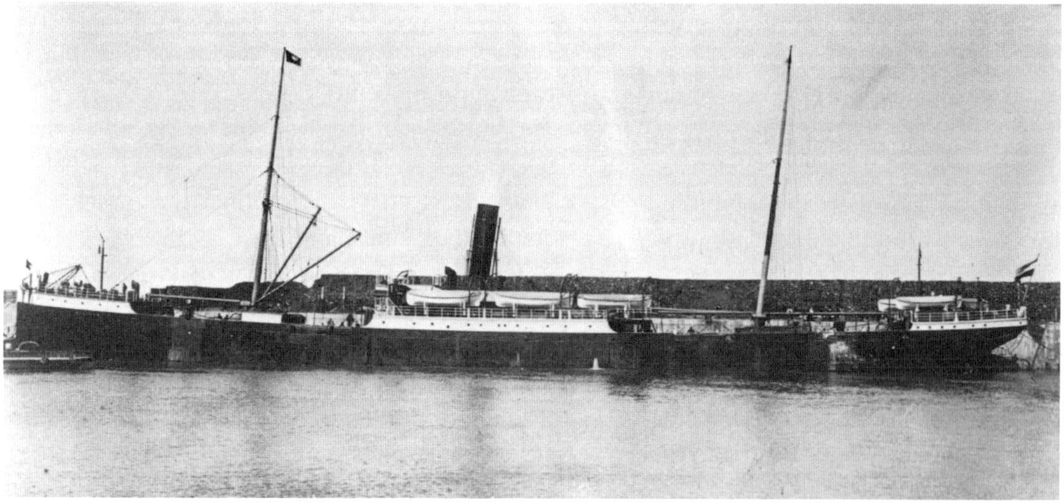

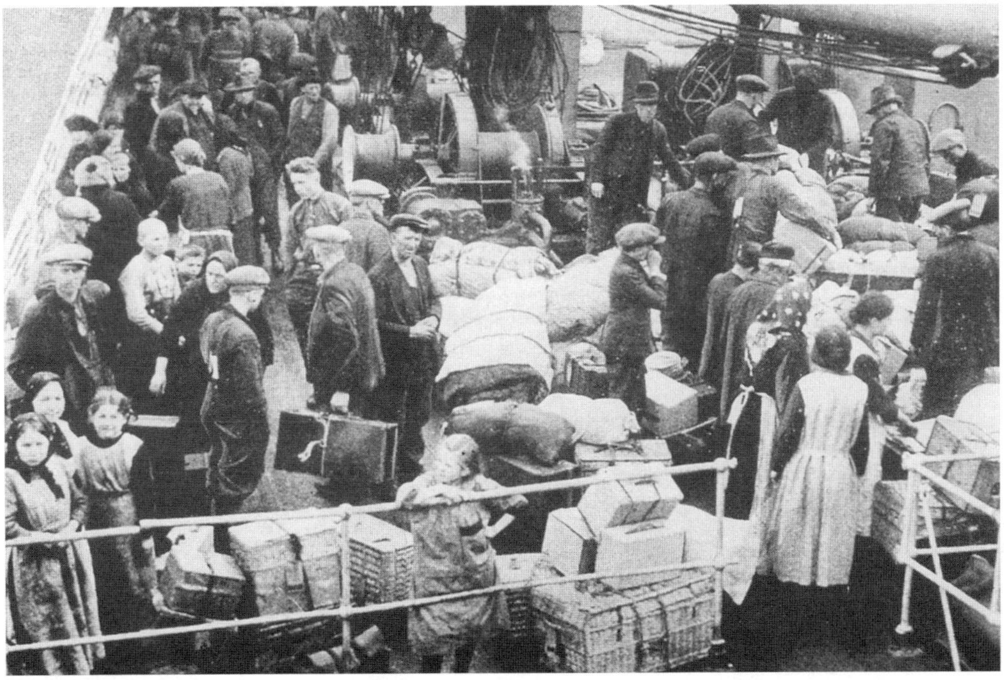

Ellis Island. Steerage passengers, circa 1890 Courtesy of the Ellis Island Immigration Museum

While he was waiting at Ellis Island, Varaztad learned from newer immigrants about the horrendous acts of brutality and atrocities committed in 1895 against the Armenians in Turkey by the government of Sultan Abdul Hamid II. In 1894, inspired by the Hunchaks, the mountain district of Sasun had refused to pay protection taxes to their Kurdish neighbors. The Ottoman response was prompt and brutal: twenty-five villages were exterminated. Then on September 18, 1895, the Hunchak party staged a demonstration at Constantinople, and fighting broke out. Angered at the European pressure for long-promised reforms in the Armenian provinces, Sultan Abdul Hamid launched a merciless series of pogroms to settle the Armenian question. The massacres began on October 21, 1895.[29]

Rebecca Krikorian, an Armenian who arrived in America on August 13, 1895, recorded her feelings of anguish:

It was on the very first days of my arrival in New York City that the horrible massacres of 1895 broke out in Turkey, when about one hundred thousand of our beloved people were butchered most mercilessly . . . . Mail and telegraphic communications were cut off in my town as well as in many cities and towns in Turkey, and for days and weeks I could not hear any news from the members of my immediate family . . . but I read in daily papers of the awful accounts . . . So I did not know for a long time for whom to pray and for whom to weep."[30]

From another source we learn that the massacres of Armenians in Sivas began on November 12, 1895. The American Consul in Sivas, Milo Jewett, in a dispatch to the Department of State on November 16, 1895, reported that:

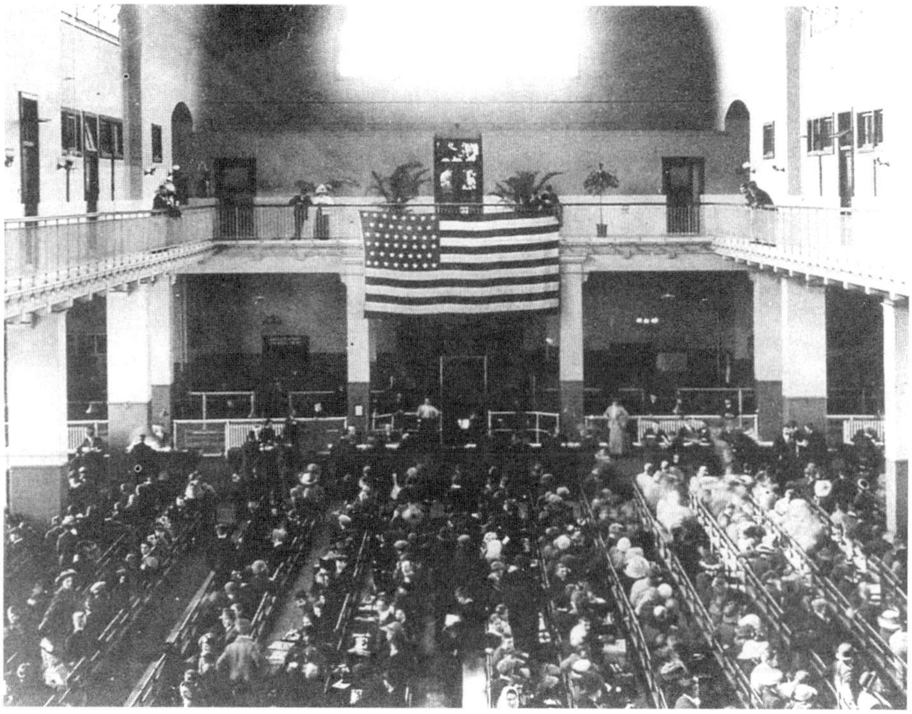

Ellis Island, the Registry Room or "Great Hall of Judgment," circa 1890. Courtesy Ellis Island Immigration Museum

> *About 11 o'clock a.m. the massacre began suddenly in the market streets devoted to shops and stores. The Mohamedans rushed upon the Armenians and began killing them and plundering the shops. The rioters were mostly of the younger rough class of Mohamedans of the city, Kars emigrants and the military force of the city. At first the rioters used their clubs chiefly, but as the soldiers and gendarmes rushed into the market and began to shoot the Armenians, the bashibazooks [wild irregulars] used their swords, daggers and firearms with terrible effect. The number killed up to date seems to be between 800 and 1,000 and about ten Turks.*[31]

Varaztad and his brothers were among the few fortunate to be on American soil, but they had no way of knowing the fate of several members of their family still in Turkey. Later they learned that their family had survived. "When we left Sivas," Dr. Garabed Hagop Paelian reminisced much later in a letter to Dr. Kazanjian, "whoever could have dreamed what the future had in store in America!" Paelian, who was born in Sivas in 1880, emigrated to America in 1906 and became a distinguished scientist and teacher. From New York, Varaztad and his fellow travelers went directly to the home of a fellow countryman in Worcester.[32]

NOTES

1 Erzincan is variously spelled as Erzingan, Erzinjan, Erzinca and Yerzinga. See Hratch A. Tarbassian, *Erzurum (Garin): Its Armenian History and Traditions*, translated from the Armenian by Nigol Schahgaldian (Garin Compatriotic Union of the U.S., 1975); *Encyclopaedia Britannica: A Dictionary of Arts, Science, Literature and General Information*, 11th ed. (Cambridge: University Press, 1910-1911, 29 v.), v. 9, p. 759. Of the 61,109 males, 11,181 were Armenians. *British Documents on Ottoman Armenians* (Ankara: Publication of the Turkish Historical Society, No. 78a, 1983), v. 2, 1880-1890, Table 1, p. 129. Major Henry Trotter reported, p. 126: "I am of the opinion that an addition of twenty to twenty-five percent of the number given will generally give a near approximation of the true number."

2 *Soviet Armenian Encyclopedia* (Erevan, Armenia: 1977), v. 3, pp. 584-585 (in Armenian). Moses Khorenatsi, *History of the Armenians*, translated by Robert W. Thomson (Cambridge, Mass.: Harvard University Press, 1978), contains the story of Saint Gregory, pp. 245-253; also, Tarbassian, *Erzurum*, p. 30.

3 Raymond H. Kévorkian and Paul B. Paboudjian, *Les Arméniens dans l'Empire Ottoman à la Veille du Génocide* (Paris: Les Éditions d'Art et d'Histoire, 1992), p. 453-454 (in French); this work contains a history of Erzincan and a collection of photographs. *Encyclopaedia Britannica*, v. 9, p. 759; *Soviet Armenian Encyclopedia*, v. 3, pp. 584-585.

4 *Encyclopaedia Britannica*, p. 759; also, *Soviet Armenian Encyclopedia*, v. 3, pp. 584-585. Ibn Batuta noted that the Armenian section of Erzincan was the largest, with neatly arranged stalls in the marketplace.

5 K. Surmenian, *Erzincan* (Cairo: Sahag Mesrob Press, 1947), p. 180 (in Armenian). The more rustic variety of coppersmithing was called in Armenian *kazantiutiune* and the more refined was called *sanagortsutiune*.

6 Ivan Sandrof, "World's Most Famous Plastic Surgeon," *Worcester Sunday Telegram*, January 12, 1958, Feature Parade section, p. 3, cols. 1-5. See also James A. Tashjian, "Dr. Varaztad Kazanjian, a Profile," *Armenian Review* 1, no. 1 (Winter 1948): 89.

7 Khorenatsi, *History*, p. 69; *Soviet Armenian Encyclopedia*, v. 3, pp. 584-585; Tashjian, "Profile." Noah Gordon, "Dr. Varaztad Kazanjian of Belmont Still Active at 80: Immigrant Boy Became 'Miracle Man' of Plastic Surgery in World War," *Boston Sunday Herald*, September 20, 1959, Section II, p. 2, quotes Dr. Kazanjian in referring to his family in Armenia: "We were fairly well off." Also personal communication with Sylvie (Tahmizian) Desteian, on December 12, 1994, Cambridge, Mass. Her father was born in Erzincan and related that the Tahmizians and Kazanjians were among the wealthiest families there.

8 Hélène K. Sargeant, Dr. Kazanjian's daughter, "Some Notes Concerning the Family of Dr. Varaztad H. Kazanjian," March 1978, preserved in Varaztad H. Kazanjian Archive in The Francis A. Countway Library of Medicine, Harvard Medical School, Boston: "Anna Seroonian's children by her first marriage were a married son, Hampartsum, a married daughter, and a young son, Haroot. Hovhannes Kazanjian's children by his first marriage were two married daughters, a married son, Jacob [Hagop], and ten-year-old twins, Alexander and Roupen." Hovhannes Kazanjian's middle name was Alexander. His wife Anna's middle name was Flora (Register of the Dental School of Harvard University Freshmen, September 25, 1902, Harvard Dental School). The other two children of this union between Hovhannes and Anna Kazanjian were another son, Yervant, and a daughter, Nouvart. In the Registration Record of the Freshman class entering September 1902, Varaztad H. Kazanjian listed his birthday as March "5" but crossed it out and entered March "18" with the notation "By new calendar."

9 Khorenatsi, *History*, p. 301. For the derivation of the name Varaztad, see Nina G. Garsoian, *The Epic Histories Attributed to Pawstos Buzand* (Cambridge, Mass.: Harvard University Press, 1989), p. 423: Varazdat, middle Persian, "given by the wild boar," i.e. the Zoroastrian god. Also, letter to the author from James R. Russell, Mesrob Mashtots Professor of Armenian Studies, Harvard University, March 2, 1995: "The name Varaztad comes from two Parthian words in Armenian; *Varaz*, 'wild boar,' the totem of the god of victory (Vahagn, the Dragon-slayer), and *dat*, 'given, created.' The name means

'gift of Vahagn.'" On King Varaztad, see David Marshall Lang, *Armenia, Cradle of Civilization* (London: Allen and Unwin, 1970), p. 162; Jacques de Morgan, *The History of the Armenian People*: translated by Ernest F. Barry (Boston: Hairenik Press, 1918), who states (p. 403) that Varaztad was King of Armenia from 374 to 378. Vahan M. Kurkjian, *A History of Armenia* (New York: Armenian General Benevolent Union of America, 1964), p. 503.

10 Carl W. Waldron, "A Testimonial to Varaztad Kazanjian," *Journal of Oral Surgery* 13, no. 2 (April 1955): 93; *Encyclopaedia Britannica*, v. 25, p. 163; Arakel Patrik, ed., *History of the Armenians of Sebastia and Neighboring Villages* (Beirut: Mesrob Press, 1974, in Armenian), pp. 605, 811, who reports that of the 1,750 craftsmen in Sivas, 1,500 were Armenians.

11 Bertha S. Papazian, *The Tragedy of Armenia* (Boston: Pilgrim Press, 1918), p. 128; *The Travels of Marco Polo,* translated by Ronald Latham (Middlesex [England] and New York: Harmondsworth, 1958), p. 47, quoted in Lucy Der Manuelian, "An Introduction to Rug Weaving in Armenia," in *Weavers, Merchants and Kings: The Inscribed Rugs of Armenia* (Fort Worth, Texas: Kimball Art Museum, 1984), p. 25.

12 Patrik, *Armenians of Sebastia*, p. 806; Papazian, *Tragedy*, p. 128.

13 *Encyclopaedia Britannica*, v. 25, p. 163; *Soviet Armenian Encyclopedia*, v. 10, p. 258; Edwin W. Martin, *The Hubbards of Sivas, A Chronicle of Love and Faith* (Santa Barbara, Calif.: Fithian Press, 1991), pp. 9, 158. Albert and Emma Hubbard were American Protestant missionaries in Sivas from 1865 to 1900. This book is a collection of their letters. The Hubbards were Edwin Martin's wife's grandparents. The book provides an invaluable view of what life was like for Armenians in Sivas.

14 C. Henry Holbrook, "Impressions of Sivas 1912," *Journal of Armenian Studies* 5, no. 1 (Winter/Spring 1990-91): 60. His paper contains a picturesque and vivid description of Sivas. The original manuscript is in the collection of the American Board of Commissioners for Foreign Missions located at the Houghton Library, Harvard University. Rev. Holbrook's service in Turkey lasted from 1911 to 1913. He was killed by a stray bullet while touring with a group of native teachers in the isolated hill country east of Sivas. Kévorkian and Papoudjian, *Les Arméniens,* contains (p. 230) a history of Sivas. The population figures for Sivas vary greatly. George H. Filian, *Armenia and Her People* (Hartford: American Publishing Co., 1896), states (p. 275) that the population was "about 30,000: one third are Christian Armenians and there are many Armenian Christian towns and villages round about, so that, if the Armenians are not more numerous than the Mohammedans, they equal them in number."

15 Patrik, *Armenians of Sebastia*, pp. 807-808, 521-528; Holbrook, "Impressions," p. 48.

16 Holbrook, "Impressions," p. 57. Also, Joseph L. Grabill, *Protestant Diplomacy and the Near East* (Minneapolis: University of Minnesota Press, 1971), p. 5; Martin, *Hubbards of Sivas,* p. 61. Sivas was in the Western Turkey mission.

17 Frank A Stone, *Academies for Anatolia* (Lantham, Maryland: University Press of America, 1984), p. 92. Stone reported on the piety of the Armenians: "The Armenian Protestants of Sivas weren't wealthy and Dr. Charles C. Tracy, after meeting with a committee of them, remarked [p. 94] that no greater amount of enlightenment and good desire, combined with humble poverty, could be brought together in one room." Holbrook, "Impressions," pp. 60, 68.

18 Waldron, "Testimonial," p. 93; Tashjian, "Profile," p. 89; letter from Florence Chakerian, Albuquerque, NM, June 4, 2001. (Her mother's paternal uncle, Aram Zartarian, was a student at the Jesuit school at the same time as Varaztad); Martin, *Hubbards of Sivas,* pp. 227-228; V. H. Kazanjian, taped interview with Robin Anderson, 1971, National Archives of Plastic Surgery in The Francis A. Countway Library of Medicine.

19 Kerop Bedoukian, *Some of Us Survived: The Story of an Armenian Boy* (New York: Farrar, Straus, Giroux, 1978), p. 5; S. M. Dzotsikian, *The Western Armenian World* (New York: 1947), p. 628 (in Armenian); Holbrook, "Impressions," p. 40.

20 Gordon, "Kazanjian Still Active," p. 1. M. Verazin, "Prof. Varaztad Kazanjian," *Hairenik Monthly*, vol. 8, no. 11 (September 30, 1930): 157 (in Armenian), identifies Hagop (Jacob) as the older brother in Samsun. He was the son of Hovhannes Kazanjian and his first wife.

21 Waldron, "Testimonial," p. 93. For a more in-depth examination of the situation of the Armenians in Turkey in the 1890s, see the following sources, which were published during this period; Edwin M. Bliss, *Turkey and the Armenian Atrocities* (New York: M. J. Coghlan, 1896); Filian, *Armenia*; Ohan

Gaidzakian, *Illustrated Armenia and the Armenians* (Boston: published by the author and B. H. Aznive, 1898); J. Castell Hopkins, *The Sword of Islam or Suffering Armenia* (Toronto, Canada: Bradley-Garretson, Ltd., 1896). Louise Nalbandian, *The Armenian Revolutionary Movement* (Berkeley: University of California Press, 1963), p. 108: Chapter V, "The Hunchakian Revolutionary Party, 1887-1896" (pp. 104-131), describes the history and philosophy of this party.

22 G. S. Graber, *Caravans to Oblivion. The Armenian Genocide, 1915* (New York: John Wiley, 1996), pp. 35-36.

23 Waldron, "Testimonial," pp. 93-94; John M. Converse, "The Extraordinary Career of Dr. Varaztad Hovhannes Kazanjian," *Plastic and Reconstructive Surgery* 71, no. 1 (January 1982): 138.

24 John W. Cooke, "Kazanjian and Harvard," *Harvard Dental Alumni Bulletin* 3, no. 2 (January 1943): 24; Waldron, "Testimonial," p. 94; Sandrof, "Famous Plastic Surgeon."

25 Converse, "Extraordinary Career," p. 138; Gordon, "Kazanjian Still Active," p. 2; Sargeant, "Some Notes."

26 Converse, "Extraordinary Career," p. 138, also Gordon, "Kazanjian Still Active," p. 2; Waldron, "Testimonial," p. 94. Victoria Stamboulian, the daughter of Paul (Boghos) Der Bedrosian, in a personal interview with author, March 6, 1995, Chelsea, Mass., reported that her father was also a member of the Hunchak party. Linda L. Avakian, *Armenian Immigrants, Boston 1891-1901, New York 1880-1897* (Camden, Me.: Pictron, 1996), lists (p. 126) Boghos Bedrossian (Bedrosian), age twenty-five, as arriving in New York from Cherbourg in April 1896 aboard the *Augusta Victoria*.

27 The line "yearning to breathe free," from the poem by Emma Lazarus entitled "The New Colossus," is inscribed on a tablet on the pedestal of the Statue of Liberty. Converse, "Extraordinary Career," p. 138; also, Gordon, "Kazanjian Still Active," p. 2. Kazanjian's application for naturalization lists March 20, 1895, as the date of his arrival in New York (Commonwealth of Massachusetts, Worcester Superior Court #2003 dated April 27, 1900). The records of the Varaztad H. Kazanjian Archive at the Countway Library of Medicine list his entry as October 1895. In a letter to the American Consul, Lausanne, Switzerland, dated June 6, 1916, Kazanjian wrote: "I was born in Armenia and went to the United States in September 1895. As I was very young at the time I do not recall the name of the boat on which I took passage, or the exact date of landing in New York City." Avakian, *Armenian Immigrants* (p. 118), records the Kazanjian name as "Castagian" and the first name of the Kazanjian brothers as Rusius (Roupen) age forty, Alescias (Alexander) age thirty, and Verastat (Varaztad) age seventeen, and their final destination as "Wolcester" (Worcester). The passenger record of the *Sicilia* lists Rusius and Alescias as blacksmiths, and Verastat as student. Courtesy of the Ellis Island Immigration Museum. The author attributes the difference in age between Roopen (40) and Alexander (30) registered in the ship's manifest as being a clerical error as they were twins.

28 Waldron, "Testimonial," p. 94; *Harvard Medical Alumni Bulletin*, v. 36, no. 3 (winter 1962): 8-10; Hagop T. Najarian, *The Story of the Armenian Communities in the Diaspora* (New York: Tankian Publishing), pp. 38-39 (in Armenian).

29 Nalbandian, *Revolutionary Movement*, pp. 121-128. See Christopher J. Walker, *Armenia: The Survival of a Nation*, (New York: St. Martin's Press, 1980), Chapter 5, pp. 121-173, for an overview of the Turkish massacres of Armenians in the 1890s.

30 Rebecca K. Krikorian, *Jerusalem* (Kansas City, Missouri: General Foreign Missionary Board Pentecostal Church of the Nazarene, 1919), p. 41.

31 Martin, *Hubbards of Sivas*, pp. 243-244.

32 Tashjian, "Profile," p. 90; Waldron, "Testimonial," p. 94; Letter from G. H. Paelian to Varaztad H. Kazanjian, June 22, 1956, Varaztad H. Kazanjian Archive in The Francis A. Countway Library of Medicine, folder C-324; also, The Alumni Association, Worcester Polytechnic Institute Biographical Records of graduates and former students, September 1970. Garabed H. Paelian graduated from Sivas Normal School in 1898 and from Anatolia College in 1903. He earned an M.A. from Oberlin College in 1907, a B. S. from Worcester Polytechnic Institute in 1911, and a Ph.D. from New York University in 1936. He went on to a distinguished career as a scientist with the Western Electric Company and with the Bell Telephone Laboratories and as a teacher.

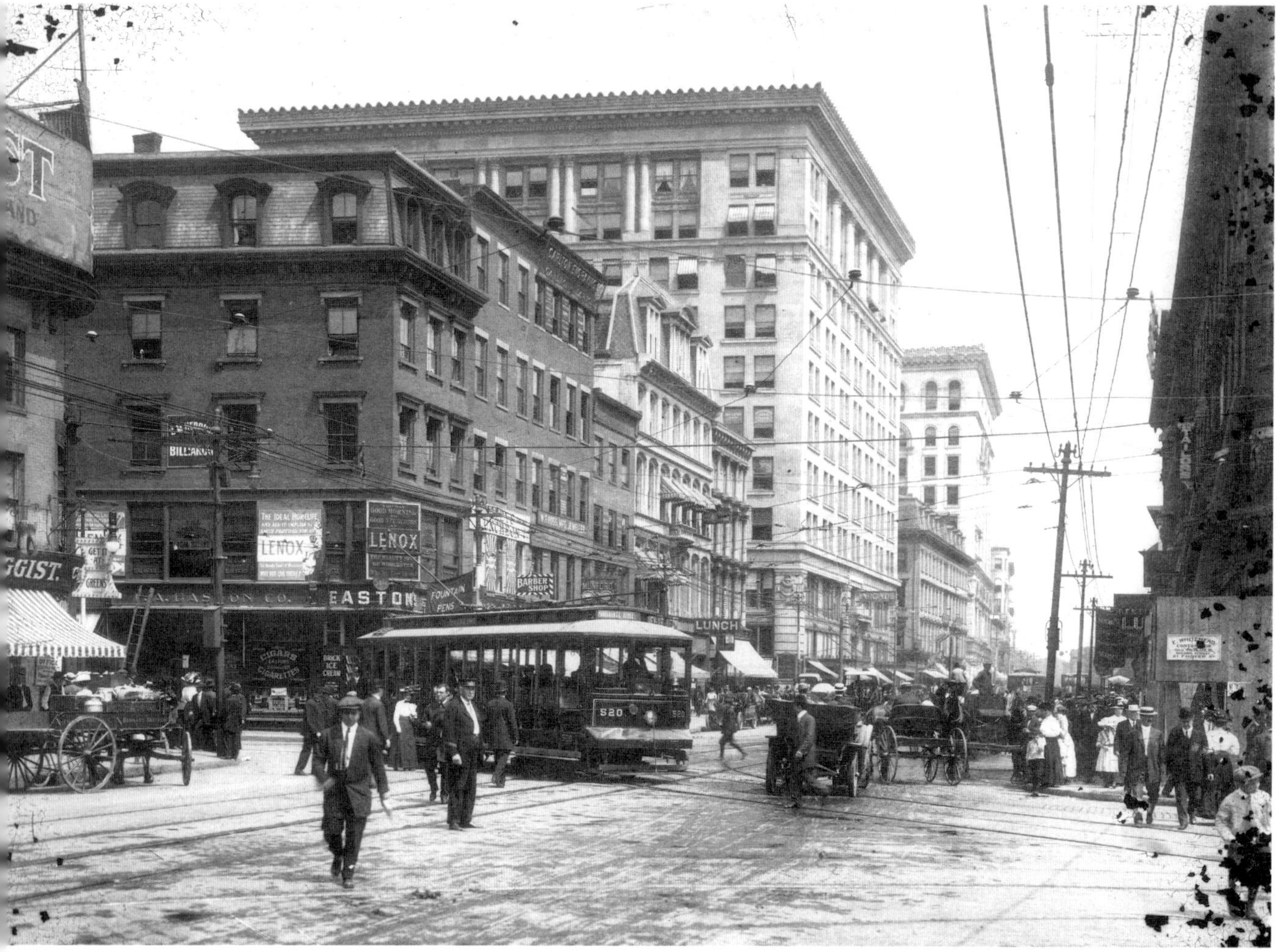

Harrington Corner, Worcester, Mass. as it appeared at the turn of the century
Courtesy Melikian Studio

CHAPTER TWO

Worcester, Massachusetts, the Armenian Capital of America

The industrial city of Worcester, in central Massachusetts, midway between Boston and Springfield, has fostered the largest colony of Armenians in America in the nineteenth and early twentieth centuries. It harbored approximately 700 by 1893, and with the number continually growing, it was soon to become known as "the Armenian metropolis of the country."[1] To the Armenian immigrant, Worcester was synonymous with America. He would not believe that he was in the United States until he set foot in Worcester. A likely dialogue at Ellis Island between the Armenian immigrant and the immigration official at the turn of the century has been recorded as follows:

Official: "What is your destination?"
Armenian: "America."
Official: "You are now in America."
Armenian: "No, no. Worcester is America."[2]

Like a magnet, Worcester drew Armenians to her, including the Kazanjian brothers.

At the turn of the century Worcester was one of the most ethnically diverse cities of its size in the United States. With a population of 118,421 in 1900, it was not so large a city as to bewilder immigrants and make them uncomfortable. Worcester had acquired wide experience with immigrants since 1826 when the Irish arrived to work on the Blackstone Canal connecting Worcester to Providence, Rhode Island, which contributed much to the city's industrial growth. When the Armenians arrived later, they were assured of a job and a place to stay in an Armenian setting. The first Armenian churches in the United States were established in Worcester: the Apostolic Church of Our Saviour was consecrated in January 1891, and the Church of the Martyrs, an Armenian Evangelical Protestant Church, was organized in 1892, the church building being dedicated in 1901.[3]

"Worcester is an unlikely industrial city," historian Roy Rosenzweig has observed. "Lacking the usual prerequisites of . . . industrial and urban development, a navigable body of water, water power and raw material, it nevertheless developed into a major industrial center, the twenty-eighth largest city in the United States by 1880." Worcester also developed and maintained "its distinctive pattern of local ownership." The largest single employer of Armenians in Worcester was the Washburn & Moen Manufacturing Company, "the wire mill," as it was to become known. This was the era of the opening of the west. Barbed wire was needed to fence off the ranges, as stiffeners in women's hooped skirts, for pianos, for telephones and electric lights, and for a great many other purposes. Washburn & Moen became the largest wire mill in the world. On its payroll by 1888 were 265 Armenians, about one-third of Worcester's Armenians.[4]

The three Kazanjian brothers applied for work in the wire mill, but only the two older brothers were initially hired. Varaztad, who was only sixteen, had to settle for less. "I got a job in a factory making springs," he recalled. It was

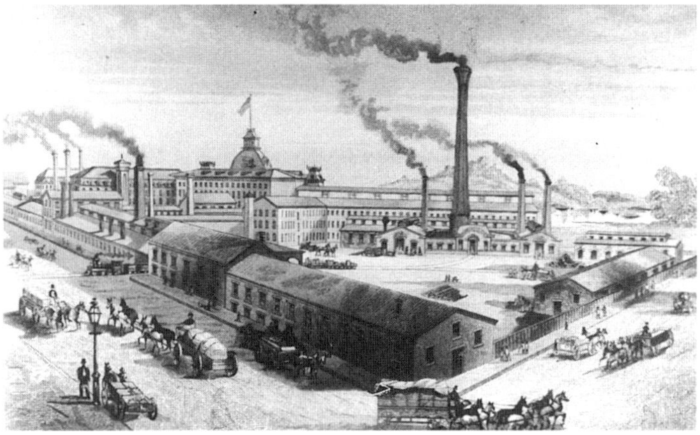

The American Steel & Wire Company was the successor of Washburn & Moen Manufacturing Company, circa 1895
Courtesy Worcester Historical Museum

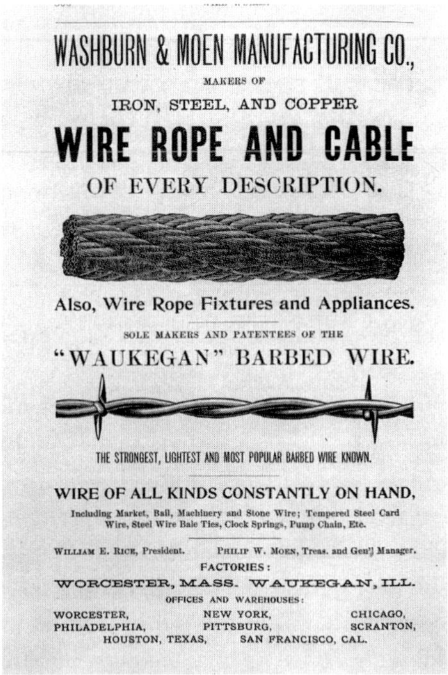

Products of the wire mill, circa 1895
Courtesy Worcester Historical Museum

piece-work, and, since he did not understand English well nor the system for recording time and wages, his first week's pay in America was ninety cents. He quickly learned the system and his next week's pay was three dollars, which soon escalated to six dollars per week for a ten-hour day. "The working conditions were unsanitary, the machinery was dangerous and there was no protection from dust and dirt." This job lasted for six months, whereupon he joined his brothers in "the wire mill," in the wire-drawing room. His affiliation with the wire mill would continue intermittently for eight years. By working overtime, he earned as much as twenty dollars a week.[5]

The Armenians at the mill were primarily wire-drawers, and this was true of the Kazanjian brothers. The process of wire-drawing consists of taking a coarse wire rod and drawing it white hot through a hole of smaller diameter than the rod, in an iron or steel plate, and repeating the operation until the rod is reduced to wire of the required size. The reduction is effected by stretching the wire, and not by removing the metal. It was one of the most difficult jobs in the mill, and industrial accidents were common. Lost fingers were commonplace long before the advent of industrial insurance and workmen's compensation, and Dr. Sherman Santoian related the tragedy of an Armenian wire worker who was killed when his clothing became enmeshed between the flywheel and leather belt of his machine.[6]

In 1896, only Roupen among the Kazanjian brothers was listed in the *Worcester Directory*. He worked at 96 Grove Street, which was the address of the wire mill, and lived at 16 Arch Street in "Little Armenia," on Laurel Hill, within walking distance of the mill. All of Arch Street was occupied by Armenians. The Armenians had difficulty in renting houses due to prejudice and economic constraints and gravitated toward run-down areas. Again, in 1897, Roupen alone was listed in the city

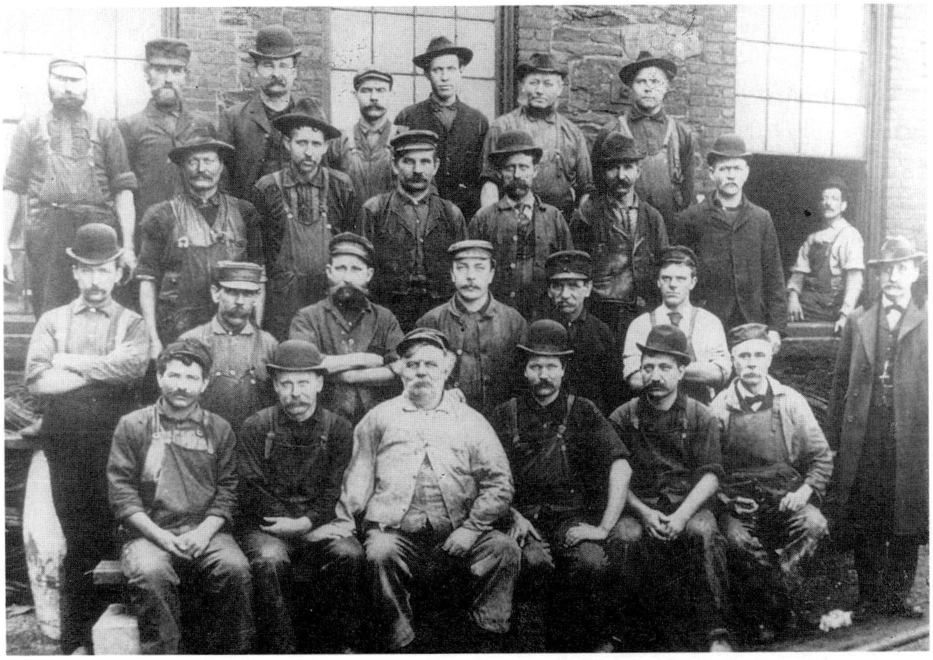

Workers at the wire mill, circa 1895
Courtesy North Works Restaurant, Worcester, Mass.

directory, as a wireworker who boarded at 179 Park Avenue, no longer in "Little Armenia," but in another Armenian enclave, "Big Armenia."[7]

No mention is made in the *Worcester Directory* of 1896 and 1897 of Varaztad, who had reached the age of eighteen on March 18, 1897. One of the first Armenian families to establish a home in a better section of Worcester was that of Mr. and Mrs. M. S. T. Nahigian who, in 1891, built a house at 62 Uxbridge Street. Nahigian had been in Worcester since 1883 and the Nahigian home was a frequent first stop for Armenian immigrants arriving in the city. There is a strong possibility that 62 Uxbridge Street was Varaztad's first place of abode in America and that M. S. T. Nahigian helped the Kazanjian brothers obtain work in the wire mill. Dr. Mark B. Constantian, a plastic surgeon in Nashua, New Hampshire, related that his grandfather, Maghak Berberian and Varaztad Kazanjian lived on the Tomajan Farm in Paxton, Massachusetts (a suburb of Worcester) "when they were both working as teenagers at the wire mill."[8]

For the first time in 1898, Roupen, Alexander, and Varaztad were all listed as wireworkers boarding at 13 Fountain Street in "Little Armenia." The proprietor of the boarding house was recorded as Jacob [Hagop] Kazanjian, the older half-brother who had arrived from Samsun in 1896. The 1899 *Worcester Directory* listed Alexander and Varaztad as living and working as they did the previous years, but Roupen was not listed, having returned to Sivas. Boghos Der Bedrosian, the friend from Sivas, was identified for the first time as a wireworker who also boarded at 13 Fountain Street. Der Bedrosian's daughter related an anecdote that on one occasion that, when her father was living with the Kazanjian brothers in Worcester, the three were so poor that they had only fifty cents among them, which they used to purchase a bushel of apples that they shared. In 1899, the American Steel & Wire Company bought Washburn & Moen; later it became part of United States Steel Corporation. [9]

About three years after his arrival in Worcester, Varaztad became ill. Body and brain had been driven too hard, and he was forced to rest for a time. In 1899, there was a brief summer interlude when Varaztad was employed in shoe factories in Berlin and Nashua, New Hampshire. "I found out there was no evening school, so I quit and went back to my less lucrative work in Worcester," at the wire mill. Thinking back on his summer employment in Nashua, he wrote, "I do recall that all the Armenians in Nashua worked in the same factory where I was employed, and there were a good many French-speaking workers, so I felt quite at home as I spoke better French than English at the time."[10]

The 1900 *Worcester Directory* reported Alexander and Varaztad as wireworkers living at 16 Thomas Street. That was the year that Nouvart (Nevart) Kazanjian, Varaztad's sister and Alexander's half-sister, arrived in Worcester. The city directory for 1901 listed Alexander and Varaztad as wireworkers who boarded at 14 Market Street, at which address Vartanis Donigian operated a rooming house. Boghos Der Bedrosian moved to Boston in 1901. Varaztad was listed in Worcester for the last time in 1902. He and Alexander, wireworkers, dwelled at 6 George Street Court.[11]

Many years later, Varaztad still recalled, with trepidation, "those days of early colonization, their complete sense of isolation, their ignorance of the language, their helplessness, their hardships, their nostalgia for their homeland, their longings to return." Initially, Varaztad was tempted to return to Armenia to defend the homeland. Fiery orators aroused the immigrants. On one occasion the "listeners were so carried away that they rose up to the last man, and demanded to leave at once and fight against the Turks." Parsek Roopenian, Varaztad's friend, who had been in Worcester before 1900, was among those who returned to Turkey and became a "freedom fighter." When he came back to America, he married Varaztad's sister, Nouvart.[12]

On Sunday evenings, a lyceum or "national meeting," often secular in nature, was held in the hall of the Church of Our Saviour. The function of these meetings was to assist the Armenians to adjust more readily to life in America. On February 7, 1897, on the topic "Reading and the Love of Reading," one of the speakers was Varaztad, barely eighteen years of age. "It is by reading that man is able to appreciate beauty, the sublime and the truth," he proclaimed. "It improves his mind, refines his taste, and ennobles his soul. Therefore, read papers and books as the only means of your advancement," he advocated.[13]

Varaztad would take books with him to work, and whenever time allowed, there would be one open in his lap. He was perceived by his fellow workers as being different from them. He was ambitious and goal-oriented. Years later, with great pride, his former fellow workers would point out to friends and relatives the wire mill window where he was assigned working space. It was in a long, low building. "Every time I'd walk by that particular window, I would think of Kazanjian once working in there," Harold Gregory wrote, "and I would marvel about how his life developed."[14]

Operating the machine next to Varaztad at the mill was a fellow Armenian, Krikor Aroian, who had arrived in 1900. Ruth Aroian, his daughter, related the following exchange between the two workers which occurred in 1902 when Varaztad was about to move to Boston. "This is slave work. It will kill you," Varaztad complained. "Go to school," he advised. Krikor replied that this was impossible: "I have five brothers, a sister and my parents in the old country and I must bring them to America." Through hard work, Krikor was able to do just that. His daughter could never forget how her father's hands looked as she sat at the dinner table. They were so badly cut that it made her sick.

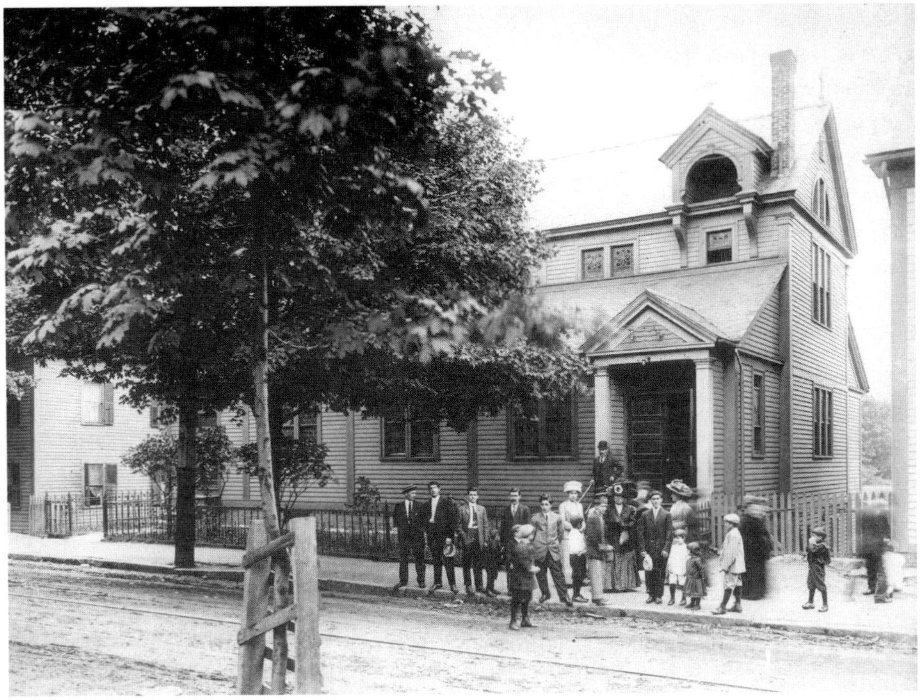

The Armenian Church of Our Saviour, Worcester, Mass. where Varaztad Kazanjian delivered his talk on "The Importance of Reading," in 1897
Courtesy Melikian Studio

Krikor had become an expert at "pulling" fine wire.[15]

About eighty percent of the Armenians in Worcester came from Kharpert (or Harpoot) province, known officially as Mamouret ul Aziz, which was located adjacent to the province of Sivas. Worcester seemed to attract the villagers rather than the more worldly urban dwellers. As a result, Worcester was sometimes called "Little Kharpert."[16] The Kazanjian brothers were different, having come from the city of Sivas, by way of Samsun.

The Armenians who had lived under oppression in Turkey arrived with a very humble, almost servile attitude. They were taken advantage of easily. To the factory owners the Armenians represented an excellent source of labor; they were industrious, reliable, and willing to put up with atrocious working conditions. One visitor to Worcester who toured the Washburn & Moen mill in 1891 complained that "The heat is unbearable. A worker can stand near his oven only a couple of minutes. The place is dense with acrid smoke. I left suffocating after a few minutes. I had had my bellyful . . . bade the place farewell forever." That same year a correspondent from Worcester wrote in the New York Armenian Journal *Haig*: "For God's sake tell them not to come here! Tell our people over there and elsewhere not to come here. The streets are not lined with gold nor is there a heaven here. Come here and be buried." Bishop M. Seropian, writing in 1913, dramatically and graphically described the working conditions in the mill:

The mill sucked the blood and flesh of the workers. It was as if they were condemned to be sacrificed. Even the smiles on their faces expressed the bitterness of death. Worcester's reputation was built on this factory with its prevailing odor of death and emaciation. The Armenian workers who journeyed from the remote provinces poured their blood and sweat into the deafening machines for the purpose of creating a platform of gold for the owners of the [mill] trust.[17]

Their willingness to work for low wages made the Armenians unpopular with the other workers, who labeled them "scabs," or strike breakers, believing that "the Turks [as Armenians were called] have come to take our jobs away." The labor movement held no interest for them. "My father was beaten almost every day by the other workers because he was Armenian," recalled John Aroian, the son of one of the early arrivals. "When I brought him lunch from mother, he would give me a dime to see a Chaplin movie. He did not want me to see him when he looked so bad from the work."[18] The immigrants lived a frugal, drab life but, no matter how little they earned, money was always sent abroad to help support families at home and to bring friends and relatives to America.

The early Armenian settlers complained that they could not walk the streets of Worcester alone at night and were often denied police protection. They had no redress and had to be mutually protective. Called "God-damned Armenians" or "Turks," they were thought to be non-Christian or Muslim. In 1886, for the first time, an Armenian sought redress in the courts for being insulted and called a "God Damn Turk." The Armenian won the case and the guilty party was required to pay a ten dollar penalty, but the harassment continued. Their children were mocked and had snowballs thrown at them as they came home from school. Sometimes it must have seemed to the immigrants that they had left one form of subjugation in Turkey for another in America. Even when they went grocery shopping, they went in a group for self-protection. But they were admonished by their elders back home, who had sent them to America, never to waver but to be as stalwart as their legendary Mount Ararat. The *Dictionary of Worcester*, published in 1893, reported that, as a rule, the Armenians are industrious and worthy and *many* are skilled artisans. Nonetheless, "They have been subjected to persecution and some brutal treatment in Worcester." But despite their deplorable living conditions, the Armenians never became public charges; they were too proud. The Associated Charities office in 1897 reported that not a single one had been known to have asked for bread or money.[19]

Varaztad Kazanjian's passion for knowledge was so intense and insatiable that immediately upon arrival in Worcester, he began night school at Dix Street School. He would later admit that, for seven years, "I did not miss a single night." It was a very difficult transition from work to school. Classes in the evening school began at 7 p.m. but most students did not leave work until 6 or 6:30 p.m. Their homes were often a mile or more away. It was therefore usually impossible to go home, eat, and arrive at school on time, but Varaztad had the motivation and perseverance. He also took correspondence courses at the International Correspondence School, attended lectures, and took private tutoring in English. "There was one teacher—I'm ashamed to say I don't remember her name," Varaztad recollected. "At the wire mill I worked ten to twelve and a half hours a day, and she used to wait for me to teach me English after work. There are some nice people who want to help others."[20]

Varaztad later attended night school with a class of Armenians at Belmont Street School. One teacher in the night school was a fellow worker at the wire mill, Simon Pazeian, who knew English well. (Later Pazeian would become a classmate of Kazanjian's at the Harvard Dental School class of

1905.) Varaztad also attended the Worcester Evening High School, from which he received certificates for completing courses in chemistry and English literature, dated March 16, 1900; Latin and physics, dated March 15, 1901; and geometry and advanced French, dated March 20, 1902.[21]

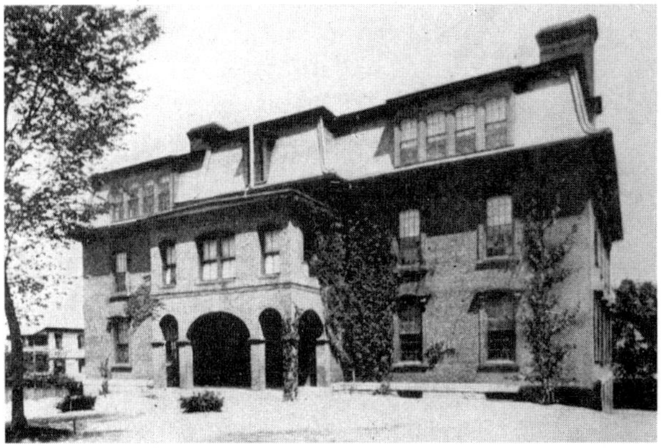

Dix Street School, circa 1895
Courtesy Worcester Historical Museum

Among these "nice people" who greatly influenced him was the Reverend Kachadour G. Benneyan, who served as pastor of the Protestant Armenian Church of the Martyrs in Worcester from 1896 to 1904. Meeting Varaztad one day at the post office, he urged the young homesick wire worker to renounce the idea of returning to what was left of Armenia and advised him to become an American citizen. "My son, give up this foolish idea of going back to Turkey; go to evening school, learn the English language, and settle down. This is a wonderful country." Varaztad listened and thereafter participated even more fully in the life of his new country. He considered the Reverend Benneyan to be "one of our wisest leaders" who understood the plight of the Armenian immigrant. It was neither appropriate nor desirable for them to be isolated from the life of the American community, Benneyan urged. "I was tempted to go back to Armenia," Varaztad admitted, "but Reverend Benneyan prevented me from doing so." For many years thereafter he considered Mr. Benneyan to be "one of my most esteemed friends." "As soon as I decided to make this country my home," he later revealed, "I determined to understand the American psychology, a resolution which proved invaluable to me in my final adjustment to my new environment."[22]

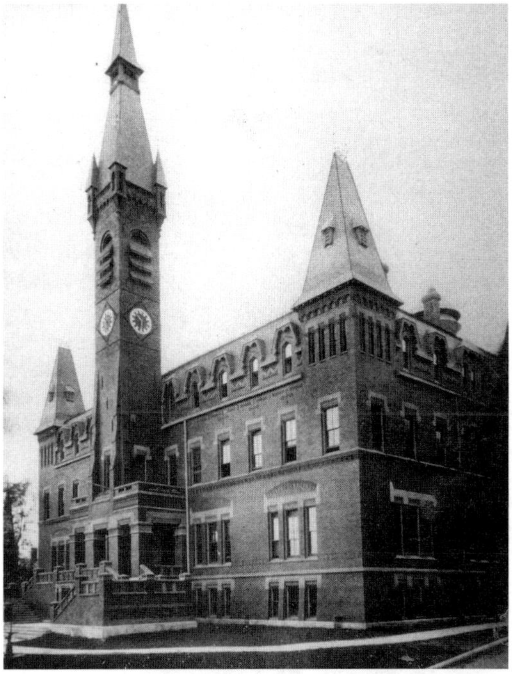

Worcester Evening School held in Worcester English High School where Dr. Kazanjian attended evening school, circa 1895
Courtesy Worcester Historical Museum

His application for citizenship was recorded in the Worcester Superior Court on April 27, 1900. It attests that he was born in "Yerzinga" [Erzincan] on March 5, 1879, and that he arrived in New York, on March 20, 1895. These dates are at variance with previously recorded information, which indicated that he was born on March 18, 1879, and that he arrived in New York in November 1895. The witnesses were Kevork B.

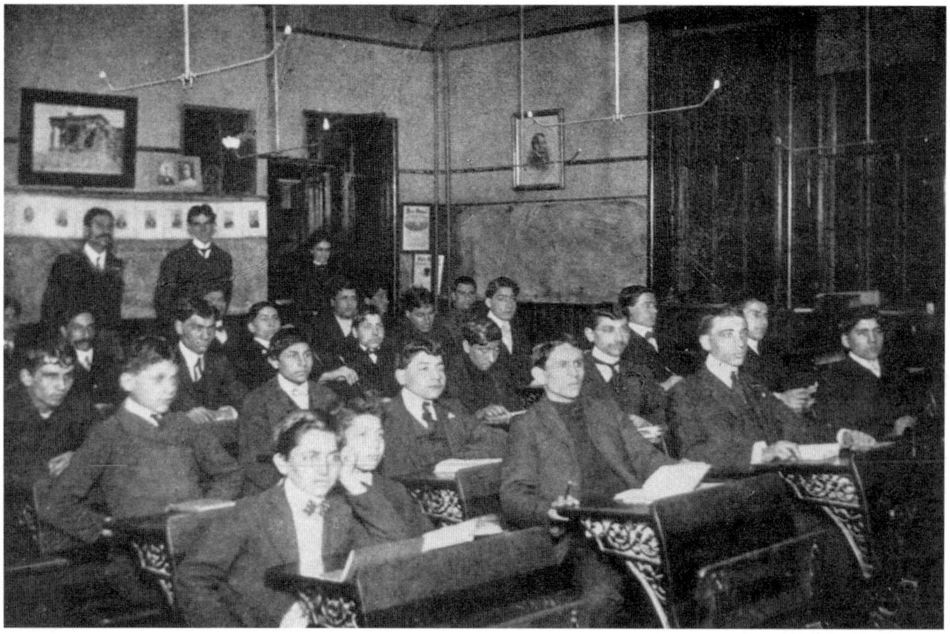

Armenian class, Belmont Street Evening School, ca. 1900
Photograph from the Worcester Magazine, *April 1903*
Courtesy Worcester Historical Museum

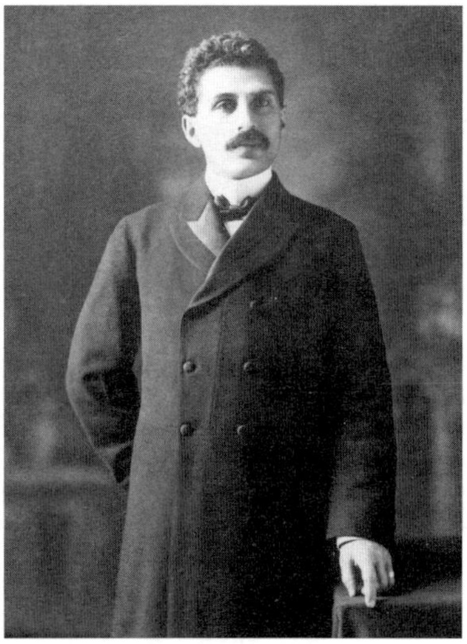

The Reverend Kachadour G. Benneyan, pastor of the Evangelical Armenian Church of the Martyrs, who greatly influenced Varaztad H. Kazanjian to stay in America. He became a lifelong friend.
Courtesy Armenian Church of the Martyrs

Thomajanian, proprietor of the Star Men's Furnishing Store, and Krikor Markarian, a tobacconist. Both were leaders in the Armenian community. The application lists Varaztad Kazanjian as twenty-one years of age and a wire drawer who resided at 16 Thomas Street. Later in the year, on October 15, 1900, he swore that he would "absolutely and entirely renounce and abjure all allegiance and fidelity" to Abdul Hamid, Sultan of Turkey, and became a citizen of the United States. This acquisition of citizenship marked a great turning point in his life.[23] Commenting on the Americanization process years later (1933), Kazanjian wrote:

> *The Armenians are among the most recent of the newcomers to America. They too have been subject to the melting pot which is the strongest factor in effecting the unification of the American culture. I hope the future generations of Armenians will maintain the traditional industry and high ideals of the Armenian race. The merging of the old and the new is the tried method of continuing progress.*[24]

An Armenian bicycle club was organized in Worcester in 1895, with an initial membership of thirty men. It became increasingly popular, and Varaztad became a cyclist. Ivan Sandrof has recorded one bicycling incident:

> *Once he [Varaztad Kazanjian] shot down Belmont Street toward Lincoln Square, [and] was horrified to find when he squeezed his foot brakes for control that there wasn't any. A streetcar lurched by under his nose and other traffic. Kazanjian, eyes popping like flying saucers, made a turn on a dime, abandoned his bicycle and clutched the neck of a man walking by. Everyone was very surprised.*[25]

On a Sunday afternoon bicycle outing in 1900, the subject of careers was being discussed by the young workers of the wire mill. Varaztad was uncertain about his future. He knew that he did not want to work in the wire mill for the rest of his life. Yet, he was over twenty-one and still in night school, and he did not have even a high school diploma. He was seriously considering mechanical engineering, but on this particular outing, one of his wiser and more worldly friends urged him to consider dentistry as his lifework. "You take dentistry," the friend said, "that's a good profession."[26]

That piece of advice remains an extraordinary career suggestion made by a fellow worker whose identity is unknown. He saw in Varaztad a gifted man with an untapped potential. After much thought, the idea took firm root in Varaztad's mind. Commenting on this choice, he admitted, "I always enjoyed working with my hands." True, he had inherited his father's manual skills and had become dexterous in "pulling" fine wire. Dentistry would provide for him a sense of security, the satisfaction that comes from being self-employed, and allow him to work with his hands and achieve professional status in life. Once he had made the decision to become a dentist, he characteristically concentrated his efforts in fulfilling his goal, but first there were family obligations to meet.

His fourteen-year-old sister, Nouvart, came to America from Sivas in 1900, settled in Worcester and attended school. Soon thereafter, in 1903, she married Parsek Roopenian, a close friend of Varaztad Kazanjian. They lived in Worcester until 1920, when they moved to the Boston area. By 1900, his half-brother, Roupen, had returned to Sivas. Varaztad had saved $300 but gave the money to Roupen for his return trip. It was a gesture typical of his generous nature. Roupen and his family disappeared during the 1915 massacres in Sivas.[27] In 1916, Varaztad, then an officer in the British Royal Army Medical Corps, was greatly concerned and, in an attempt

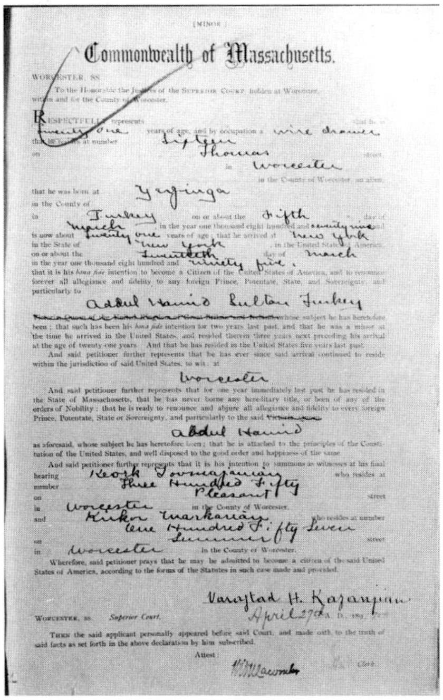
[MINOR]

Commonwealth of Massachusetts.

WORCESTER, SS.

To the Honorable the Justices of the Superior Court, holden at Worcester, within and for the County of Worcester.

RESPECTFULLY represents that he is twenty one years of age, and by occupation a wire drawer that he resides at number fifteen on Thomas street in Worcester in the County of Worcester, an alien, that he was born at Yegringa in the County of in Turkey on or about the fifth day of March, in the year one thousand eight hundred and seventy nine and is now about twenty one years of age; that he arrived at New York in the State of New York, in the United States of America, on or about the fourteenth day of March in the year one thousand eight hundred and ninety five; that it is his *bona fide* intention to become a Citizen of the United States of America, and to renounce forever all allegiance and fidelity to any foreign Prince, Potentate, State, and Sovereignty, and particularly to Abdul Hamid Sultan Turkey [illegible] whose subject he has heretofore been; that such has been his *bona fide* intention for two years last past, and that he was a minor at the time he arrived in the United States, and resided therein three years next preceding his arrival at the age of twenty one years. And that he has resided in the United States five years last past.

And said petitioner further represents that he has ever since said arrival continued to reside within the jurisdiction of said United States, to wit: at Worcester

And said petitioner further represents that for one year immediately last past he has resided in the State of Massachusetts, that he has never borne any hereditary title, or been of any of the orders of Nobility; that he is ready to renounce and abjure all allegiance and fidelity to every foreign Prince, Potentate, State or Sovereignty, and particularly to the said Abdul Hamid as aforesaid, whose subject he has heretofore been; that he is attached to the principles of the Constitution of the United States, and well disposed to the good order and happiness of the same.

And said petitioner further represents that it is his intention to summons as witnesses at his final hearing Keork Toumajanian who resides at number Three Hundred Fifty on Pleasant street in Worcester in the County of Worcester, and Kirkor Markarian who resides at number One Hundred Fifty Seven on Summer street in Worcester in the County of Worcester.

Wherefore, said petitioner prays that he may be admitted to become a citizen of the said United States of America, according to the forms of the Statutes in such case made and provided.

Varaztad H. Kazanjian

WORCESTER, ss. Superior Court. April 27th A. D. 1900

THEN the said applicant personally appeared before said Court, and made oath to the truth of said facts as set forth in the above declaration by him subscribed.

Attest: W. W. Macomber Clerk.

Application for citizenship,
April 27, 1900
Worcester Superior Court

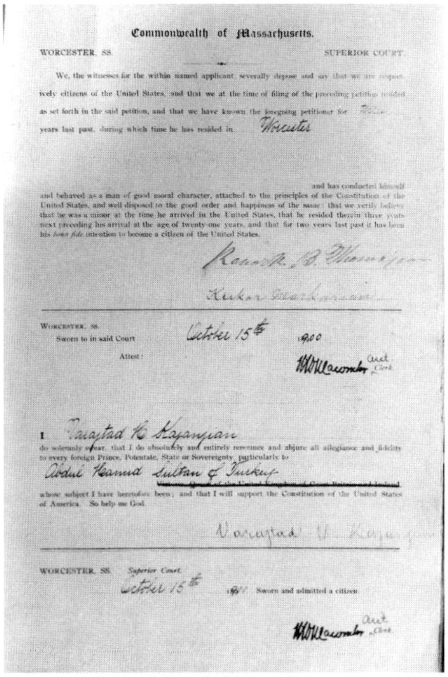
Commonwealth of Massachusetts.

WORCESTER, SS. SUPERIOR COURT.

We, the witnesses for the within named applicant, severally depose and say that we are respectively citizens of the United States, and that we at the time of filing of the preceding petition resided as set forth in the said petition, and that we have known the foregoing petitioner for [illegible] years last past, during which time he has resided in Worcester and has conducted himself and behaved as a man of good moral character, attached to the principles of the Constitution of the United States, and well disposed to the good order and happiness of the same; that we verily believe that he was a minor at the time he arrived in the United States, that he resided therein three years next preceding his arrival at the age of twenty-one years, and that for two years last past it has been his *bona fide* intention to become a citizen of the United States.

Keork B. Toumajanian

Kirkor Markarian

WORCESTER, SS. Sworn to in said Court October 15th 1900

Attest: W. W. Macomber Asst. Clerk.

I Varaztad H. Kazanjian do solemnly swear, that I do absolutely and entirely renounce and abjure all allegiance and fidelity to every foreign Prince, Potentate, State or Sovereignty, particularly to Abdul Hamid Sultan of Turkey [illegible] whose subject I have heretofore been; and that I will support the Constitution of the United States of America. So help me God.

Varaztad H. Kazanjian

WORCESTER, SS. Superior Court. October 15th 1900 Sworn and admitted a citizen.

W. W. Macomber Asst. Clerk.

The granting of citizenship,
October 15, 1900
Worcester Superior Court

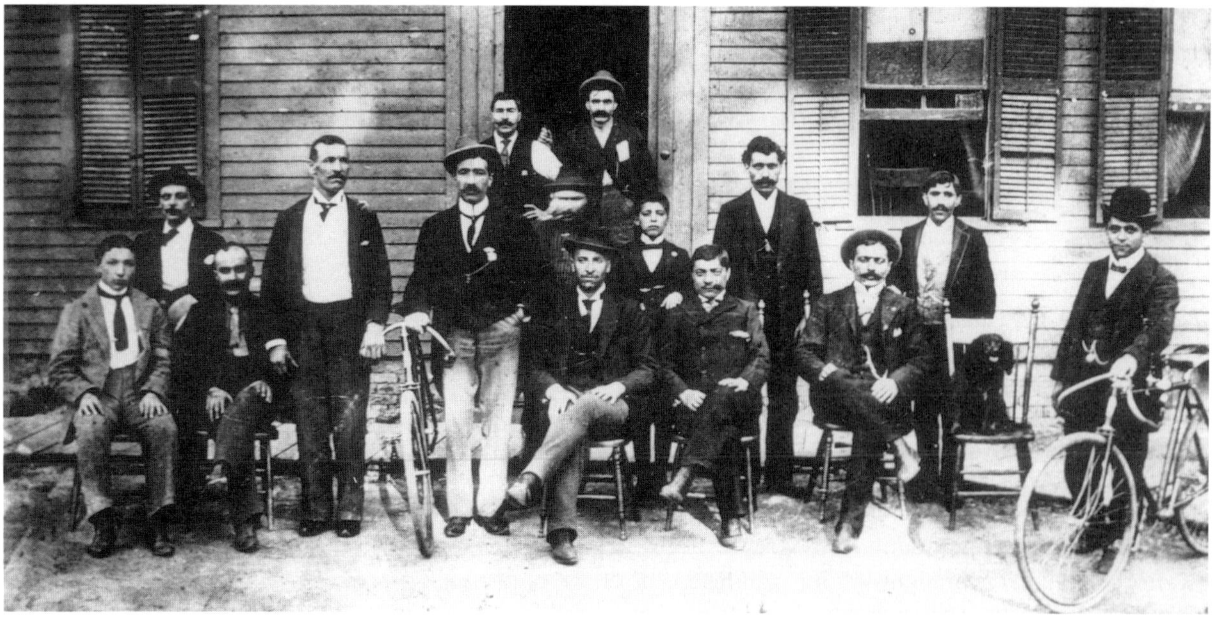

Armenian Bicycle Club, circa 1902
Courtesy Melikian Studio

to seek answers and offer help, wrote a letter of inquiry to an unnamed official or a relief agency such as the Red Cross on his half-brother's behalf:

> *I have a brother in Sivas, Turkey, where he has lived for many years. He is a merchant, with wide dealings, and well known to both American missionaries and Armenians. Since the war, I have been unable to get into communication with him, although I have written many times. As we are Armenians, I am greatly concerned as to his safety . . . . He is fifty years of age and a dealer in copper. We last heard from him in May 1915. He has a wife and children . . . . It is my wish, if my brother and his family are safe, and if they desire to, to arrange for their transport to America, or give any necessary aid at home.*[28]

It was for naught. Nothing was heard from Roupen and his family after 1915.[29]

No matter what his salary, Varaztad had never failed to send money to support his mother, Anna, and his brother, Yervant, who were still in Sivas. By 1909, both arrived in Worcester, Yervant being the last of the brothers to leave Sivas. They moved to the Boston area in 1918. Anna died later that year. She had been the mainstay of her family for over twenty-five years, since her second husband, Hovhannes, had died in 1891. She was "a kind and unassuming lady."[30]

"When I was freed of family responsibilities," Varaztad said, "I left Worcester for Boston." The six years in Worcester had been the struggling and bitter years of the new immigrant. He not only had survived these experiences but had been motivated to broaden his horizon and become a professional. As soon as he had saved $400, he moved to Boston, where there were two dental schools, at Harvard and Tufts. Nonetheless, the memory of Worcester, his first home in America, would vividly remain with Varaztad for the rest of his life.[31]

NOTES

1 Franklin P. Rice, *Dictionary of Worcester and its Vicinity* (Worcester, Mass.: F. S. Blanchard, 1893), p. 8; Eldridge Mix, "The Armenians of Worcester," *The Worcester Magazine*, (August 1902), p. 58; Bishop Moushegh Seropian, *The American-Armenian Annual Yearbook* (Boston: Cilicia Press, 1913), p. 40 (in Armenian). The first permanent Armenian settler arrived in Worcester in 1877. For a comprehensive history of the Worcester Armenians, see Hagop Martin Deranian, *Worcester Is America, The Story of the Worcester Armenians: The Early Years* (Worcester, Mass: Bennate Publishing, 1998), where some of the material in this chapter appeared earlier.

2 John H. Aroian, *Mountains Stand Firm* (New York: Green Hill Publishing, 1977), p. 3.

3 Jessie May Thornton, "Character, Composition and Distribution of the Southeastern Europeans in Worcester," Unpublished M.A. thesis, Clark University, 1934, p. 46; Morris H. Cohen, "Worcester Ethnics," *Holy Cross Quarterly* 5, nos. 3-4 (1973): 42; James H. Tashjian, *A Bicentennial History of the Armenian Community of America* (Watertown, Mass.: *The Armenian Review,* 1976), p. 7; *Worcester Telegram*, January 19, 1891, p. 1, col. 7, and July 15, 1901, p. 10, col. 3. The total population of Worcester in 1890 was 84,655; by 1900 it had increased to 118,421. See Rose Zeller, "Changes in the Ethnic Composition and Character of Worcester's Population," Ph.D. dissertation, Clark University, Department of Geography, 1940, table 10; Population Increases of Worcester, 1790 to 1930, p. 77.

4 Roy Rosenzweig, *Eight Hours For What We Will: Work and Leisure in an Industrial City, 1870-1920* (Cambridge, England: Cambridge University Press, 1983), pp. 11, 14; Franklin P. Rice, ed. *The Worcester of Eighteen Hundred and Ninety-eight* (Worcester, Mass.: Blanchard Co., 1899), pp. 457-458; Michael T. Neary, "Industrial Development of the American Steel & Wire Co.," M.A. thesis, Clark University, 1933. Orreal L. Stone, *History of Massachusetts Industries* (Boston: S. J. Clarke, 1930), v. 2, estimates (p. 123) that by 1888 over 150,000 tons of wire had been produced. The Armenians called it "the vire mill." Charles E. Stevens, *Worcester Churches 1719-1889* (Worcester, Mass.: Lucius Paulinus Goddard, 1890), states that the Armenians began to be employed at the wire mill as early as 1882 (p. 158).

5 James A. Tashjian, "Dr. Varaztad H. Kazanjian, a Profile," *Armenian Review* 1, no. 1 (Winter 1948): 90; Noah Gordon, "Dr. Varaztad Kazanjian of Belmont Still Active at 80," *Boston Sunday Herald*, September 20, 1959, Section II, p. 2; Carl W. Waldron, "A Testimonial to Varaztad Kazanjian," *Journal of Oral Surgery* 13, no. 2 (April 1955): 94. Waldron, states that the overtime wages were fifteen dollars a week. H. Martin Deranian, "With a Passion for Humanity," *Harvard Dental Alumni Bulletin* 38, no. 3 (1978): 44, sets the figure at twenty-five dollars a week.

6 A. Grace Aharonian, "Early Armenians in Worcester," Industrial Museum Case 7, April 5, 1937, folder DCB987, American Steel & Wire Collection, Baker Library, Harvard Business School; Charles G. Washburn, *Industrial Worcester* (Worcester, Mass.: Davis Press, 1917), p. 144; Dr. Sherman Santoian, personal interview with author, July 15, 1987, Harwich, Mass.

7 *Worcester Directory* (Worcester, Mass.: The Drew Allis Co., 1896 and 1897). In December 1987, *The Messenger,* a news sheet issued by the Church of Our Saviour, reported that many houses in this area were demolished to make way for the Interstate 290 Expressway. "Little Armenia" was in Worcester's East Side, primarily Ward 2 with a portion in Ward 3. It encompassed Laurel Hill, in an area bounded roughly by Belmont and Summer Streets with an extension to Lincoln Square and Thomas Street. "Big Armenia" was in the vicinity of City Hospital and Chandler Street and its intersection with Park Avenue. For descriptions of Big Armenia and Little Armenia see Marion Der Kazarian, "My Recollections of the Laurel Street Church," *The Messenger*, May 1987. U. S. Bureau of the Census. *Thirtieth Census of the United States*, 1910, Bulletin Population. Massachusetts (Washington: Government Printing Office, 1911-1912) lists sixty-one Armenians living on Arch Street. Also, Manug K. Jizmejian, *Kharpert ev ir Zavagnera* [Kharpert and Her Children] (Fresno, Calif.: 1955), pp. 198-199 (in Armenian).

8 John G. Eresian, "A History of the Tomajian and Eresian Families," Chevy Chase, Maryland, January 30, 1993, unpublished manuscript; interview with Marion Ogasapian, May 30, 1995, Worcester, Mass., who was M. S. T. Nahigian's granddaughter; interview with Edward Rustigian, April 6, 1990, Worcester. Mass., who confirms that Varaztad Kazanjian lived with the Nahigians; also Letter from Dr. Mark B. Constantian to the author, February 17, 2000, in the author's possession. Varaztad Kazanjian resided at the farm of Charles and Pepron Tomajan in Paxton, a town adjacent to Worcester. He was related to Pepron, who was the daughter of Hagop Kazanjian. The date cannot be precisely verified, but it is believed to be circa 1899—1901. He shared a room with Maghak G. Berberian, who was related to Charles Tomajan. Maghak G. Berberian became the maternal grandfather of Dr. Mark B. Constantian of Nashua, New Hampshire, a distinguished practitioner of plastic surgery, teacher and contributor to the literature of his specialty.

9 *Worcester Directory*, 1898; Gary E. Swan, "Ichabod Washburn Made Worcester World Center of the Wire Industry," *Worcester Sunday Telegram,* July 16, 1972, p. 31A, cols. 1-8. Hélène K. Sargeant, "Some Notes Concerning the Family of Dr. Kazanjian" (March 1978, preserved in Varaztad H. Kazanjian Archive in The Francis A. Countway Library of Medicine, Harvard Medical School, Boston), records that Hagop (Jacob) Kazanjian arrived in the United States in 1896 and that "Roupen returned to Sivas in the early 1900s, and he and his family disappeared during the 1915 massacres." The *Worcester Directory,* 1899, also records Roupen's return to Armenia. According to Linda L. Avakian, *Armenian Immigrants, Boston 1891-1901, New York 1880-1897* (Camden, Me.: Pictron, 1996), p. 140, Hagop Kazanjian (Hagob Kazanojian) arrived in New York on September 21, 1896, from LeHavre aboard the French ship, *La Gascogne*. Hagop Kazanjian's grandson, Zareh Thomajan, founded Zareh's, a noted men's furnishings store on State Street in Boston. He died in 1978 at the age of 77. Zareh's father, Jacob Thomajan, operated clothing stores at 158 and 228 Front Street in Worcester. In the author's interview on March 6, 1995, with Victoria Stomboulian, who was Boghos Der Bedrosian's daughter, she stated that her father worked in the wire mill. Dr. Kazanjian was the best man at the wedding of Mr. and Mrs. Boghos Der Bedrosian on April 1, 1905, in Boston and was the godfather at the christening of their daughter, Victoria, in 1910.

10 Waldron, "Testimonial"; Ivan Sandrof, "World's Most Famous Plastic Surgeon," *Worcester Sunday Telegram*, January 12, 1958, Feature Parade section, p. 3, cols. 1-5; Mary Murray O'Brien, "Boston's Famous Plastic Surgeon Once Worked for Ninety Cents a Week," *Boston Sunday Globe*, March 16, 1952, p. 16A, cols. 1-8. See also letter from V. H. Kazanjian to Russell Cole, March 20, 1952, Kazanjian Archive, folder C-80. Cole recorded in an earlier letter of March 18 that when he was a young man, he worked in the office of Estabrook Anderson Shoe Co. "We hired on a number of Armenian young men, and I took a personal interest in them."

11 *Worcester Directory*, 1895, 1900, 1901, 1902. Boghos Der Bedrosian is listed as the operator of the boarding house at 16 Thomas Street in 1900. George Street Court is not in "Little Armenia." Sargeant, "Some Notes," uses the spelling of "Nouvart" for Varaztad's sister. According to one anecdote, Varaztad had so little money that, for one year, he was in debt to the proprietor of one of the boarding houses where he was staying. (H. Martin Deranian, "With A Passion for Humanity," *Ararat Quarterly* 76, no. 4 (1978): 4). In a letter to the author dated November 7, 1988, Diana Der Hovanessian relates that her maternal grandfather, Hagop Israelian, and Varaztad Kazanjian were roommates and went to night school together. The two men did not keep in touch, except once during the Depression, when the parents of a child needing surgery appealed to her grandfather to call his friend for help. Dr. Kazanjian did the surgery without a fee. In a personal interview by author with Grace Deradoorian on September 10, 1989, Belmont, Mass., she reported that Varaztad Kazanjian worked with her father at the wire mill. She was also recalled that Kazanjian would deliver groceries to her family home on Ormond Street.

12 Tashjian, "Profile," p. 90; M. Verazin, "A Famous Oral and Plastic Surgeon," *Hairenik Daily*, May 8, 1930 (in Armenian). Parsek Roopenian arrived in Ellis Island on February 1, 1892, according to Avakian, *Armenian Immigrants*, p. 69. See also John Hughes, "The

Eye of Armenia," *Orange County Register* (Dec. 8, 1996), Accent section, p. 8.

13 Church of Our Saviour, Worcester, Mass., Records, February 7, 1897 (in Armenian). Courtesy of Harry Sogigian.

14 Deranian, "With a Passion for Humanity," p. 44; Personal interview by the author with John Kassabian, December 22, 1993, Worcester, Mass., who related stories told to him by his father and uncle; *The Messenger*, December 1987. Harold Gregory, *The Messenger*, September 1989, identified his cousin, Nazareth Keljikian, as the one who pointed out Varaztad Kazanjian's work place in the mill.

15 Ruth Aroian, personal interview with author, April 19, 2001; also, *Worcester Sunday Telegram*, April 22, 2001, Section B, p. 8, cols. 4-8.

16 Tashjian, *Bicentennial History*, recorded on p. 8: "The first Armenian to arrive from Kharpert and to work in the wire mill was Aaron Yenovkian, who was here between 1878 and 1880." Also, Seropian, *Yearbook,* 1913, p. 43. Both of the author's grandfathers were from Kharpert province; both were in Worcester as sojourners before the turn of the twentieth century; both worked in the wire mill; both returned to Armenia and perished during the inferno of 1915.

17 Seropian, *Yearbook,* 1913, pp. 41, 250-251. Also Tashjian, *Bicentennial History*, p. 9; "The Armenian Colony: Recent Additions, Though Many Here Out of Employment," *Worcester Telegram*, July 31, 1887, p. 6, col. 1.

18 Jezmejian, *Kharpert,* p. 198; Aroian, *Mountains*, p. 3. Seropian, *Yearbook*, 1913, p. 45, relates that as the Armenians emerged from Congregational Sunday services at Summer Street Chapel, they were beaten. "A Multimillionaire in Making Friends," *Armenian Reporter* (August 23, 1973).

19 Seropian, *Yearbook,* 1913, p. 46; "Armenians' Mass Meeting: Numerous Instances Where Police Protection Was Denied, Say They Were Insulted and Assaulted and Have No Redress, Form an Organization for Mutual Protection," *Worcester Telegram*, September 7, 1891. Also, *The Armenians in Massachusetts*, American Guide Series (Boston: Armenian Historical Society, written and compiled by the Federal Writers Project of the Works Progress Administration, 1937), pp. 31-32; Jezmejian, *Kharpert,* p. 198; Rice, *Dictionary*, p. 8; "Armenians Find Haven of Safety in Worcester," *Worcester Sunday Telegram*, January 26, 1919, p. 4, cols. 3-4; also, *Worcester Evening Post*, January 12, 1897.

20 Gordon, "Kazanjian Still Active"; Tashjian, "Profile," p. 91; Sandrof, "World's Most Famous," pp. 3-4.

21 Aharonian, "Early Armenians." *Worcester City Documents, 1900*, p. 158, lists Simon V. Pazeian as a teacher. In a letter to Eugene H. Smith, Dean of the Harvard Dental School, July 13, 1903, Pazeian wrote: "I have been teaching in the Worcester Evening School for seven years" (records of the Harvard Dental School in the Harvard Medical Archives in The Francis A. Countway Library of Medicine). See also Certificates from the Worcester Evening High School signed by the chairman of the School Committee, Superintendent of Schools, Chairman of Committee on Evening Schools, and Principal; these certificates are preserved in the Kazanjian Archive, folder M-4.

22 For a biographical sketch of the Reverend K. G. Benneyan see the Armenian-language weekly *Gotchnag*, December 31, 1960; *75th Anniversary Memorial Booklet* (Worcester: Church of the Martrys, 1892-1967), p. 5. Also Avedis Derounian, "Noted Surgeon Prescribes Industry," *Armenian Spectator*, February 7, 1935; Verazin, "Plastic Surgeon." The friendship between Benneyan and Kazanjian continued long after Benneyan left Worcester in 1904, when he became editor of an Armenian weekly, *Gotchnag*, in New York. The dialogue between Benneyan and Kazanjian was recorded by Tashjian, "Profile," p. 90, Professor Branislav Dimitrijevic, of Belgrade, Yugoslavia, writing to the author on November 10, 1991, presented a differing view of Kazanjian's failure to return to Armenia: "Every Scotsman, every Irishman has a dream to visit his native city, country, village. But the world's most famous plastic surgeon lost that dream . . . One empire fell forever, during Dr. Kazanjian's life . . . he lost his country, and was obliged to change one civilization of 4,000 years' duration for another one of only 200 years! . . . Nobody understood him."

23 Recorded in Superior Court, Worcester, Mass., v. 34, petition. no. 203. Original preserved at Massachusetts Archives, 220 Morrissey Boulevard., Boston, Massachusetts. A copy

preserved in the New England Regional National Archives, 380 Trapelo Road, Waltham, Mass.

24 Foreword, Boston Historical Society, *The Armenians in Massachusetts.*

25 *Worcester Telegram*, May 5, 1896, p. 1, col. 4; Sandrof, "World's Most Famous."

26 Waldron, "Testimonial," p. 94: also, Gordon, "Kazanjian Still Active"; Sandrof, "World's Most Famous"; O'Brien, "Boston's Famous Plastic Surgeon"; John W. Cooke, "Kazanjian and Harvard," *Harvard Dental Alumni Bulletin 3*, no. 2 (January 1943): 24.

27 Letter from Louise Roopenian to the author, August 11, 1972, in the author's possession. *The Worcester Directory,* 1899, refers to Roupen for the last time. See also Waldron, "Testimonial," p. 94; Sargeant, "Some Notes."

28 Letter preserved in the National Archives of Plastic Surgery in The Francis A. Countway Library of Medicine signed "V. H. Kazanjian, 20th General Hospital, B[ritish] Ex[peditionary] F[orce], France." The date would have to be 1916. The addressee is not identified.

29 Sargeant, "Some Notes"; also Verazin, "Plastic Surgeon," states that Roupen was deported and killed.

30 Tashjian, "Profile," p. 90; Sargeant "Some Notes." *Worcester Directory,* 1918; Letter from Betty Topjian, Watertown, Mass., to the author, March 1, 1991, in the author's possession. Betty Topjian's mother and Anna Kazanjian "would run into each other at the beach called City Point, in South Boston." Yervant Kazanjian died on April 23, 1968.

31 Hagop T. Najarian, *The Story of the Armenian Communities in the Diaspora*, (New York: Tankian Publishing), p. 39 (in Armenian); Deranian, "With A Passion for Humanity," p. 44; Personal letter from V. H. Kazanjian to the author, dated February 21, 1958, inviting him to luncheon at the Harvard Club in Boston on February 27, 1958. During our conversation, he expressed great interest in Worcester in general and the condition of the Armenians in particular.

CHAPTER THREE

Brave New World[1]
Matriculation at Harvard Dental School, and First Years in Dental Practice

Upon his change of residence from Worcester to Boston in 1901, still lacking a high school diploma, Varaztad Kazanjian enrolled in the freshman class of English High School. He later recalled, "I was a man then and at first felt embarrassed when I saw the children who were my classmates, but I soon said 'What of it?' The main thing is to improve my English."[2]

In 1902, after one year at English High School, he approached Dr. Eugene Hanes Smith, dean of the Harvard Dental School, concerning admission requirements. He was informed that he must pass satisfactory examinations in English, physics, Latin or French; as well as in German, algebra, plane geometry, and botany or chemistry. Graduation from high school was not a requirement for admission to the Dental School until 1904. An examination was scheduled to be given in two weeks, and Kazanjian was encouraged by Dean Smith to take it. For the examination in English, he was required to read Shakespeare's *Julius Caesar*, George Eliot's *Silas Marner*, James Russell Lowell's *The Vision of Sir Launfal*, Scott's *Ivanhoe*, and Tennyson's *The Princess*. He was also required to present an exercise book containing compositions or other written work. To his great astonishment, he was admitted. There was a condition in French. "My best language was French," he said, "but I had trouble translating into English." He passed the admission examination in English and general chemistry and geometry, and was "admitted conditionally."[3]

During the summer of 1902, Kazanjian worked at the wire mill to earn his tuition. In

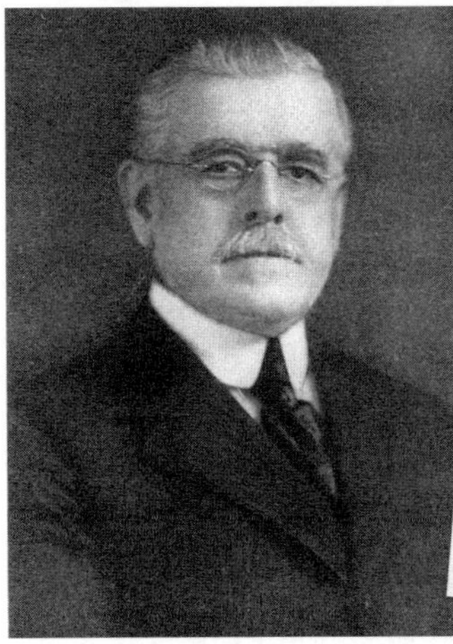

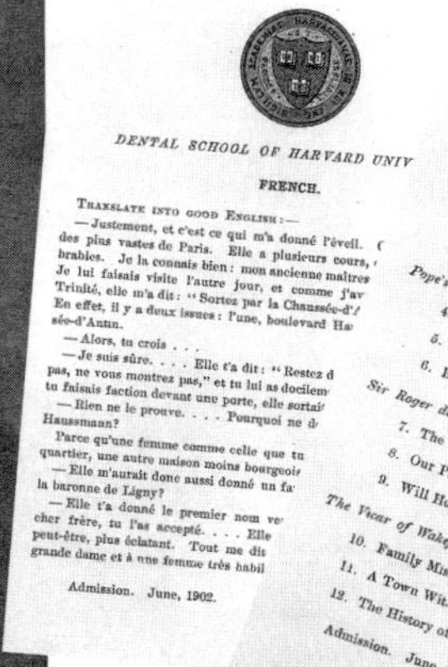
DENTAL SCHOOL OF HARVARD UNIV

FRENCH.

TRANSLATE INTO GOOD ENGLISH:—

—Justement, et c'est ce qui m'a donné l'éveil. (des plus vastes de Paris. Elle a plusieurs cours, brables. Je la connais bien: mon ancienne maîtres Je lui faisais visite l'autre jour, et comme j'av Trinité, elle m'a dit: « Sortez par la Chaussée-d' En effet, il y a deux issues: l'une, boulevard Ha sée-d'Antin.

—Alors, tu crois . . .

—Je suis sûre. . . . Elle t'a dit: « Restez d pas, ne vous montrez pas," et tu lui as docilem tu faisais faction devant une porte, elle sortai

—Rien ne le prouve. . . . Pourquoi ne d Haussmann?

Parce qu'une femme comme celle que tu quartier, une autre maison moins bourgeois

—Elle m'aurait donc aussi donné un fa la baronne de Ligny?

—Elle t'a donné le premier nom ve cher frère, tu l'as accepté. . . . Elle peut-être, plus éclatant. Tout me dit grande dame et à une femme très habil

Admission. June, 1902.

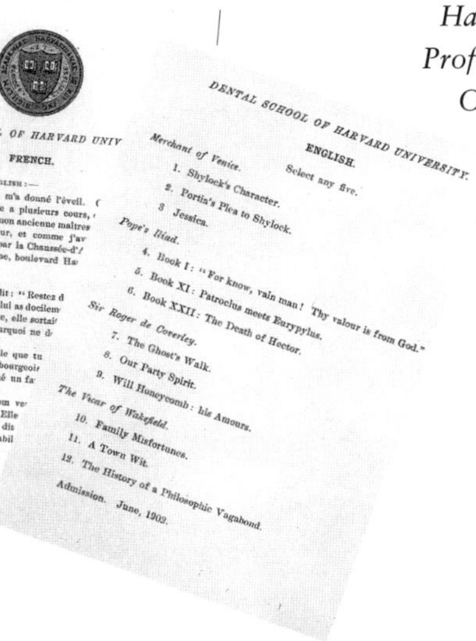
DENTAL SCHOOL OF HARVARD UNIVERSITY.

ENGLISH.

Select any five.

Merchant of Venice.

1. Shylock's Character.
2. Portia's Plea to Shylock.
3 Jessica.

Pope's Iliad.

4. Book I: "For know, vain man! Thy valour is from God."
5. Book XI: Patroclus meets Eurypylus.
6. Book XXII: The Death of Hector.

Sir Roger de Coverley.

7. The Ghost's Walk.
8. Our Party Spirit.
9. Will Honeycomb: his Amours.

The Vicar of Wakefield.

10. Family Misfortunes.
11. A Town Wit.
12. The History of a Philosophic Vagabond.

Admission. June, 1902.

Left: Dr. Eugene Hanes Smith, Dean of Harvard Dental School (1895-1924), Professor of Mechanical Dentistry and Orthodontia, an extraordinary supporter of Dr. Kazanjian
Hapgood, p. 68
Center: Examination questions for admission in French
Right: Examination questions for admission in English
All images left courtesy of The Harvard Medical Library in the Francis A. Countway Library of Medicine

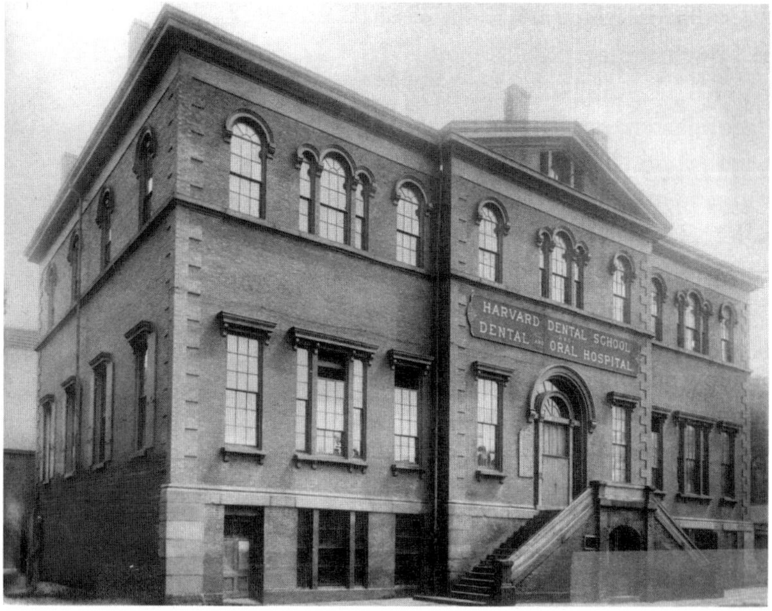

Home of the Harvard Dental School from 1883 to 1909
The Harvard Medical Library in the Francis A. Countway Library of Medicine, Hapgood, p. 48

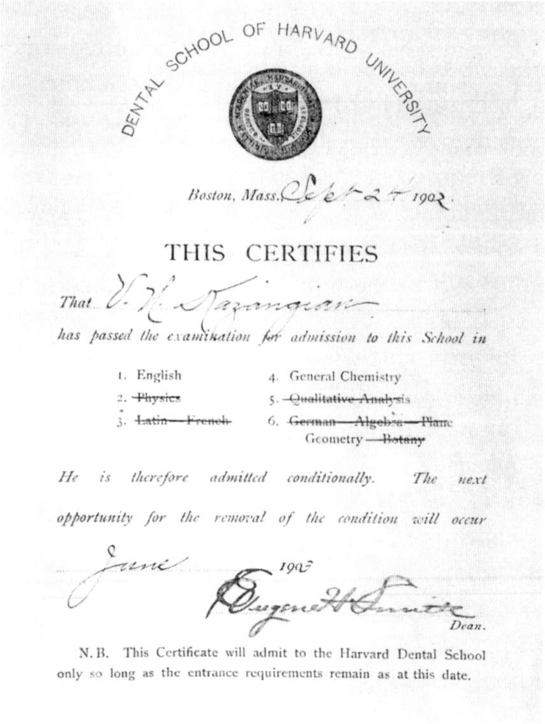

DENTAL SCHOOL OF HARVARD UNIVERSITY

Boston, Mass. Sept 24 1902

THIS CERTIFIES

That V. H. Kazanjian

has passed the examination for admission to this School in

1. English
2. ~~Physics~~
3. ~~Latin — French~~
4. General Chemistry
5. ~~Qualitative Analysis~~
6. ~~German — Algebra — Plane~~ Geometry — ~~Botany~~

He is therefore admitted conditionally. The next opportunity for the removal of the condition will occur

June 1903

Eugene H Smith
Dean.

N.B. This Certificate will admit to the Harvard Dental School only so long as the entrance requirements remain as at this date.

Certificate of Varaztad Kazanjian of conditional admission to the Dental School of Harvard University September 24, 1902
The Harvard Medical Library in the Francis A. Countway Library of Medicine

October, he matriculated at the Harvard Dental School as a member of the class of 1905, an amazing feat. "This accomplishment is all the more remarkable," an earlier biographer commented, "when one is reminded that almost until the day of his entrance into dental school, Kazanjian's associations were almost entirely with members of his own race."[4]

At the time Varaztad Kazanjian began his course of study at the Harvard Dental School in 1902, the school was in its thirty-fourth year of existence. Founded at the urging of Nathan Cooley Keep, the first president of the Massachusetts Dental Society, who became its first dean, it enrolled its first class in February 1868 and opened its doors the following November with sixteen students and a full corps of teachers, all of whom held the M.D. degree.[5] Like the recent founding of the Massachusetts Dental Society itself, Keep's plea for the establishment of a dental school by Harvard was an attempt to upgrade a profession through controlled training, regulation and standards. Dentistry had become tainted by a crowd of low-level and irregular practitioners. Although the Harvard Dental School was the eleventh dental school to be founded in the United States, it was the first such institution to be connected to a classical university. (The

Baltimore College of Dental Surgery, founded in the year 1840, was the first bona fide dental school in America, while some of the others, also proprietary in nature, were short-lived.)

During the early years of the Harvard Dental School's existence, no admission requirements were thought to be necessary. The course was short—two terms of four months, one in each of the two years required, and men who had been in practice for five years were considered second-year students. The degree of D.M.D. (Dentariae Medicinae Doctor) was conferred upon the graduates. In 1891, the curriculum of the school was extended to three years, with a term of five months in each year, which was the situation that prevailed at the time Varaztad Kazanjian commenced studying there. Tuition was $200 for the first year and $150 for each of the second and third years.[6]

Dr. Eugene Hanes Smith became Dean of Harvard Dental School in 1895. Also, as its Professor of Mechanical Dentistry and Orthodontia, he brought to the school "a highly developed administrative ability. He had not enjoyed luxury and ease in his youth and was . . . dependent upon unremitting toil for all that he achieved . . . a prominent position among Boston practitioners . . . he was aggressive, clear-thinking, with common sense."[7] From the start, Smith understood Kazanjian and would remain his ally and support during the remainder of his deanship, until 1923.

Of the twenty-three students who registered on September 25, 1902, in the Class of 1905, two students were from Australia, two from Nova Scotia, and one from Germany. The matriculants ranged in age from eighteen to twenty-nine. There were only two members of the class with bachelor's degrees: one from Dartmouth and the other from Bowdoin, while a third had attended Bates College. Kazanjian listed his local address as 15 Highland Park Avenue, Roxbury, his birthplace as Yerzinga, Armenia, Turkey, and his home as Sivas, Turkey.[8]

The first year course of the three-year program was identical with that of Harvard Medical School and included instruction in anatomy-dissection, physiology, histology and embryology, and physiological chemistry. "It could not have been easy," a later biographer observed, for "Thomas Dwight was then the Professor of Anatomy, and while Kazanjian's fingers obeyed his commands with dexterity, his efforts with written and spoken English were a constant struggle." He was spurred on when he received a good grade in one subject. He did well even though he did not have a high school diploma. Because of his unusual dexterity, he was given the task on weekends of making casts and models for the school.[9]

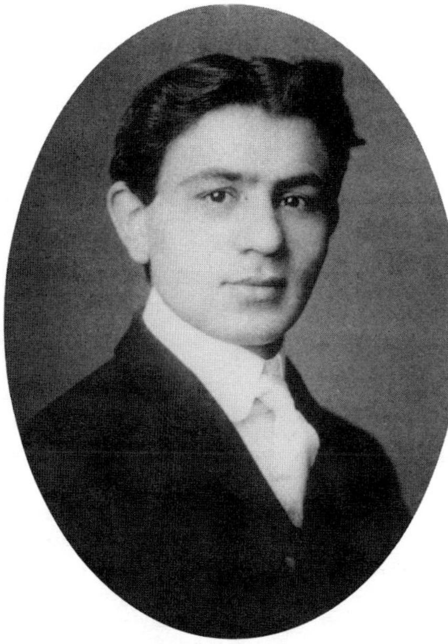

Varaztad H. Kazanjian, while a student at Harvard Dental School, Class of 1905
The Harvard Medical Library in the Francis A. Countway Library of Medicine

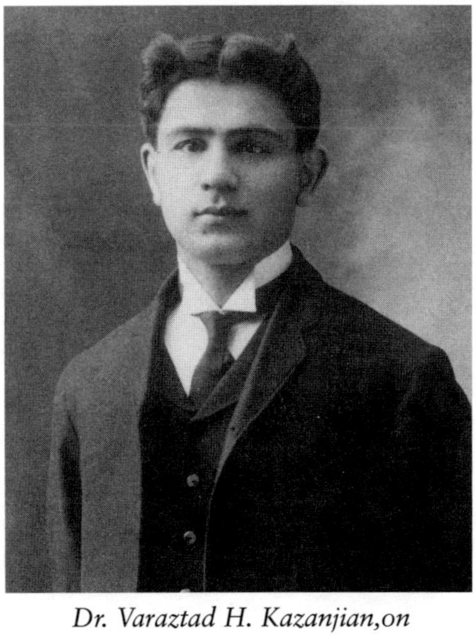

Dr. Varaztad H. Kazanjian,on receiving his DMD in 1905
The Harvard Medical Library in the Francis A. Countway Library of Medicine

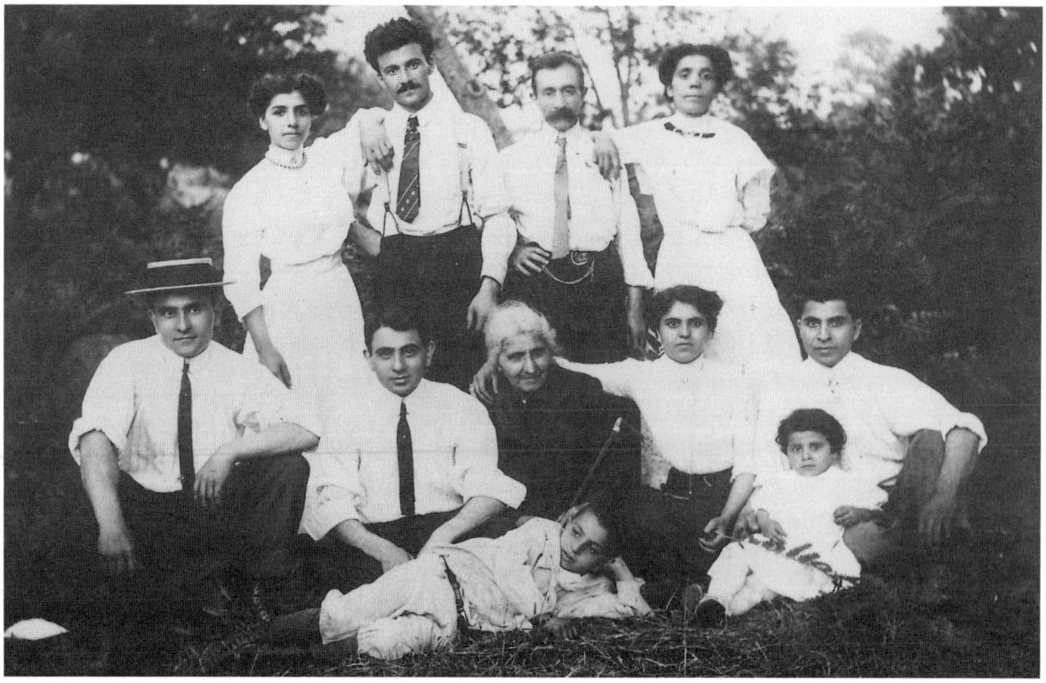

Dr. Varaztad H. Kazanjian and his family circa 1913-14
Adults seated, left to right: Yervant Kazanjian [V.H.K.'s brother],Dr. V. H. Kazanjian, Anna (Seroonian) Kazanjian [V.H.K.'s mother], Nouvart Kazanjian Roopenian [V.H.K.'s sister], Parsek Roopenian [Nouvart's husband]. Standing back row, left to right: Satenig (Aroian) Payelian [niece of Hripsime (Roopenian) Markarian], Hagop Boronian [Satenig Payelian's brother-in-law], Markar Markarian and Hripsime (Roopenian) Markarian [Parsek Roopenian's sister and wife of Markar Markarian]
Children in front: Flora Roopenian Ohanessian and Deran Roopenian [children of Parsek and Nouvart Roopenian]
Courtesy Melikian Studio

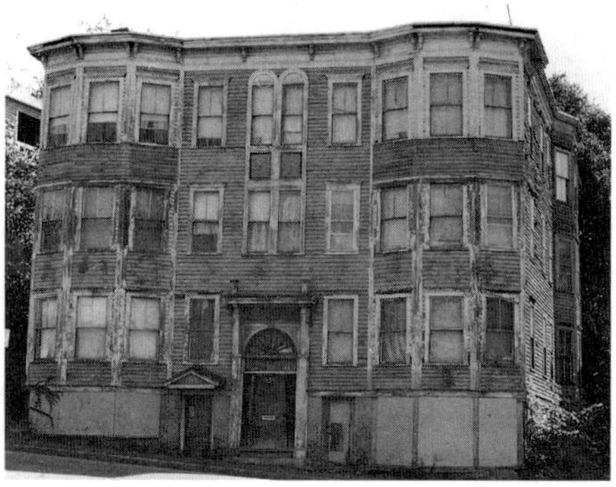

130 Belmont Street, Worcester, Mass. where Kazanjian listed his "present address" in 1904
Photograph by Melikian Studio, Worcester, Mass. 1999

When the class of 1905 first assembled, Robert Scott Catheron, class president later recorded, "It would have taken wiser men than we to pick out the man who, a quarter of a century later, would have deservedly outstripped his classmates." He doubted that "Kazanjian would have been selected among the first ten, handicapped as he was by unfamiliarity with the language and, . . . by being a foreigner."[10] At the end of the first year, in June 1903, Kazanjian returned to Worcester and to the wire mill so that he could earn tuition money for his second year of study.

The second year at Harvard Dental School began on October 1, 1903. There were now twenty-nine members of the class. Among the new

members was Simon V. Pazeian who had been a co-worker at the mill and an instructor at the night school in Worcester. He was a transfer student and had spent the first year at Tufts Dental School. "Along in the second and third years when we were wrestling with dentistry at the old school on North Grove Street," Dr. Catheron later wrote, "we became more aware of the little dark-eyed fellow who was always good natured and busy as the proverbial bee. It was apparent in talking to him that his existence had not followed the conventional lines in which most of us were cast and his modes of thought were different, often refreshingly so." During the summer between his second and third years, Kazanjian earned money by doing laboratory work for one or two dentists.[11]

For the third or last year, which began on September 29, 1904, the Class of 1905 had expanded in registrants because of transfers of forty-three students, including two who had received dental degrees from other schools. In registering for that year, Kazanjian listed his "present address" as 130 Belmont Street, Worcester. His brother, Alexander, and his sister, Nouvart, and her husband, Parsek Roopenian, lived at that address. Kazanjian still maintained his links to Worcester, no matter how tenuous. For three years he was so busy that night was merged into day for him. He had financial difficulties, often without money in his pocket.[12]

"When I was a student," Kazanjian later reminisced, "we used to see such things as cleft palates in children and adults. At that time prosthetic appliances were preferable to surgery because surgery wasn't advanced enough. Yet many of the patients with prosthetic devices could talk as well if not better than those who had surgery." This early interest in the treatment of unusual facial and jaw deformities, either congenital or acquired, by means of prosthetic appliances gave his future life its singular direction. His

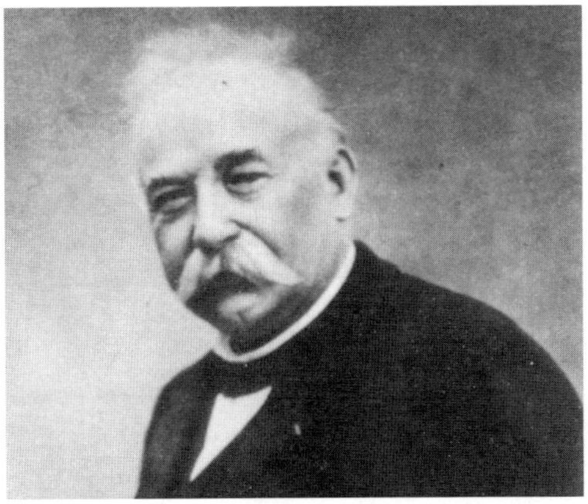

Dr. Claude Martin, (1843-1911)
Photograph from the personal collection of Dr. Charles Freidel

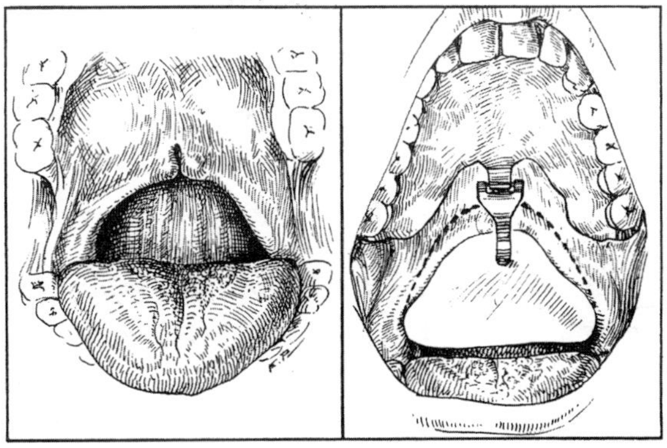

Fig. 5.—Posterior border of metal base plate carries a hinged joint to which a soft rubber obturator is attached

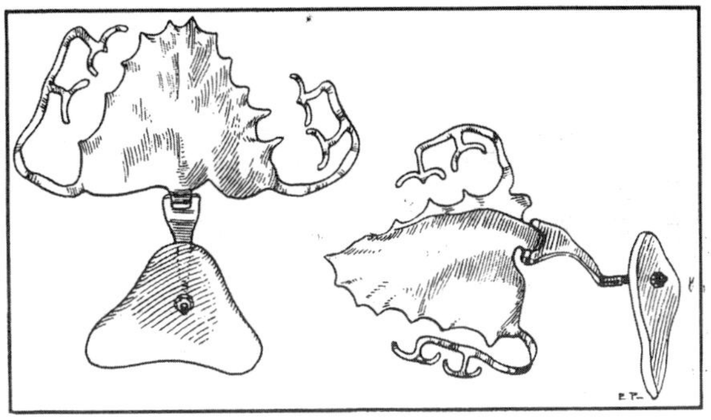

Cleft Palate Prosthetic Appliance
V. H. Kazanjian, Prosthetic Restoration of Congenital and Acquired Deformities of Hard and Soft Palate, Journal of Oral Surgery, *5 (July 1947): 188*

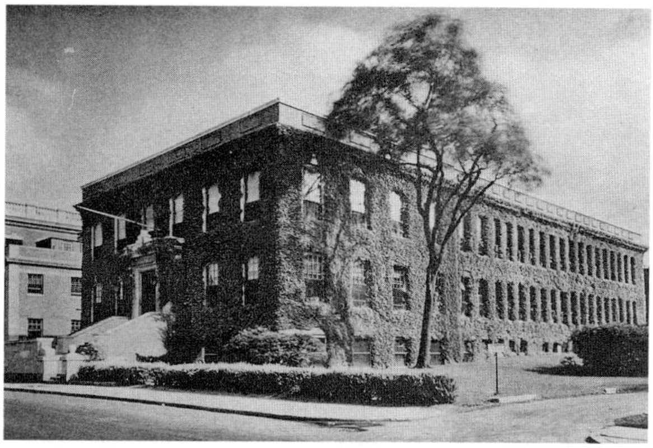

Harvard Dental School, Longwood Avenue, Boston, Mass, circa 1930. Built in 1909
The Harvard Medical Library in the Francis A. Countway Library of Medicine, Hapgood, p. 100

classmates would laugh at him for treating these difficult cases, saying, "Why bother? There is no money in it." But for him it was a challenge. "I always enjoyed problem cases," he said.[13]

Kazanjian became interested in the creative work of Dr. Claude Martin (1843-1911), a French dentist, whose book, *De la Prosthèse Immédiate, Appliquée à la Résection des Maxillaires*, had appeared in 1889. His ambition was "to vie with nature, and his ceramic reproductions and prosthetic reproductions proved him to be a true creator . . . his restorations of the esophagus, the pharynx, the palate, the velum, the nose, were nothing short of marvelous." Although the two men never met, Kazanjian's life had some similarities with that of Claude Martin, of whom it was said: "His cordiality, kindness, unselfishness, devotion, and above all, his rare modesty, won him every heart . . . and his fame added a most remarkable page to the book of honor of dentistry." Later, during World War I, while stationed in France, Kazanjian travelled to Lyon, France, to see Martin's collection of ingenious prostheses and to pay homage to his memory. Martin's principle of supplying a temporary framework to restore the lost part of the jaw was never forgotten.[14]

On June 28, 1905, Kazanjian received the degree of "Dentariae Medicinae Doctor."[15] The impossible dream, which originated on the bicycle outing in Worcester five years before, had been realized. He entered dentistry at a time when it was emerging from a practice into a profession, when it was striving desperately for dignity and recognition, but with the heavy shadow of the charlatan still hovering over it.

PRE-WAR PRACTICE

Varaztad Kazanjian opened his dental office in the Pelham Building at the corner of Boylston and Tremont Streets (74 Boylston Street) in Boston, where the present Little Building stands.[16] It was a modest endeavor. His initial attempts to establish a practice were disappointing, and his financial situation was guarded. He survived by performing dental laboratory procedures for his classmates. His patients were his own countrymen, theatrical people, those sent by other tenants in his office building, and transients. "Some of them were unusual and interesting," Dr. Catheron has recorded, "but on the whole not the material from which a practice worthy of his ability would be made."[17]

His fees for dental services were low: extraction $1.00; gold inlays $6.00; amalgam fillings $1.50 to $2.00; cleanings $1.00; full upper denture $15.00 and treatment of fractured jaws $30.00. Kazanjian spent his spare time in the company of other young dentists, such as Dr. Robert Catheron, among whom he was known for his interest in political matters "more on the theoretical than the practical side."[18]

Dr. Kazanjian's teaching career began in 1906 when he was appointed Assistant in Mechanical Dentistry at Harvard Dental School. In the following year he became Assistant in Prosthetic Dentistry, the colorful new title given to Mechanical Dentistry at Harvard. The introduction of the casting process and the expanded use of rubber vulcanite as a base for dentures transformed the department. Kazanjian's abilities were quickly recognized, and he became Demonstrator of Prosthetic Dentistry in 1909. That year, the Harvard Dental School moved to its new building on Longwood Avenue, its present location, adjacent to the Medical School, which also had recently transferred from its Boylston Street location to the new medical complex on the old Francis Farm. The newly elected Harvard University president, A. Lawrence Lowell, accepted the building on behalf of the University on December 8, 1909. For its time it was a modern dental infirmary with laboratories and clinical facilities but with no lecture halls. For lectures, the facilities of the adjacent Harvard Medical School were used.[19]

Kazanjian's part-time teaching positions were performed "for no great compensation." Therefore "Money came hard and went easily, because there were always relatives who needed help." Thus began a teaching career that would span his entire professional life. "Our first few years after graduation were for all of us a struggle in getting established," Dr. Catheron recalled. "Those of us who had families with whom we lived thought ourselves fortunate that our financial and other difficulties were properly cushioned. In the light of our later experiences we may doubt our good fortune and recognize the value in toughened fiber that the hard years gave to those like Kazanjian who were on their own."[20]

Kazanjian's practice increased and gradually brought him relief from his financial difficulties. His reputation as a maxillofacial prosthodontist[21] grew, and dentists began referring their difficult cases to him. In 1913 or 1914 he moved his office to 157 Newbury Street in the more fashionable Back Bay area of Boston. He shared office space with Dr. Harry A. Stone, as well as a dental assistant, Miss Wynifred Shaw, who recalled those lean days:

> *I was his first dental assistant in an office on Newbury Street near Dartmouth. [He and Stone] were both struggling young dentists . . . and I worked for $6 a week, the then Massachusetts minimum wage. It was all they could pay, I assure you. But they were wonderful to me, and we had a very happy year. I often wonder how different my life would have been if I had accepted his offer to give up the idea of marriage and let him train me as his assistant.*[22]

Dr. Kazanjian made an extensive tour of Europe in the summer of 1909 for four months, visiting London, Paris, Switzerland, Italy, Constantinople, Berlin, and Holland, and concentrated his attention on activities related to dentistry. He did not travel alone. His companion was a close Armenian friend, M. Vartan Malcom, who was born in Sivas and was a graduate of Amherst College and Harvard Law School.[23]

Scarcely two years after his graduation from dental school, Kazanjian gave a clinical demonstration at the Harvard Dental Alumni Association's thirty-sixth annual meeting on June 24, 1907. His topic was "A Bridge for Leaning Anterior Teeth," which was in keeping with his interest in prosthetic dentistry.[24] Thereafter, he was proposed for membership in March 1908 in the Harvard Odontological Society, during the term of Dr. Harold DeWitt Cross as president. His sponsors were Dr. John A. Furbish, his classmate and an instructor in Prosthetic Dentistry at Harvard, and more importantly, Dr. Waldo Boardman, a Yankee who was a highly placed and influential leader in the dental community both locally and nationally. Boardman had served as president of the American Dental Association in 1904-05, and his endorsement not only assured Dr. Kazanjian's acceptance by the Society, but signified that he was beginning to receive the nod of approval from his colleagues with power in dental circles.[25]

The Harvard Odontological Society chose its essayists by lot, and Dr. Kazanjian's selection "caused him no little concern and anxiety." He was

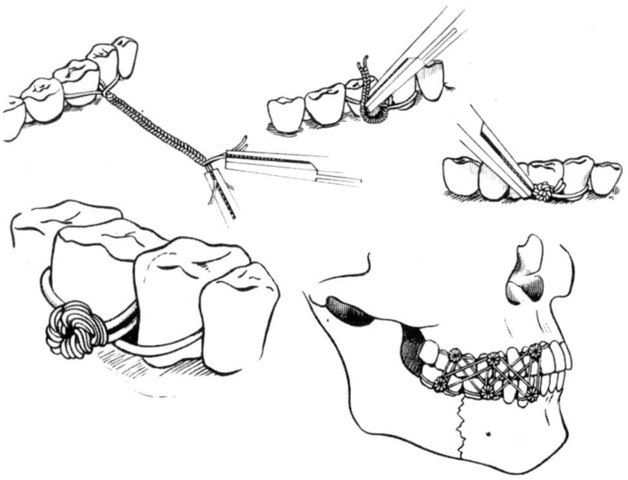

Kazanjian Button
Modified from P.D. Wilson, Management of Fractures and Dislocations, *(Lippincott: Philadelphia, 1938) p. 478. Illus. Robert H. Albertin*

encouraged to accept this important assignment by the head of the Prosthetic Department and his chief, Dr. Harold DeWitt Cross, "a kindly man whom Kazanjian remembers with honor." Dr. Cross was also a member of the Administrative Board of the School. Kazanjian's friend, Dr. Catheron, "edited the painstakingly prepared" paper that Kazanjian delivered early in 1910 "with credit." It was his first formal presentation before a professional meeting and was meritorious enough to be accepted for publication in the *Journal of Allied Dental Societies*. It appeared in 1911 and was the first of his more than 120 contributions to the dental and medical literature. Among his early works was an extensive article in Armenian entitled "What Is the Value of the Teeth?" published in the 1913 *Armenian American Almanac*. Presented in the form of questions and answers, the article is an extremely well-organized and well-written educational article on the care of the teeth. It went over the relationship between the teeth and the rest of the body, the anatomy and function of the teeth, the cause of dental caries, and the care of the teeth.[26]

Fractures of the jaws in those days were treated in the Harvard Dental School's Prosthetic Department rather than in the Department of Oral Surgery or in a hospital—no hospital facilities existed for this "dirty work." This was before the hazards of automobile accidents, and most broken jaws were the result of "drunken altercations on holidays and weekends." These patients were described as being "unkempt people . . . and people, poor souls, who could not even be offered . . . bed care at the dental school because there were no beds." General surgeons had neither "the interest or the knowledge to assume the responsibility for jaw fractures." The mouth was "an educational no man's land." Upper jaw fractures were rare. Marshall in 1902 recorded that they were "the result of great violence—like the passage of the wheel of a carriage over the face—the kick of a horse—a gunshot wound—a moving elevator."[27]

With little financial remuneration, no one seemed to want to treat these unfortunate patients—no one except Dr. Kazanjian. Under these adverse conditions, he treated over 400 cases of jaw fractures in the Dental School Clinic. He even helped innovate the technique of treatment. He was one of the first, although not the

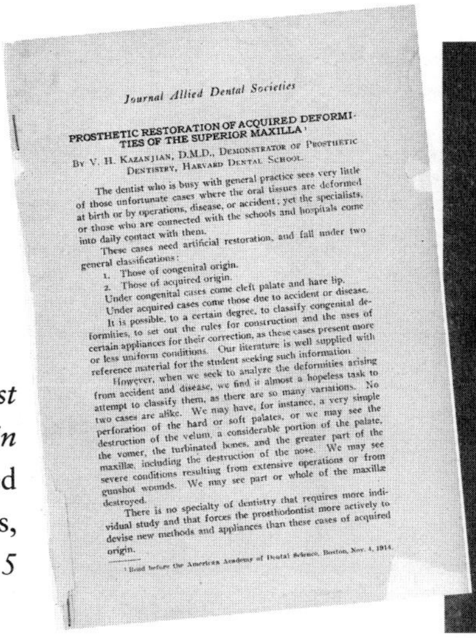

Journal Allied Dental Societies

PROSTHETIC RESTORATION OF ACQUIRED DEFORMITIES OF THE SUPERIOR MAXILLA[1]

By V. H. Kazanjian, D.M.D., Demonstrator of Prosthetic Dentistry, Harvard Dental School.

The dentist who is busy with general practice sees very little of those unfortunate cases where the oral tissues are deformed at birth or by operations, disease, or accident; yet the specialists, or those who are connected with the schools and hospitals come into daily contact with them.

These cases need artificial restoration, and fall under two general classifications:

1. Those of congenital origin.
2. Those of acquired origin.

Under congenital cases come cleft palate and hare lip.

Under acquired cases come those due to accident or disease.

It is possible, to a certain degree, to classify congenital deformities, to set out the rules for construction and the uses of certain appliances for their correction, as these cases present more or less uniform conditions. Our literature is well supplied with reference material for the student seeking such information.

However, when we seek to analyze the deformities arising from accident and disease, we find it almost a hopeless task to attempt to classify them, as there are so many variations. No two cases are alike. We may have, for instance, a very simple perforation of the hard or soft palates, or we may see the destruction of the velum, a considerable portion of the palate, the vomer, the turbinated bones, and the greater part of the maxillæ, including the destruction of the nose. We may see severe conditions resulting from extensive operations or from gunshot wounds. We may see part or whole of the maxillæ destroyed.

There is no specialty of dentistry that requires more individual study and that forces the prosthodontist more actively to devise new methods and appliances than these cases of acquired origin.

[1] Read before the American Academy of Dental Science, Boston, Nov. 4, 1914.

Dr. Kazanjian's first published article in the Journal of Allied Dental Societies, *10:14, 1915*

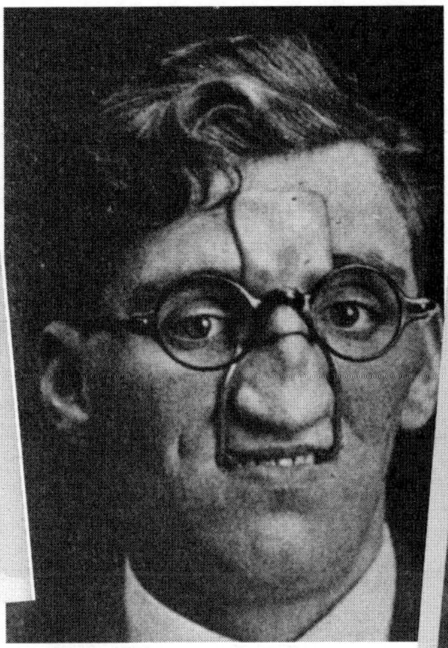

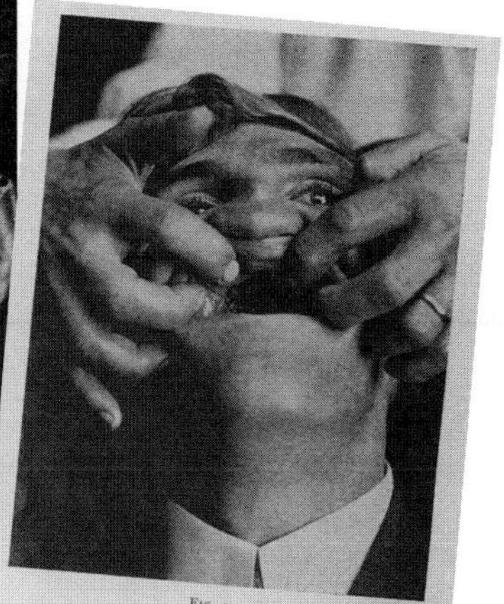

Fig. 11

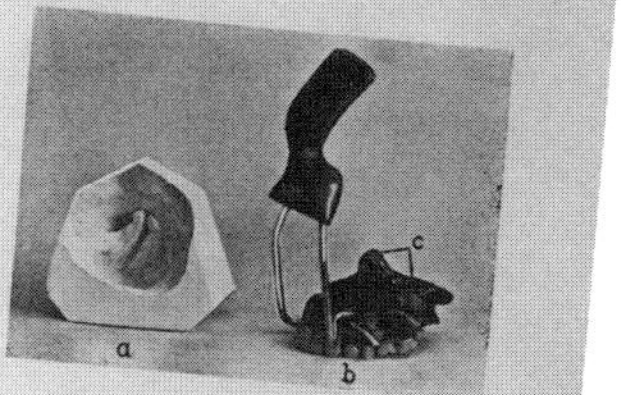

Fig. 12

The case reported by Dr. Kazanjian in his paper read before the American Academy of Dental Science in 1914, in which the patient lost his entire maxilla, and extra-oral retention was necessary V. H. Kazanjian, "Prosthetic Restoration of Acquired Deformities of the Superior Maxilla," Journal of Allied Dental Societies, *10:14, 1915, unpaged. Figure 1, 2, and 3*

first, to eliminate the cumbersome and uncomfortable interdental splint made of vulcanite rubber and to substitute the simpler intermaxillary wiring method in which dislodged fragments of the jaws were joined together with wire during healing. "We began to use intermaxillary wiring of the upper and lower teeth into adequate occlusal relationship in harmony with the normal occlusion of the patient's teeth," he reported. His patients improved in spite of everything they "could do to prevent it, and, in many instances, they did a lot." The years at the wire mill were remembered and applied. "Had the road up been smooth," John Cooke has suggested, "Kazanjian might well have avoided the results of those weekend and holiday altercations, and could not have acquired the background which later carried him far in France."[28]

To the Dental School Clinic also came people with congenital and acquired deformities of the face and jaws for treatment by the construction of artificial prosthetic appliances. Among these were patients with cleft palates who required such appliances, often in preference to surgery. As an example, Kazanjian reported the case of an elderly woman who was born with a cleft palate, whom he examined in 1926. At the age of eight, she had been taken to a dentist in

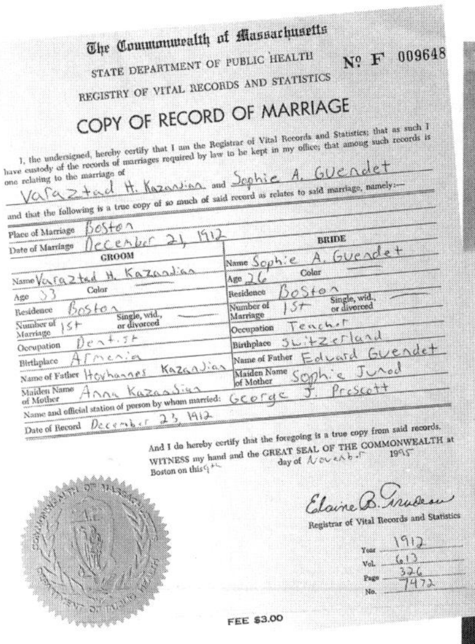

The Commonwealth of Massachusetts
STATE DEPARTMENT OF PUBLIC HEALTH
REGISTRY OF VITAL RECORDS AND STATISTICS
№ F 009648

COPY OF RECORD OF MARRIAGE

I, the undersigned, hereby certify that I am the Registrar of Vital Records and Statistics; that as such I have custody of the records of marriages required by law to be kept in my office; that among such records is one relating to the marriage of Varaztad H. Kazanjian and Sophie A. Guendet and that the following is a true copy of so much of said record as relates to said marriage, namely:—

Place of Marriage Boston
Date of Marriage December 21, 1912

GROOM		BRIDE	
Name	Varaztad H. Kazanjian	Name	Sophie A. Guendet
Age	33	Age	26
Color		Color	
Residence	Boston	Residence	Boston
Number of Marriage	1st	Number of Marriage	1st
Single, wid., or divorced	—	Single, wid., or divorced	—
Occupation	Dentist	Occupation	Teacher
Birthplace	Armenia	Birthplace	Switzerland
Name of Father	Hovhannes Kazanjian	Name of Father	Edward Guendet
Maiden Name of Mother	Anna Kazanjian	Maiden Name of Mother	Sophie Junod

Name and official station of person by whom married: George J. Prescott
Date of Record December 23, 1912

And I do hereby certify that the foregoing is a true copy from said records.
WITNESS my hand and the GREAT SEAL OF THE COMMONWEALTH at Boston on this 9th day of November 1995

Elaine B. Trudeau
Registrar of Vital Records and Statistics

Year 1912
Vol. 613
Page 326
No. 7472

FEE $3.00

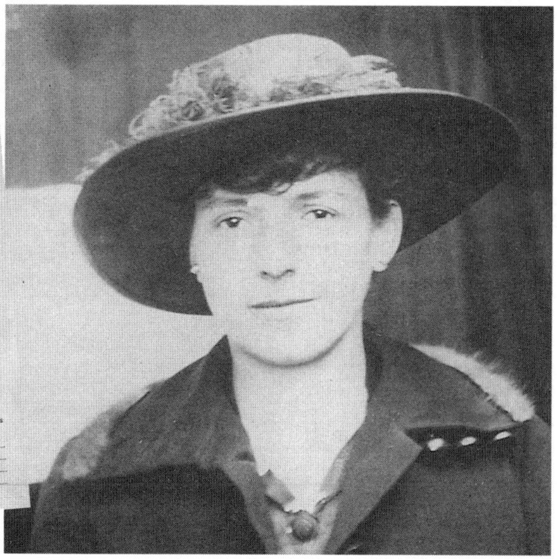

Left: Certificate of marriage, Boston, December 21, 1912 between Varaztad H. Kazanjian and Sophie A. Cuendet Commonwealth of Massachusetts, Registry of Vital Records—Statistics No. F009648

Right: Sophie A. Cuendet, World War I era photograph The Harvard Medical Library in the Francis A. Countway Library of Medicine

Berlin who made her a denture with an obturator which she had worn since then. It had been so skillfully constructed that "she had been married for over fifty years and neither her children nor her husband knew of her deformity."[29]

Patients also came with missing portions of the face and jaws due to injury or following cancer surgery. For them, like a sculptor, Dr. Kazanjian fashioned artificial noses, eyes, ears, and other facial tissues, often defying detection. In those days, prosthetic appliances were used to replace defects of the jaws. "Let us hope that the proportions of surgical failures," one authority on the prosthetic treatment of cleft palate urged, "will be greatly lessened in the future." The same authority went on to explain, "Surgeons depended mostly upon artificial devices for the restoration of defects of the nose, eyes, palate, and even of defects of the soft tissues of the face." Yet in spite of the marvels he effected, Dr. Kazanjian had no official hospital appointment.[30]

The American Academy of Dental Science was born in 1867, about the same time that the Harvard Dental School came into existence. It was the first honor society for dentists and originally drew its members from dental educators. It took the position that "dentistry is a specialty of the science of medicine" and should "be placed on an equality with other specialties of medicine." Fellowship was by invitation, and the presentation of an original paper or invention was required.

On November 4, 1914, Dr. Kazanjian read before the Academy his paper "Prosthetic Restorations of Acquired Deformities of the Superior Maxilla," which was published and which prompted an invitation to fellowship in the Academy.[31]

"A sailor on a warship lost his entire upper jaw in an accident," he reported on the major case in his article. "I was asked to make a denture for him. It took me six months, but I finally devised a way which involved an apparatus which was held in place by rods and wires leading to the upper part of the face. I was very proud. Then someone wrote to Robert "Believe It or Not" Ripley about it, and he published it: 'Believe it or not—Dr. Kazanjian made a man chew with his eyebrows.'"[32] More than any other, it was his successful treatment of this patient that presaged his wartime services.

Kazanjian's creative work in maxillofacial prosthetics and jaw fractures was a bridge to medicine.[33] Thus, in 1911, he quietly entered the Medical School at Boston University. He was given credit for the first year and successfully completed the second year in 1912.[34] In the interim, he continued his dental practice and his teaching. Many dentists of the period held both medical and dental degrees. There were those who believed that, since dentistry was a branch of medicine, all dentists should have the medical degree. Dr. Kazanjian never returned for his third year at Boston University Medical School, due to his increased duties at Harvard and perhaps partly because it was then a homeopathic institution, and holding its degree would stigmatize his position as a physician.

Dr. Kazanjian was appointed head of Harvard's Prosthetic Dentistry Department in the fall of 1912 after his mentor, Dr. Harold DeWitt Cross, "who rendered invaluable services in developing prosthetic teaching," resigned from the faculty to assume the directorship of the Forsyth Dental Infirmary for Children. Dr. Kazanjian was in charge of lectures and demonstrations to the senior classes while Dr. Fred A. Beckford was in charge of the junior class. His new duties were so challenging and time-consuming that, according to one source, he was forced to lay aside his goal of completing his requirements for an M.D. degree. Teaching had become of paramount interest to him, and he was willing to make the necessary sacrifices. He never forgot the support and encouragement that Dr. Cross gave him.[35]

Some time after 1907, Kazanjian met Sophie Augusta Cuendet, who was living in Boston. She was a "beautiful, lovely woman," and "sweet and so attractive." A native of Sainte-Croix, Switzerland, she had three sisters, two of whom, Ida and Georgine, lived in Boston and were teachers. Ida was married in 1909 to a Belgian born into a noble family, Victor de Bellefroid, who was a riding master. They operated a riding academy.[36] Varaztad H. Kazanjian and Sophie A. Cuendet were married on December 21, 1912, in Boston by the Reverend George J. Prescott, who was Rector of the Episcopal Church of the Good Shepherd.[37] Kazanjian was thirty-three years old and his bride was twenty-six. Sophie's sister, Georgine, and M. Vartan Malcom were married on October 26, 1912, in Montclair, New Jersey, with Kazanjian serving as best man.[38]

The year 1912 marked a turning point in the life of Varaztad Kazanjian. For the first time, his life had reached a level of comparative ease. He was married, his practice was becoming more lucrative, he was making his mark in his profession and was a department head in his alma mater. He was recognized as one of the best men in the country in his specialty.[39] His family had safely arrived in America with the ominous exception of Roupen, who was still in Sivas. He was in his prime, and he had found his place in the sun. But the success he now enjoyed was to last less than three years.

NOTES

1 William Shakespeare, "The Tempest," Act V, Scene 1.

"O, wonder!
How many goodly creatures are there here!
How beautious mankind is. O, brave new world,
that has such people in it!"

2 Mary Murray O'Brien, "Boston's Famous Plastic Surgeon Once Worked for Ninety Cents a Week," *Boston Sunday Globe*, March 16, 1952, p. 16A, cols. 1-8.

3 Ibid.; Carl W. Waldron, "A Testimonial to Varaztad Kazanjian," *Journal of Oral Surgery* 13, no. 2 (April 1955): 94. Richard Locke Hapgood, in *History of the Harvard Dental School* (Peterboro, N.H.: Transcript Printing Co., 1930), p. 75, writes that "the official catalogue of 1899-1900, for example, illustrative of the years from 1895 to 1904, gives these provisions as the requirements for admission. The prospective student must pass satisfactory examinations in (1) English, (2) physics, (3) Latin or French, and (4) German, algebra, plane geometry, botany or chemistry." Kazanjian passed his condition in French on re-examination in 1903, according to the Report of September Entrance Examination by William H. Potter, Sept. 30, 1903. His certificate of admission is dated September 24, 1902, Varaztad H. Kazanjian Archive in The Francis A. Countway Library of Medicine, folder M-5.

4 John W. Cooke, "Kazanjian and Harvard," *Harvard Dental Alumni Bulletin* 3, no. 2 (January 1943): 25. A letter from Dr. John W. Cooke to Dr. Jerome Webster, October 14, 1946, preserved in the Webster Collection, Health Services Library, Columbia University, states, "For several years I have been working off and on preparing a biography of Kazanjian." His manuscript was never completed.

5 For biographical information about Nathan Cooley Keep, see M. D. Ring, "The Early Life of Nathan Cooley Keep, Monumental Figure in American Dentistry," *Bulletin of the History of Dentistry* 38 (October 1990): 15-18; Hapgood, *Harvard Dental School*, pp. 15-18.

6 Hapgood, *Harvard Dental School*, p. 63; Harvard University, *Catalogue*, 1903 (Cambridge, Mass.: Harvard University, 1903), "The Dental School," p. 606.

7 Hapgood, *Harvard Dental School*, p.67. For a biographical sketch of Dean Eugene H. Smith, see pp. 235-238.

8 Register of the Dental School of Harvard University, Freshmen, September 1902 to June 1903, handwritten record listing students entering September 25, 1902. The Harvard University *Catalogue* 1904-1905, (p. 175) lists Varaztad Kazanjian as a third year student residing in Worcester, Mass.

9 Harvard University, *Catalogue*, 1902, p. 606; Cooke, "Kazanjian and Harvard," p. 24; Waldron, "Testimonial," p. 95.

10 Dr. Robert S. Catheron, Unpublished account included as a part of Dr. Ferdinand Brigham's longer manuscript on the Dental Unit of the First Harvard Unit during World War I. The section is headed, "Dr. Robert Catheron wrote the following appraisal of Kazanjian." It is in the author's private collection and was given to him personally by Dr. Brigham, whom he interviewed in Cambridge in the 1960s.

11 "Register of the Dental School of Harvard University, Juniors, October 1903 to June 1904," and letter from Dean Smith to Simon V. Pazeian, July 18, 1903, preserved among the records of the Harvard Dental School Archive in The Francis A. Countway Library of Medicine; Catheron, Unpublished account; Cooke, "Kazanjian and Harvard," p. 24.

12 Harvard University, *Catalogue* 1904-05, p. 174; *Worcester Directory,* 1905, lists Alexander Kazanjian on p. 360, Parsek Roopenian on p. 561. *Worcester House Directory,* 1908 (Worcester, Mass. Drew Allis), v. 2, p. 49, also lists both Alexander Kazanjian and Parsek Roopenian as living at 130 Belmont Street. In the *Worcester Directory* for 1912, Alexander Kazanjian is listed (p. 381) as "remitted to Boston." Also, M. Verazin, "A Famous Oral and Plastic Surgeon, *Hairenik Daily*, May 8, 1930, (in Armenian).

13 *Harvard Medical Alumni Bulletin*, 36, no. 3 (Winter 1962): 9; V. H. Kazanjian,

"Remembrance of Things Past," *Plastic and Reconstructive Surgery* 35, no. 1 (1965): 5; V. H. Kazanjian, taped interview with Robin Anderson, 1971, National Archives of Plastic Surgery in The Francis A. Countway Library of Medicine.

14 Claude Martin, *De la Prosthèse Immédiate, Appliqué à la Résection des Maxillaires* (Paris: G. Masson, 1889); "Obituary of Dr. Claude Martin," *The Dental Cosmos* 53 (1911): 497-498. F. Helme, "Le Docteur Claude Martin, de Lyon: Un Technicien de Génie," *La Presse Médicale* 925, no. 95 (Nov. 27, 1909). Kazanjian, "Remembrance," p. 7.

15 Twenty-seven candidates were awarded the D.M.D. degree in the Harvard dental class of 1905. Kazanjian's best grades were in histology and operative dentistry.

16 Another occupant of the office building at 74 Boylston Street was Aram Kazanjian, who was a photographer (*Boston Directory*, 1911, p. 1642). It is the author's belief that Aram and Varaztad were first cousins, their fathers being brothers. Aram Kazanjian had been a painter in Paris when he learned that his father had been killed in Armenia. He came to Boston, where he apprenticed himself to an Armenian photographer. He married a Bostonian, Leah Davis, and lived in the Boston area for seven years before moving to New York. Their daughter, Arlene Francis Kazanjian, born in Boston on October 23, 1908, went on to a distinguished career in stage, screen, and radio under her stage name, Arlene Francis. Her father and Dr. Kazanjian were strong influences on her life. See Arlene Francis (with Florence Rome), *Arlene Francis, A Memoir* (New York: Simon and Shuster, 1978). Arlene Francis died in 2001 and is remembered as "one of the busiest personalities on television in the 1950s." Obituary, *The Boston Globe,* June 2, 2001.

17 Waldron, "Testimonial," p. 95; Catheron, Unpublished account.

18 "Dental Practice Records 1909-1914," Kazanjian Archive, folder PS-2; Catheron, Unpublished account.

19 Harvard University, *Catalogues,* 1906-07, p. 31; 1907-08, p.36; also *Boston Sunday Globe*, November 21, 1915, which related that Dr. Kazanjian "was grabbed by Dean Smith as an instructor in prosthetics for the Dental School"; Hapgood, *Harvard Dental School*, pp. 80-105.

20 Cooke, "Kazanjian and Harvard," pp. 23-24; Catheron, Unpublished account.

21 Maxillofacial prosthetics is that dental specialty that deals with the fabrication of artificial substitutes for those parts of the oral cavity, face, and adjoining structures that have been lost to disease, surgery, trauma or congenital malformation.

22 *Boston Directory* 1913 (Boston: Sampson and Murdock, Association of American Directory Publishers, 1913) records his office at 157 Newbury Street and his home address as 538 Newbury Street. The Boston directories for 1906 to 1912 list his office at 74 Boylston Street. During this time, he had several home addresses: 1906, 594 Tremont Street; 1908, 534 Tremont Street; 1909, 555 Tremont Street; 1910, 5 Newbury Street; 1912, 85 St. Botolph Street. A letter from Dr. Kazanjian dated April 30, 1914 on the letterhead lists 157 Newbury Street as his office address. Miss Shaw went on to marry Frank P. Foisie, Harvard '12, and had four children, one of whom, Jack Foisie, became a newspaperman and Nieman Fellow at Harvard. See Letter from Jack Foisie to Dr. Kazanjian, December 18, 1946, Kazanjian Archive, folder C-153.

23 *Gotchnag*, February 23, 1918, pp. 1771-1772 (in Armenian); Letter from M. Vartan Malcom's son, Dr. Edward Malcom, of Boothbay, Maine, to the author, November 28, 1994. M. Vartan Malcom (Malcom Vartan Malconian) wrote *The Armenians in America* (Boston: Pilgrim Press, 1919). His autobiography appears on p. 24. He arrived in America in 1892.

24 Announcement of the Harvard Dental Alumni Association thirty-sixth annual meeting and banquet, June 24, 1907, Young Hotel, Boston. The Association was established in 1887 and organized in 1891 "to advance the cause of dental education, to promote the interest and increase the usefulness of the Harvard Dental School and to promote mutual acceptance and good fellowship among all members of the association." Harvard Dental School Archives.

25 Announcement of the Harvard Odontological Society Thirtieth Annual Meeting, Boston, March 7, 1908, in The Harvard Dental School Archives. Waldo Elias Boardman, *Biographies of the Founders, Ex-Presidents, Prominent Early*

Members and Others of the Massachusetts Dental Society (Boston: Massachusetts Dental Society, Frank D. Brown, 1914) contains a biographical sketch of Dr. Boardman, pp. 108-110. The Harvard Odontological Society was organized in 1878 by graduates of the Harvard Dental School "for promoting the Art and Science of Dentistry." See Hapgood, *Harvard Dental School,* pp. 214-221, for a history of the Harvard Odontological Society, and pp. 242-243 for additional material on Dr. Boardman.

26 Cooke, "Kazanjian and Harvard," p. 23. Kazanjian's article was titled "The Retention of Artificial Dentures," *The Journal of Allied Dental Societies* 6 (1911). The Armenian article appeared in Moushegh Seropian, *The American-Armenian Yearbook, 1913*, pp. 433-444.

27 Cooke, "Kazanjian and Harvard," p. 25; Kazanjian, "Remembrance," p. 6; J. S. Marshall, *A Manual of Injuries and Surgical Diseases of the Face, Mouth, and Jaws*, 2d ed. (Philadelphia: S. S. White Company, 1902), p. 224.

28 Kazanjian, "Remembrance", p. 7. Dr. Kazanjian was not the first one to use the intermaxillary wiring method. Thomas L. Gilmer, M.D., D.D.S., published an article in the *Archives of Dentistry* (1887), pp. 388-390, on "A Case of Fracture of the Lower Jaw With Remarks on the Treatment," in which he reported the technique. For a biographical sketch of Dr. Gilmer, see Frank McDowell, *The Source Book of Plastic Surgery* (Baltimore: Williams & Wilkins, 1977), pp. 358-359. See also Cooke, "Kazanjian and Harvard," pp. 25-26.

29 Kazanjian, "Remembrance," p. 5.

30 Ibid., pp. 5-6. The quotation is from Dr. Calvin Case (1847-1923), an American dentist. Also Cooke, "Kazanjian and Harvard," p. 25.

31 H. Martin Deranian, "The First Honor Society for Dentists," a paper delivered before the American Academy of Dental Science, April 14, 1987, Boston, Massachusetts. Dr. Kazanjian became an Active Fellow in the Academy of Dental Science on April 1, 1914. Its president was Albert Jewell, its vice-president George Payne, and its secretary Waldo Boardman. Dr. Kazanjian served as its president in 1937-1938 and became an Honorary Fellow in 1949. American Academy of Dental Science, Inc., List of Fellows, 1959, p. 18.

32 V. H. Kazanjian, "Prosthetic Restoration of Acquired Deformities of the Superior Maxilla," *Journal of Allied Dental Societies* 10 no. 14 (1915), 16 pages with 16 illustrations; *Saturday Review,* July 7, 1962, p. 42. Also published in *Harvard Medical Alumni Bulletin* 36, no. 3 (winter 1962): 8-10 and reported in Tashjian, "Dr. Varaztad Kazanjian, a Profile," *Armenian Review* 1, no. 1, (Winter 1948): 91. Robert LeRoy Ripley's (1893-1949) syndicated "Believe It Or Not" columns, cartoons and features in newspapers, on radio, and in films on curiosities and oddities made him a celebrity worldwide. His column had national distribution, appearing at its peak in 17 languages in 330 newspapers in 32 countries, and brought him one million letters a year. His "Believe It Or Not" column was continued after his death and even has currency today.

33 Malvin E. Ring, "The History of Maxillofacial Prosthetics," *Plastic and Reconstructive Surgery* 87, no. 1 (1991): 174-184, traces the history of this specialty from ancient Egypt to the present.

34 Letter from Frank C. Richardson, Registrar, Boston University School of Medicine, to Dr. V. H. Kazanjian, September 6, 1912, Kazanjian Archive, folder C-607; Cooke, "Kazanjian and Harvard," p. 24.

35 Hapgood, *Harvard Dental School*, pp. 111-112. File on Harold DeWitt Cross, Harvard Dental School Archives; also, *Harvard Dental Alumni Bulletin* 3, no. 2 (January 1943): 36; Hélène K. Sargeant, "Some Notes Concerning the Family of Dr. Varaztad H. Kazanjian," March 1978, preserved in Varaztad H. Kazanjian Archive in The Francis A. Countway Library of Medicine, Harvard Medical School. M. Verazin, "Professor Varaztad H. Kazanjian: His Surgery During the Great War," *Hairenik Monthly* 8, no. 2/95 (Sept. 1930): 159 (in Armenian); *Armenian Encyclopedic Almanac* 1925 (Boston: Hairenik Press, 1925), p. 311 (in Armenian).

36 Taped interview by Robert M. Goldwyn and Madeleine W. Mullen of Louise Roopenian, Assistant to Dr. V. H. Kazanjian, November 22, 1991, of which a copy is in the National Archives of Plastic Surgery at The Francis A. Countway Library of Medicine. Sophie Cuendet was born on January 12, 1886, the daughter of Edouard Cuendet and Sophie Junod. Helen J. Lamb, *World War I, An American Nurse With the British Troops in France, Nov. 1916 - Feb. 1919* (Provo, Utah: Stevenson's Genealogical Center, 1981), p.

65. Lamb volunteered for service with the Second Harvard Unit under Dr. David Cheever's command. Her book contains short, daily entries describing life in a military hospital in Dannes-Camiers; on May 27, 1918, she was invited to tea with Major and Mrs. Kazanjian. The three Cuendet sisters appear first in the 1908 *Boston Directory*: Sophie, living at 107 Audubon Road, the other two sisters at 38 St. Botolph Street; 1909, all three sisters at 38 St. Botolph Street; 1910, all three sisters at 13 Dalton Street; 1912, all three sisters at 21 Hemenway Street. There is no mention of the name Cuendet in the 1913 *Boston Directory*. Ida Cuendet and Victor de Bellefroid were married in Beverly, Massachusetts on September 4, 1909. See the Commonwealth of Massachusetts, "Registry of Vital Records and Statistics," 1909, v. 586, p. 397. Information also provided in an interview with Dr. Edward V. Malcom by the author at Sawyer's Island, Boothbay, Maine, on August 5, 1995. Victor de Bellefroid is listed as a ridingmaster at 52 Hemenway Street, Boston, *Boston Directory*, 1906, 1907 and 1913.

37 The Commonwealth of Massachusetts, "Registry of Vital Records and Statistics," 1912, v. 613, p. 326, number 7472, Record of Marriage. Kazanjian gave his address as 66 Huntington Avenue and Sophie Cuendet as 17 Hemenway Street in Boston. Also *Boston Directory* 1912, p. 2119.

38 Certificate of marriage between Malcom Vartan Malcom and Georgine Lucie Cuendet, Montclair, New Jersey, October 26, 1912, performed by Edgar Swam Wiers, minister of Unity Church, Montclair. Among the witnesses to the wedding who signed the certificate was Hélène Bartel, another sister of the bride. Also, letter to the author from Dr. Edward V. Malcom, their son, February 27, 1996.

39 *Boston Sunday Globe*, November 21, 1915, p. 32, col. 3.

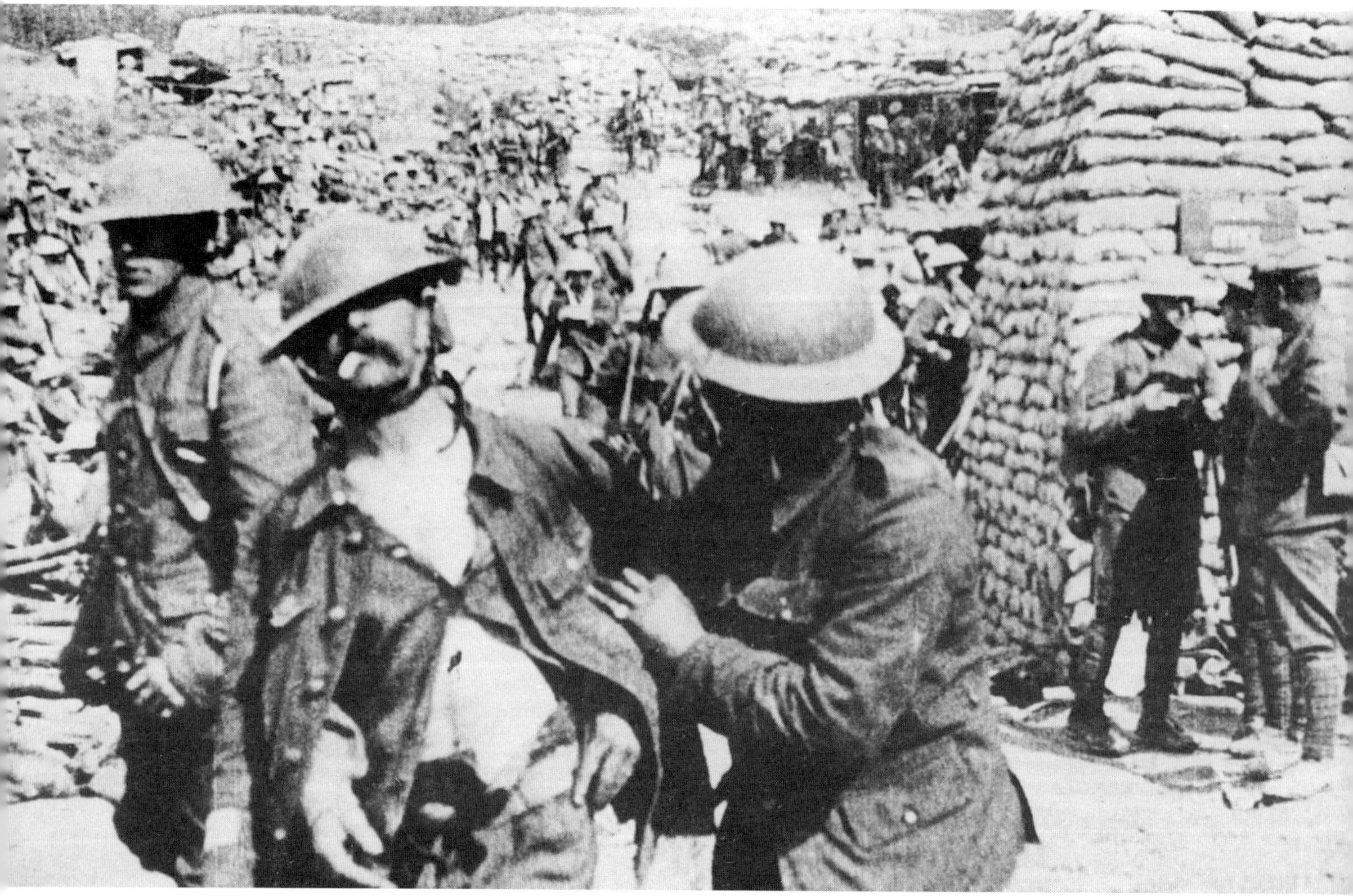

World War I photograph, Q79508, Courtesy of the Imperial War Museum, London

CHAPTER FOUR

The Great War

World War I began modestly with the firing of two pistols on June 28, 1914. Nonetheless, there was a premonition of events to come. Sir Edward Grey, England's Foreign Secretary, commented to a friend, while watching the street lamps being lit, "The lamps are going out all over Europe. We shall not see them lit again in our lifetime."[1] The English war poet Wilfred S. Owen expressed the same sentiment more imaginatively in his poem "1914":

> *War broke: and now the Winter of the world-*
> *with perishing great darkness closes in.*[2]

When the armistice was signed four years later, on November 11, 1918, ten million men had been killed and nearly twenty million had been wounded or crippled. The face of the world was forever changed.[3]

At first the United States followed a policy of neutrality, but from the start there existed intense feelings in support of the Allies (England, France and Russia) and their cause. That support was heightened and given cause on May 7, 1915, by the sinking of the British liner *Lusitania*. The 32,000-ton Cunard passenger ship had sailed on her regular run from New York to Liverpool on May 1. She carried 1,257 passengers and crew of 702. She was torpedoed by a German U-boat only a few miles off the southwestern Irish coast and sank in eighteen minutes, before life boats and life rafts could be fully loaded and lowered, with the loss of 1,195 lives, of which 128 were Americans, and thirty-five infants. Unknown at the time that the ship's cargo also included munitions, this action brought the drama of war to America and horrified the neutral people of the world.[4]

The Canadian-born physician, Sir William Osler, then Regius Professor of Medicine at Oxford and one of the most influential teachers of medicine in his day, reflected the strong ties that many of the people of the United States still held to Britain. In April 1915, he urged that Harvard and two other American universities supply health professionals to staff a much-needed base hospital in France or England to care for casualties sustained by the British Expeditionary Force(BEF) and to relieve over-taxed British physicians.

"Do you think that Harvard University," Sir William wrote to Harvard President Abbot Lawrence Lowell on April 3, 1915, "would offer to staff a British war hospital for 1,040 beds?" In his effort to attain this goal, Osler was assisted by Robert Bacon, an A.B. graduate of Harvard College (1880) with whom he conferred in London, and by Sir James Bryce (1838-1922), who had been the British ambassador at Washington from 1907 to 1913.[5] "The plan arose in the fertile brain of Sir William Osler," Dr. David Cheever wrote, "who at once consulted with Dr. Harvey Cushing." Cushing, who was in France in April 1915, reported that Sir William and Robert Bacon gave him "a dossier of documents and letters on the subject to present to the Harvard authorities," and asked him "to get first-hand information." Nonetheless, despite his

English heritage, Lowell, a fair-minded man, said, "If Germany should make a similar request, I should make my best to furnish a similar unit."[6]

The Geneva Conventions comprised an international agreement established in 1864 and supplemented afterwards to improve the condition of wounded and captured soldiers of armies in the field. One clause provided that a neutral nation "may send sanitary and medical aid to a belligerent nation without breaking the neutrality of the persons in that service, providing that the nation to whom the aid is sent shall notify its enemy. It was under this clause . . . that . . . American citizens went to aid the wounded of the British Expeditionary Force." Initially, Columbia University and Johns Hopkins agreed to join Harvard in the enterprise, each institution responsible for providing personnel for three months of service, with Harvard being the first. There was an alarming need for such aid, for in the single month of May 1915, the number of sick and wounded troops returning to England from the Western Front was 42,000.[7]

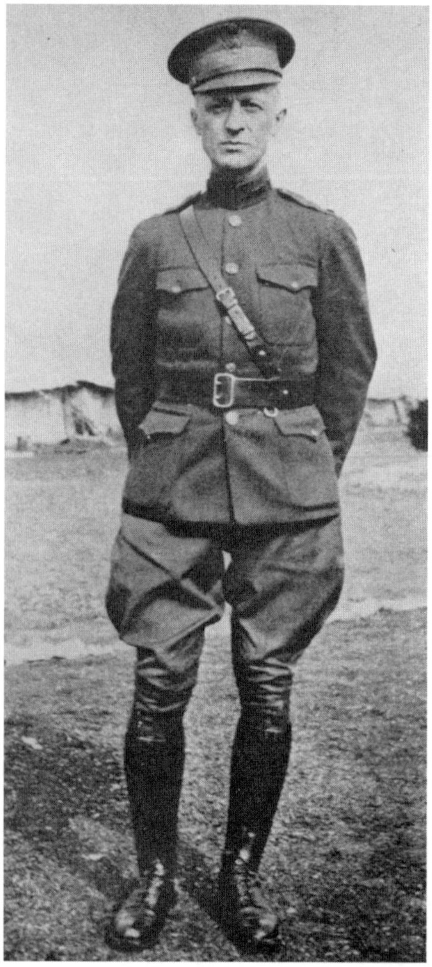

Dr. Harvey Cushing, Yale University. Harvey Cushing/John Jay Whitney Medical Library

Harvard already had volunteer medical personnel serving in Europe. The American Ambulance, located at Neuilly-sur-Seine, a suburb of Paris, was a military hospital and ambulance service established by the former American ambassador, Robert Bacon. The French government had allowed them the use of a school, Lycée Pasteur. The first wounded soldiers arrived on September 7, 1914. [8]

With Dr. Harvey Cushing as chief, a surgical unit from Harvard Medical School served at the American Ambulance hospital from April to July 1, 1915. The surgical unit was one of the first agencies of American aid. There were thirteen physicians in the unit, many of them Americans living in Europe. It was funded by a gift of $10,000 through the generosity of William Lindsay, of Boston. At the time, it was called the First Harvard Unit, which led to later confusion when the First Harvard Surgical Unit was formed.[9]

There was a dental department at the American Ambulance hospital for the treatment of dental, jaw and facial wounds. The department was under the care of Drs. George B. Hayes and William Davenport, American dentists practicing in Paris. From November 1914 to February 1915 they were joined temporarily by Dr. William H. Potter, Professor of Operative Dentistry at the Harvard Dental School, who was visiting in France. Upon his return to Boston, Dr. Potter undoubtedly informed Dr. Kazanjian of the great need for his specialized services in France. When Dr. Cushing arrived in April 1915, he expressed regret "that we could not have brought a capable dentist with us." He pointed out that the work in

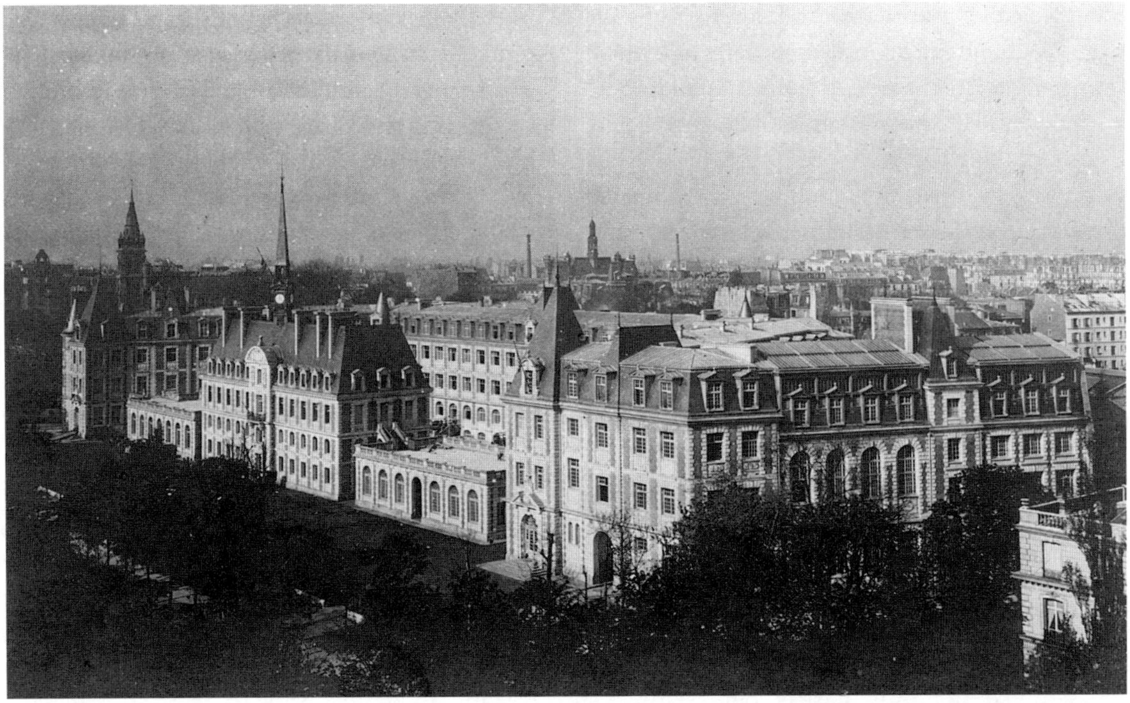

American Ambulance, Lycée Pasteur, Neuilly-Sur-Seine
The Harvard Medical Library in the Francis A. Countway Library of Medicine

the dental department was "doubtless the most impressive work we have thus far seen—new, ingenious, effective."[10]

It was predicted on both sides that the war would be a short one. "You will be home before the leaves have fallen from the trees," the Kaiser told his departing troops. "We were in a hurry," Dr. Ferdinand Brigham said, "because most authorities estimated that the war would be over and the Germans defeated in four weeks. Despite initial optimism, attaining that objective took four prolonged years." By the end of 1914 the opposing armies became trapped below ground level in muddy trenches along a virtually stationary line extending 1,656 miles from Switzerland to the North Sea. The front never advanced more that ten miles in either direction. Only a hundred yard "no man's land" separated the enemies at some points.[11]

Life for the soldiers in the trenches approached and often exceeded the limits of human endurance. "We lived like swine," one soldier reported.

> *The trenches are lines, one behind the other of course, but joined together in all directions by every kind of communication trench, like the streets of a city, for a man never shows his head above the ground. There are all kinds of subterranean cells and passages; also one has to sleep under ground, wallow in the mud, eat in the mud. Our hands and faces, our uniforms, above all our feet, are caked with it all day. The sleeping quarters are fairly well protected from the rain, but the greatest hardships are the mud, the wet, the inability to wash the slightest bit, as water, except rain—is very rare—and for me who am tall, the continual necessity of stooping down so as not to get my head knocked off by the enemy snipers.*[12]

In colossal battles that ebbed and flowed, a generation of Europe's youth was forever lost or maimed and its aristocracy virtually annihilated.[13]

The Harvard Unit that Sir William Osler had proposed was a surgical unit on a much larger scale than previously organized and was intended to staff a field hospital of 1,000 beds. It was rapidly organized in May 1915 under the professional direction of Dr. Edward H. Nichols, "one of the most prominent Boston physicians," who practiced at 294 Marlborough Street and who was an associate professor at the Harvard Medical School. Herbert H. White, head of the Harvard University Press, in Cambridge, was appointed as business manager. Provision was made originally for thirty-two physicians and surgeons and seventy-five nurses. Later, positions were added for three dentists, who were Harvard graduates. A fourth dentist, Dr. Samuel A. Hopkins, also joined the Unit. The Unit was assembled not only hastily but seemingly cursorily.[14]

Varaztad Kazanjian first learned of the formation of the Harvard Unit, according to Dr. John M. Converse, as "the result of a chance encounter on Commonwealth Avenue in Boston." Events were unfolding early in 1915 in Ottoman Turkey, one of the Central Powers, which may have influenced Dr. Kazanjian to volunteer his services to the Allied war effort. Beginning on February 19, 1915, British naval forces sought to break through the Dardanelles and to seize Constantinople. "On March 19, the Germans and Turks were prepared to retreat to Anatolia and leave Constantinople at the mercy of the British," Henry Morganthau, American Ambassador in Turkey, recorded. "The Allies abandoned the attack at the precise moment when complete victory was in their grasp." The subsequent Allied land campaign at Gallipoli similarly ended disastrously several months later, with the heaviest casualties sustained by the British and the Australian-New Zealand Army Corps (ANZAC). After one month of action, the Allied navy almost achieved its objective, but hastily withdrew after seven ships struck mines, three of them having sunk.[15]

Soon thereafter, on April 24, 1915, some 200 unsuspecting Armenian intellectuals and leaders in Constantinople were aroused from their sleep, imprisoned, tortured and killed. Dr. Kazanjian was well aware of these and other new atrocities before he joined the Harvard Unit. They were reported in *The New York Times* beginning in early April.[16] His brother, Roupen, was in Sivas, his fate at the time uncertain. Kazanjian may have felt that serving the Allied cause was also service to his beleaguered people.

"Dr. Edward Nichols took some good advice and offered the job [as chief dental officer] to Kazanjian," Dr. John Cooke wrote , adding "It was Bob Catheron who told the truth about what Kazanjian could do." This was another instance of Dr. Catheron's loyalty and support of Dr. Kazanjian, dating back to their student days as members of the Harvard dental class of 1905. Dr. Kazanjian himself stated that "Dr. Nichols asked me to join and take charge of the dental surgery as a part of the hospital." Anxious to participate in some form of war service, perhaps sensing the possibilities that such service would offer in the future and development of maxillofacial prosthetics and the treatment of jaw and facial wounds, Dr. Kazanjian reported, "I accepted the offer and chose for my assistants Ferdinand Brigham and Frank Cushman, who were both seniors at the school." Dr. Brigham, who was President of the Class of 1915, had received an A.B. from Tufts University and Dr. Cushman a B.S. from Dartmouth. "The Unit left two days before commencement, so that ceremony was denied me," Brigham later lamented, "and I never saw my diploma and my state license for four years." He volunteered for the unknown out of a sense of adventure.[17]

Initially, the roles that the dentists were to perform were ill-defined. Dr. Kazanjian joined as "the prosthetic dental expert;" but the dentists

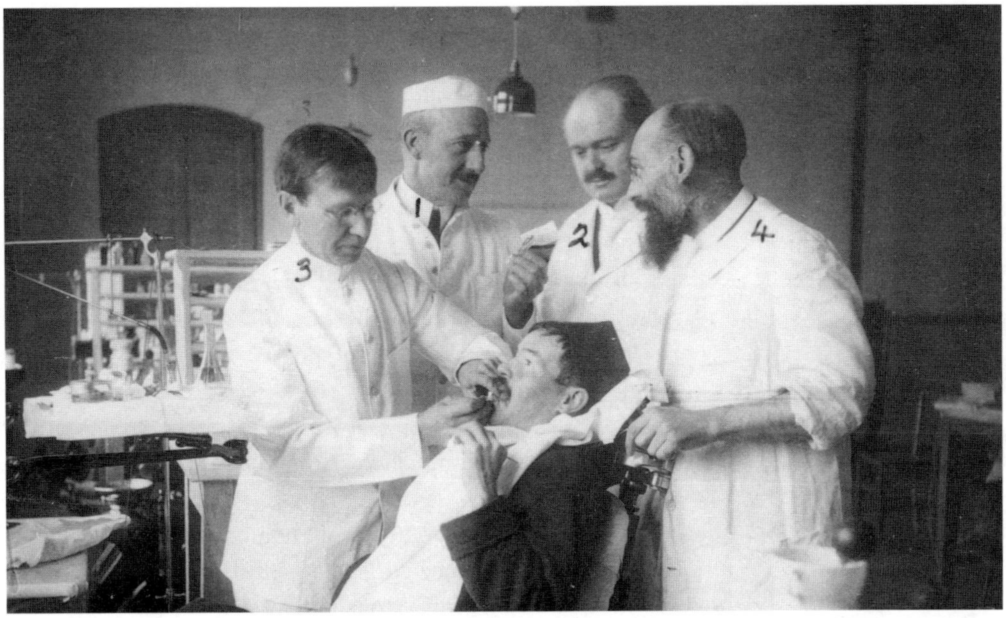

Officers of the Dental Department of the American Ambulance: 1. Dr. George B. Hayes; 2. Dr. William Davenport, Jr.; 3. Dr. William H. Potter; 4. Dr. Choquet
The Harvard Medical Library in the Francis A. Countway Library of Medicine

had no idea what they were to do in warfare. For a time, Dr. Samuel A. Hopkins, M.D., D.M.D. (neither degree from Harvard) was nominated as "chief dental consultant of the Harvard Unit." As Brigham reported,

> *Dr. Hopkins was the richest of the Back Bay dentists . . . and with his two degrees had the ear of the Medical Faculty . . . Dr. Smith, Dean of the Harvard Dental School, worried about the imaginary future trouble between his quiet, unknown knight and the polished, sophisticated campaigner . . . Dr. Kazanjian showed no concerns . . . he simply told the Dean, "Let's wait until we get to work."*

"At least he could have chosen a Harvard dentist," Dr. Smith grumbled.[18]

Dr. Brigham wrote in his memoir that "He [Dean Smith] sensed that it was the most dramatic event in the history of the School, and he intended to make the most of it."

> *He chose Dr. Kazanjian with instinctive judgment, based on all his experience in choosing men and shaping dental events. Dr. Smith knew that his quiet, unassuming manner, which confounded many from that day to this into thinking that he was timid or unmethodical, cloaked a thorough-going ability to forge ahead, an ease in organizing, an imagination in meeting the unknown. Then, as now, Dr. Kazanjian had the knack of making it look as though the other fellow really organized the job; that he had just happened to be around at the time. It is to heap praise on a friend one admires. Other things he was not. He was not of the elite Back Bay dentists, his reputation as a teacher did not yet go far beyond Harvard's door, he was not an M.D. as well as a D.M.D., he had not been in the position to know medical members of the Unit well, he had not yet gained the prestige with the University and Medical School that*

older dentists enjoyed. I am not sure that Dr. Smith considered any other candidate than Dr. Kazanjian. He could have chosen someone whose reputation had gone farther among the profession, he might have chosen a personal associate, or someone prone to enhance his personal position, but he had the interest of the School at heart. He read the future carefully.[19]

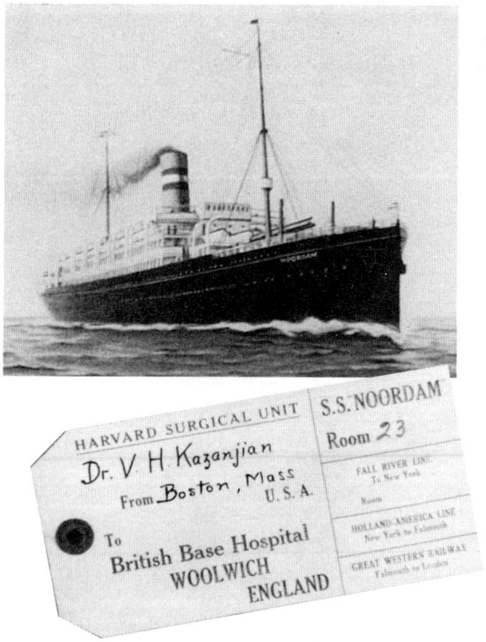

Above: *S. S. Noordam, Holland-American Line, the ship that carried the First Harvard Unit to England*
Below: *Dr. Kazanjian's baggage tag*
The Harvard Medical Library in the Francis A. Countway Library of Medicine

"I was present," Dr. Catheron later wrote, "when Dr. Harvey Cushing spoke at the Harvard Dental School to the alumni. The hearty and prolonged applause when Dr. Cushing spoke of Kazanjian as the school's representative showed that the alumni were solidly behind the appointment." It proved to be a major turning point in the life of Dr. Kazanjian. The recruitment of the members of the Harvard Unit had to be accomplished with extraordinary care and caution on account of "the degree of German spies securing service in the Royal Army Medical Corps." It was mandated that "no person whose loyalty to the Allied cause could be held in doubt should be enlisted as an officer or sister [nurse] in the Harvard Unit."[20]

An incident occurred just before sailing which demonstrated Kazanjian's memory and clear thinking. A list was needed of dental instruments and supplies for immediate use during the initial three-months stay. From sheer memory and without any omissions, he compiled the list, a remarkable feat, as the number of instuments and supplies was very large. The dental equipment, which was purchased in this country and paid for by the Unit, included ordinary instruments for amalgams and cement fillings, a complete set of extracting instruments, a laboratory set, including a foot-lathe, gasoline blow-pipe, German silver and wire and plate metal, vulcanite rubber, a good supply of Novocain, and material for the treatment of maxillary fractures.[21]

President and Mrs. Lowell tendered a reception at their Quincy Street home in Cambridge on June 18 for the doctors of the Unit. The entire Unit assembled at Boston's South Station on June 25, 1915, and travelled to New York by the Fall River Boat. There they boarded the S. S. *Noordam*, a neutral ship of the Holland-American Line, which sailed on June 26. Drs. Brigham and Cushman shared a stateroom. "Our party is a jolly one," Brigham wrote to Dean Smith just before sailing, "at least so far."[22]

It was a rough fifteen-day crossing with great heaps of marvelous Dutch food left uneaten. Near the British Isles, the ship took a zig-zag course to avoid reported German submarines. For Dr. Kazanjian this eastward crossing of the Atlantic was markedly different from his westward crossing twenty years earlier. This time he travelled in a first-class cabin rather than in steerage. As the ship

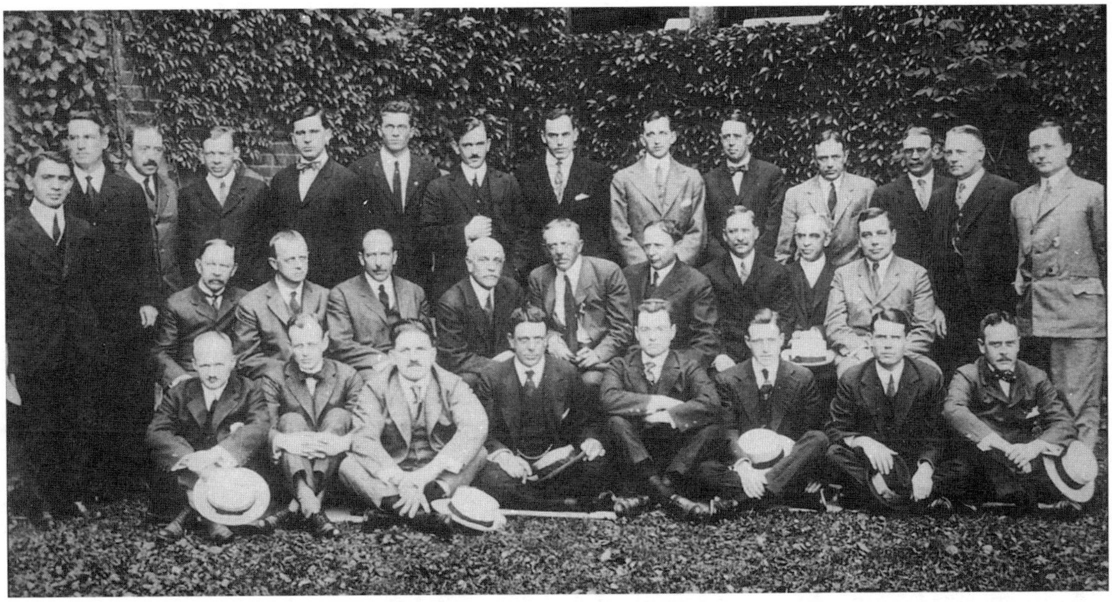

Members of the First Harvard Unit, prior to sailing on June 26, 1915
Dr. Kazanjian is the first one standing on the left.
The Harvard Medical Library in the Francis A. Countway Library of Medicine

approached England on July 4, the passengers sang "The Star Spangled Banner" and "Fair Harvard," indicating the shared allegiances that motivated them to undertake this enterprise.[23]

They docked at Falmouth and were placed on a train on the Great Western Railway for London. En route, they received their first remuneration from the British in the form of gold coins of the realm, which included wages from the time they volunteered plus a uniform allowance. Their arrival caused something of a stir. The British War Office did not know what to do with them; there was no precedent to follow. Their chief, Dr. Nichols, resolutely refused to allow them to take the oath of allegiance to the British Crown with its traditional "So help me God" response. They were officially listed in the British Gazette as officers of the Royal Army Medical Corps with equivalent rank, and they drew the appropriate pay, but their uniform was cock-eyed. It contained no pips (stars) and no insignia indicating rank on shoulder straps or wrists, but the name HARVARD was embroidered on the shoulders. "On the street all ranks looked at us in curiosity and amazement," Dr. Brigham recorded, "and we were considerably embarrassed."[24]

They were rightfully designated the First Harvard Unit, in contrast to Dr. Cushing's group at the American Ambulance hospital in Paris. The Army Register officially listed Dr. Nichols' group as the Harvard Unit and the officers had identification disks with the lettering "H.U."[25] The remainder of their clothes consisted of the standard khaki uniform of a British officer of World War I, including the Sam Browne belt[26] and puttees. "A soldier's length of service," Dr. Brigham wrote, "and in fact his neatness, character, type and everything can be interpreted in his puttees."[27]

The four dentists in the Unit were granted the specially created rank of Honorary Lieutenant in the Royal Army Medical Corps, a remarkable deference to American dentists since their British colleagues were not commissioned in the British Army at the time. For their chief, Dr. Nichols, the commission of temporary Lieutenant Colonel was created. While the Unit was waiting in London "pending final disposition" of their services, they visited various military hospitals. Dr. Kazanjian observed that "special maxillofacial centers for the British Army were not perfected in organization, and patients with gunshot wounds of the face and jaws were not confined to hospitals especially equipped for their treatment.[28]

The Unit was graciously entertained on July 10, 1915, at Warwick Castle, which had been leased that summer to Henry W. Marsh, a Chicago insurance man and a Harvard graduate. He assisted the Unit and became an assistant to Herbert H. White, who was the manager of all of the Harvard units during their stay in France. The Unit was kept in London for over ten days, "doing nothing and waiting patiently. They do not hurry here very much." Lieutenant Kazanjian used the time to inquire into the dental situation in the British Army.[29]

On July 17, 1915, about one year after the war had begun, the Harvard Unit sailed for France. When they crossed the English Channel, their ship was convoyed by torpedo boats, and they were required to wear life preservers. Their destination was Dannes and Camiers, two hamlets situated fourteen miles south of Boulogne-sur-Mer on the Channel coast. There they took over General Hospital No. 22, which was one of a group of five base hospitals located adjacent to one another, containing a combined total of about 10,000 beds. It was situated a quarter-mile from the joint railroad station, Dannes-Camiers, which was on the main rail line from Boulogne to Paris.[30] The site of the hospital had been a "soggy field" and the conditions were described in verse as,

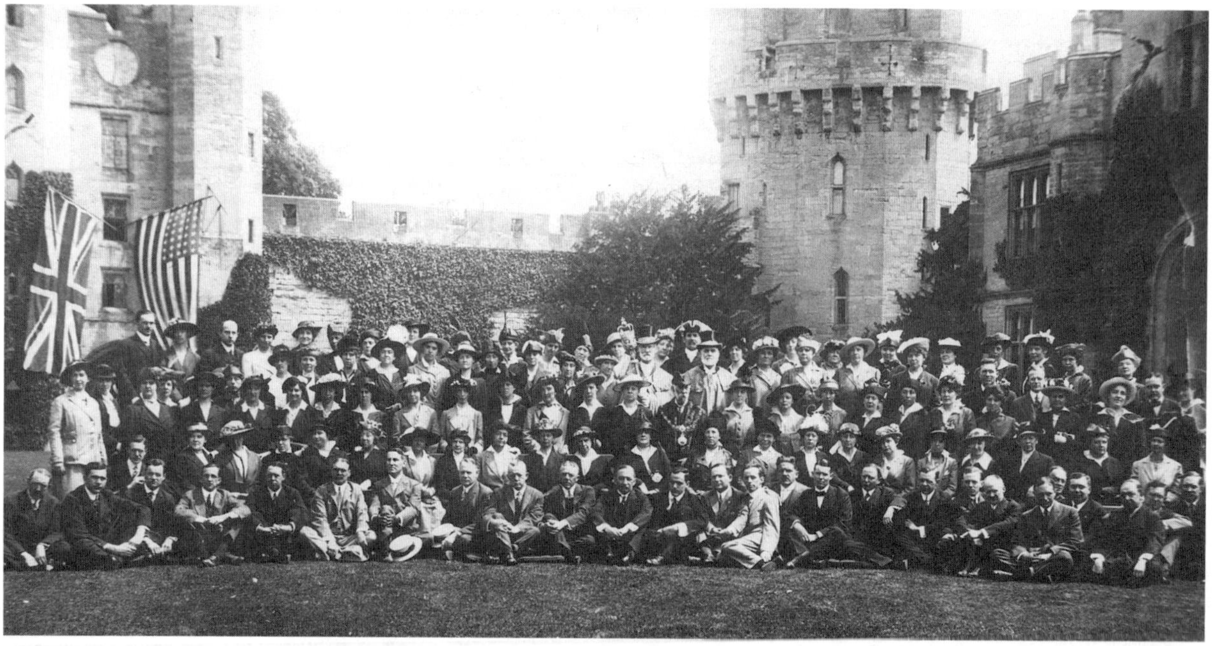

Harvard Unit entertained at Warwick Castle, England, July 10, 1915
The Harvard Medical Library in the Francis A. Countway Library of Medicine

In Camiers by the sea. . .
In mud up to my knees, and it's mud we get at tea,
The stretchers, I found, came hard up from
the ground,
You had to hustle, use all you muscle,
And the nurses wore a frown.[31]

Except for a few buildings where surgery was performed, the facilities of General Hospital No. 22 were under tents erected by the Royal Engineers. "Our hospital was situated in a field in northern France," Dr. Kazanjian wrote. "We have no luxuries such as hospital buildings, gas and electricity or running water. Everyone is arranged under tents." A few months later he reported, "It is more or less a lonesome place, and living conditions are far from ideal."[32] Dr. Kazanjian's ability to speak French fluently, which he had learned in Sivas, was a major asset.

Each British general hospital unit was a self-contained village, with its own commanding officer and administration. There was an interchange of services among hospitals. The arrival of the Harvard Unit relieved British doctors to perform other duties. However, the administrative functions remained with the Royal Army Medical Corps. The British doctors and nurses stepped out of the hospital, and the Americans stepped in. The British commanding officer was Sir Allan Perry, "straight out of Kipling's pages, swagger, titled . . . who maintained good old-time discipline, spit and polish. He was formerly governor of Ceylon."[33]

In addition to the officers, there was a staff of seventy-five nurses, under the supervision of a matron, and some 200 orderlies and clerks headed by a sergeant major. Officers were assigned a manservant called a batman (usually a private in

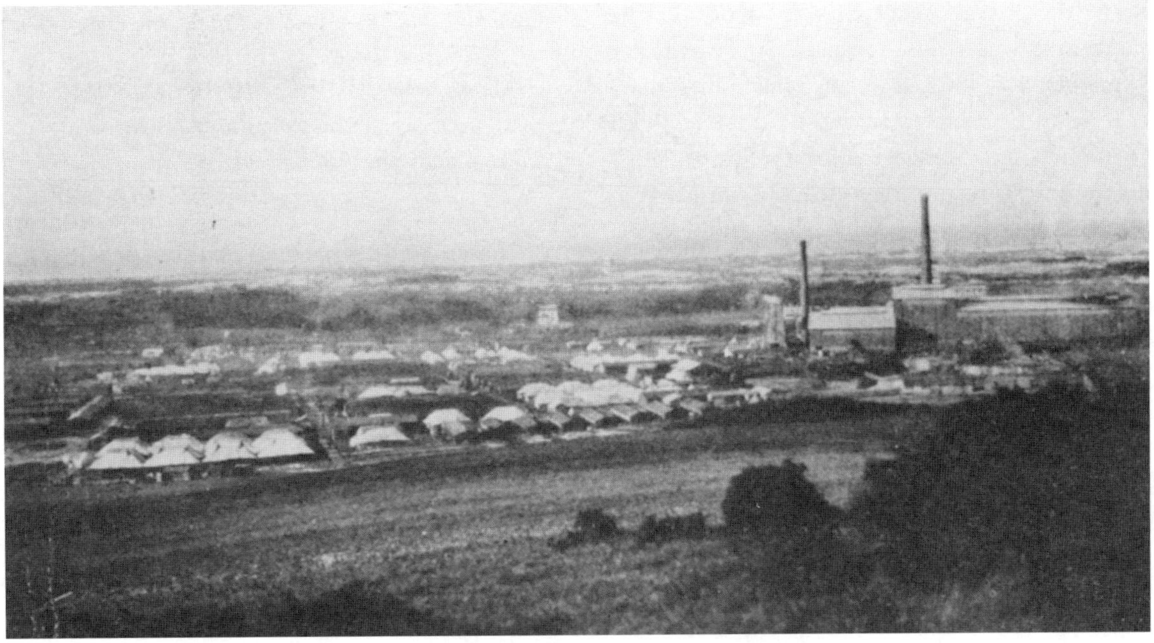

Hospitals in Dannes-Camiers, primarily under tents, 1914-1918
"At our feet lies a city of tents, spread out for miles between the dunes and the downs, white and spatter against the evening sun," Sir William Osler observed "and the scene reminds one of the descriptions of the tents of Israel in Moab." Note the cement factory in the background.
The Harvard Medical Library in the Francis A. Countway Library of Medicine, Hapgood, p. 124

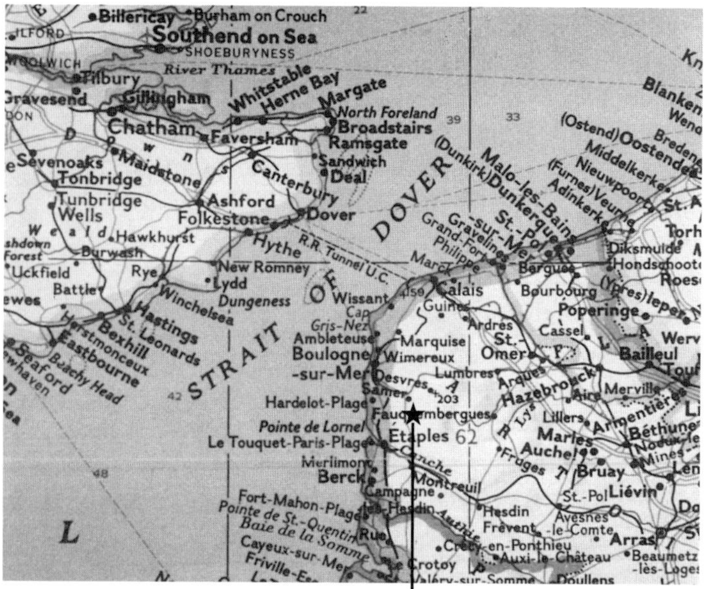

Map locating Dannes-Camiers
July-December 1915 (vol. xxviii)
Courtesy National Geographic Society

rank in the Royal Army Medical Corps). The organization was wholly British. The wards for the patients were located in large field tents (marquees) measuring twenty by eighty feet, each with four main poles. They were set three in a horizontal row and were interconnected with a central passage, with wooden floors and electric lights and with a row of thirty-five beds on each side with lockers. At first there were 1,040 beds, but the number gradually increased to 2,380.[34]

The few long permanent buildings were called huts and had a standard size of about twenty-five by 100 feet. They were made of a combination of wooden panels or uralite and cement. They were partitioned into offices, supply rooms and operating rooms for the most serious cases. Officers and soldiers were housed in bell tents, which were twelve feet in diameter and ten feet high, with wooden floors. An officer's tent was sparsely furnished, with a bed, a two-inch thick cork mattress, three blankets, a table, a washstand, a four-foot square tub, and an armchair. Tents frequently collapsed during gales, mostly at night. "You wake up in the cold February rain . . . take off your pajamas . . . grab the mallet, and in the raw, get it pegged and tied down fast."[35]

Baths were taken in the tents using pails of water. "Just put on my cap and shook two earwigs [an insect, resembling the rove beetle] out of it," Dr. Daniel Reardon, one of the surgeons of the First Unit, reported. "They were everywhere and made friends easily." He recalled chasing a "flea which had been feeding on me a good part of the day." Gourmet meals were a rarity, so doctors would often walk seven miles from camp and back to feast at a small restaurant "and thought it well worthwhile."[36]

Dr. Cushman described the adverse conditions in Dannes-Camiers in a letter he wrote home on September 29, 1915:

> *Here are Brig[ham] and I at the laboratory, though it is 11 p.m., trying to keep warm with candle, two lanterns, the sterilizer and two cigarettes going to capacity. It is cold, windy, rainy, muddy, and all else that's disagreeable outdoors, and that though you're cold and wet, there's no place at all to go where you can better your condition much.*[37]

Later, in the place of tents, chicken coops were imported and used. The men were inclined "to grouse about the small size," Dr. Hugh Cabot observed, "particularly those who require eight or ten feet of head room . . . they will be extremely glad to occupy the aforesaid chicken coop when the weather gets bad."[38]

In charge of all of the hospitals in the area of Dannes-Camiers was Colonel William Carr, whose title was Deputy Director of Medical Services and whose headquarters was in Étaples. He was able and imaginative and was to become a firm supporter of the work that Dr. Kazanjian was performing. The patients in General Hospital No. 22

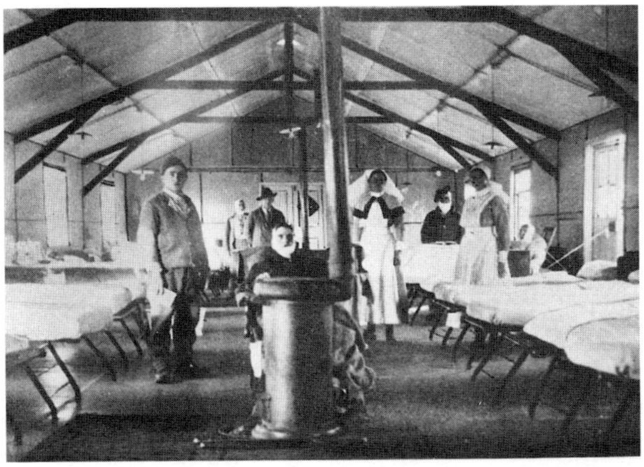

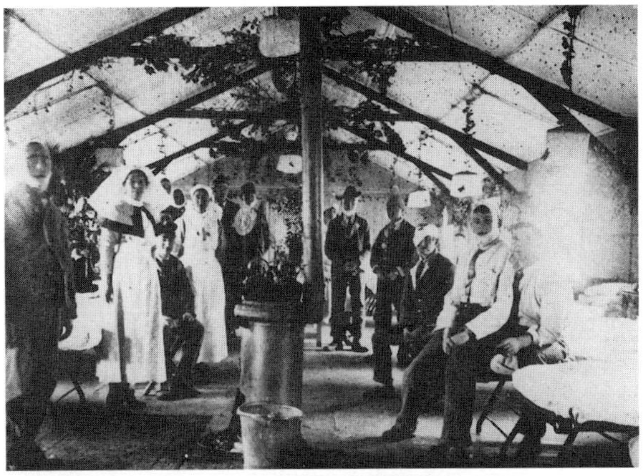

Two Views of the Dental Ward, General Hospital No. 20, Dannes-Camiers
Left, Hapgood, p. 124; right, The Harvard Medical Library in the Francis A. Countway Library of Medicine

were primarily Tommies who fought in the British-manned sector of the front about forty to sixty miles away.[39] In addition, the hospital served a few French soldiers, who were guarding the lines of communication, and the local French civilian population, as well as the staff of the hospital itself.

The soldiers were received at the hospital from one to three days after they were wounded. Initially they were transferred by ambulance to the casualty clearing station, which was from six to eight miles from the front line. From there they were transported to the vicinity of the hospital by trains and barges. The final journey to the hospital compound was made by ambulance. The trains stopped on a siding a few hundred yards from the five hospitals. The beds in the hospitals were as empty as possible in anticipation of the arrival of wounded soldiers. As a consequence, only those who would recover quickly or those who could not be moved were kept. "A base hospital under pressure can handle a thousand cases in and out, but it takes perfect organization." If walking cases predominated among the injured, it signified that "our side did not do well in the push, and did not have time to pick up our own wounded."[40]

"A few hours after we arrived here," Lieutenant Kazanjian informed Dean Smith, "I was ready for work. In fact, the dental unit was the first one to begin work. It was very fortunate that we had a complete dental outfit with us except dental chair. However, a portable head-rest came in very handy." Thus the first organized dental unit of the British Expeditionary Force in France took form and became functional under Lieutenant Kazanjian's command. The Western Front was quiet during most of the summer of 1915 while preparations were being made for a great autumn Allied offensive. As a result there were comparatively few wounded patients in the hospital. Sir William Osler observed that "in hospitals idle times and empty beds breed dissatisfaction."[41] By contrast, the primitive dental department was swamped.

"I have never seen such a group of young men with poorer teeth," Dr. Kazanjian reported, "not even at the dental school clinic." He continued:

> *The first thing I did was to depend on old fashioned dental forceps to clean the mouths. Our Novocain outfit proved very valuable. Within two weeks, we have fitted out a dental*

clinic and laboratory and put it in working order. We have extracted hundreds of useless teeth and roots: we made several plates and some cleaning and cement fillings (the latter ones done by Dr. Hopkins). By making such a good start we not only justified our existence here, but we command the respect of the medical men, the whole neighborhood and especially the English authorities.[42]

Good oral hygiene in the trenches was impossible. Tooth brushes were scarce and often passed "from mouth to mouth with contaminating effect." Disease of the gums was rampant. Among British naval recruits, 70 percent were in need of the services of a dentist and 50 percent required artificial teeth.[43]

"I am asking a few questions about teeth," Dr. Roger I. Lee reported. He was a Lieutenant Colonel in the U. S. Army Medical Corps stationed at Base Hospital No. 5. "Some [Tommies] have never cleaned their teeth. I got one gem. No, he hadn't cleaned his teeth for a long time, perhaps a dozen years; they were so bad he didn't think they would stand it." "Appalling as it seems," Dr. Cushman wrote, "a British Army order provides that no man with two teeth, one on either jaw, which occlude, shall be furnished by the government with dentures. This means, of course, that only those in the most desperate need of artificial teeth were provided with them, but even with this limitation, two laboratory men are kept constantly busy on this sort of work."[44]

Cushman added: "The original bad condition of the men's mouths . . . and the unhealthful water that the troops are obliged to drink, made it necessary during the summer to send increasing numbers back to the base hospital for dental treatment alone." Drinking water in the trenches was dear to come by. It was delivered "at the risk of men's lives," Lieutenant Coningsby Dawson of the Canadian Field Service related. "To use it carelessly would be like washing in men's blood." Lieutenant Dawson was also a poet and author who wrote about men's souls and glory in war. "In France one has to go dirty so often that the dream of being always clean seems as unrealizable as romance."[45]

There was no British military dental corps at the outset of World War I. To service all the British troops in June 1915, there were only fifteen dentists. The British Dental Society, at the outbreak of the war, offered the services of its members to the First Lord of the Admiralty and the Secretary of State for War. The formation of an Army dental corps was proposed, and was rejected. The House of Commons had discussed the matter on July 26, 1915. Instead, the War Office, beginning in 1915, employed local, civilian dental practitioners, with a very limited number of dentists given the temporary rank of Lieutenant. "England sleeps whilst other countries are thriving," the *British Dental Journal* in 1915 declared. "Canada leads the way with a special army dental service." The matter was considered to be " a disgrace for any civilized country" and a "blundering which is being perpetuated." It was pointed out that "the pity of it is that there is no expert either in the House or at the Admiralty of War Office . . . who knows about the importance of dental services for combat forces . . . to appreciate the crying evils of our present happy-go-lucky system." British dentists often served their country as fighting men.[46]

Commenting on the differences between the dental professions in England and the United States, Robinson, as early as 1850, pointed out "the need for professional organization in England." Asserting that "a dark cloud overhangs the profession," he urged the British "to imitate the noble example set them by the dentists of the United States." By contrast, it was reported that there were 500 dentists serving with the German troops in 1914. By March 1916 Germany had 800 dental surgeons in active military service. Long before 1914, Germany had appreciated the importance of the care of the teeth and had established dental school clinics where the needs of the future soldiers were met beforehand. A German hospital of 225 beds was opened at Düsseldorf in August 1914 for the treatment of gunshot wounds of the jaws.[47]

Between July 21 and October 1, 1915, Dr. Kazanjian's newly established dental clinic treated 926 patients, a staggering number: 1,519 teeth were extracted and 135 artificial dentures were supplied as well as the performance of routine fillings, cleanings, and treatment of gums. The dentists in Dr. Kazanjian's unit felt that they were making a highly important contribution to the war effort. Their unit was the only one in the five-hospital complex where regular dentistry was performed. Problems of the teeth and the feet were the most common complaints of the soldiers. Two days a week were reserved in the Dental Department for the men in nearby hospitals. During these times, the clinic was working at full capacity. Cosmetic and delicate dental procedures were "sacrificed for efficiency and durability." However, "under favorable conditions," teeth were treated and root canals and treatment of inflamed gums were performed. Ear and nose infections, arthritis and gastritis responded favorably and quickly with the removal of diseased and septic roots.[48]

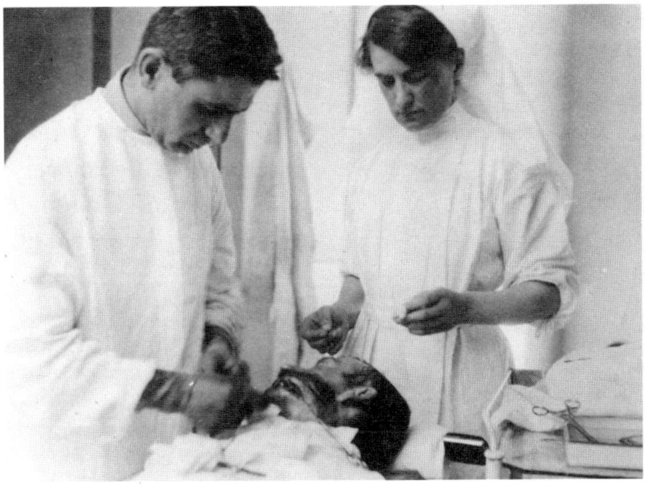

Dr. Kazanjian operating with a nurse
The Harvard Medical Library in the Francis A. Countway Library of Medicine

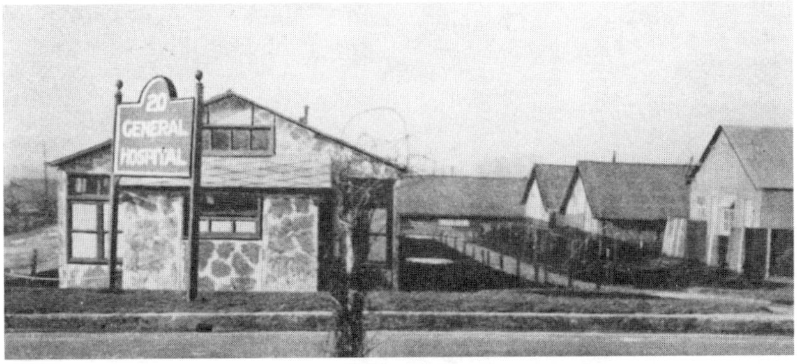

Headquarters of the Dental Department of Harvard Units, General Hospital No. 20, Dannes-Camiers, France
The Harvard Medical Library in the Francis A. Countway Library of Medicine, Hapgood, p 124

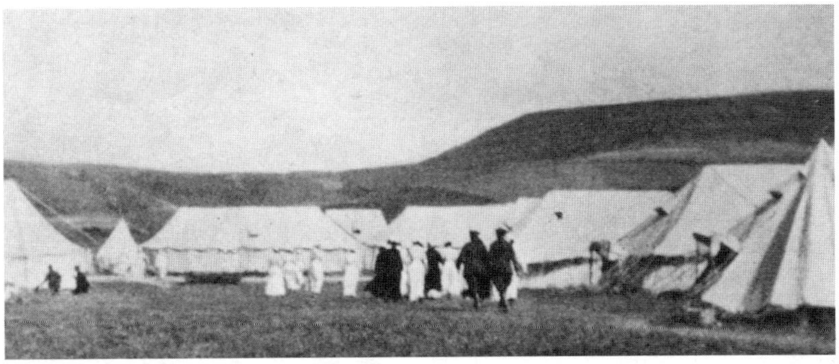

Officers' tents at General Hospital No. 20, Dannes-Camiers, France
The Harvard Medical Library in the Francis A. Countway Library of Medicine

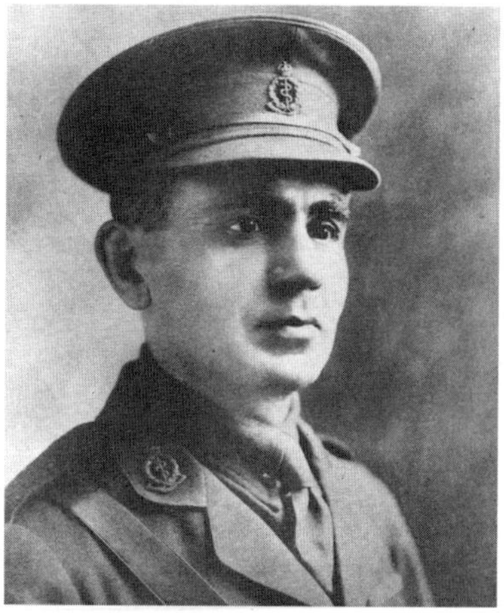

Dr. Varaztad H. Kazanjian in the uniform of an Honorary Major in the British Royal Army Medical Corps The Harvard Medical Library in the Francis A. Countway Library of Medicine

"I've got some new teeth," one soldier wrote home, "made by the American dentist here. Believe me, they're none of your rag-time dentists, but real American doctor-dentists." "The skill of American dentists holds undisputed first place," the New York Times stated in 1916, "and is particularly highly esteemed in France." Dr. Kazanjian found "an easy solution" for Dr. Hopkins and gave him the special assignment of providing routine restorative dentistry for the medical and nursing staff of the hospital. Hopkins had not extracted teeth for years and had not taken up the "new" local anesthetic, Novocain. Kazanjian's earlier comment, "Let's wait until we get to work," was prophetic.[49]

"With his usual mysterious simplicity," Dr. Kazanjian, in consultation with Sir Allan Perry, the British commanding officer, devised a plan to cope with the enormity of the need for dental services. Dentistry for British officers and nurses was prohibited, except for emergencies. Services for them was available in nearby Boulogne or Étaples. Hospital patients were directed to report their needs to the attending medical officers, who would call for a consultation

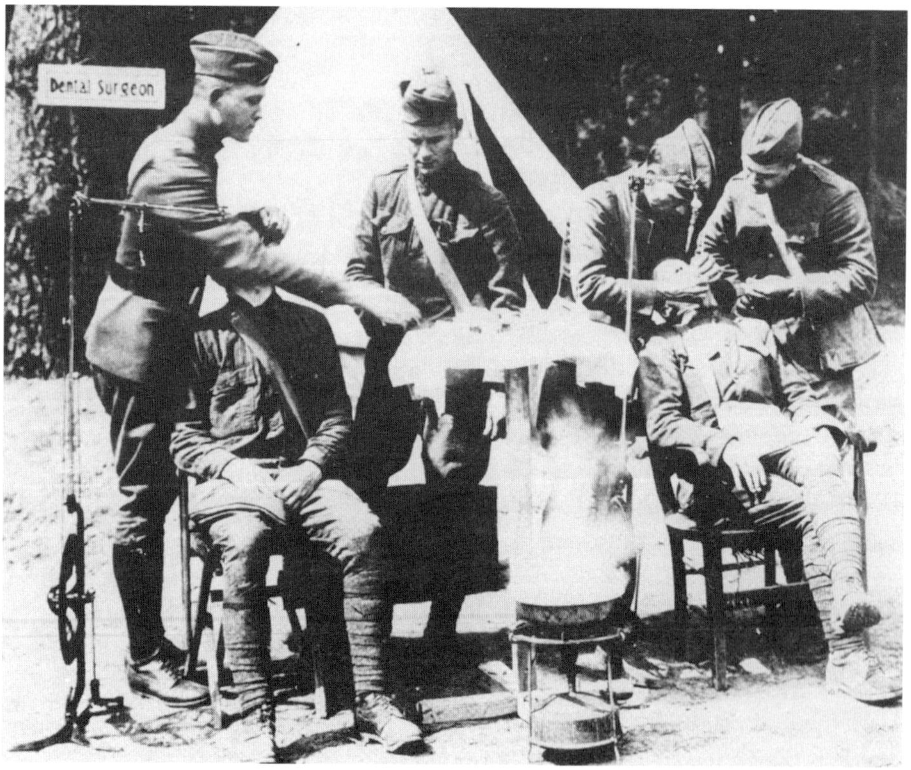

Dentistry during World War I was "performed outside to take advantage of the daylight. The boiling water is for sterilization." Photograph from Richard D. Glenner, Audrey B. David and Stanley B, Burns, The American Dentist, *(Missoula, Montana: Pictorial Histories Publication Co., 1990), p. 135*

with a dentist. The rank and file of Tommies were to report their need for dentistry at the daily sick call or sick parade. When extensive treatment was required, the responsibility for releasing dental patients for return to general duty was the responsibility of the medical officer in charge.[50]

Dr. Kazanjian always maintained a respectful and deferential stance toward Dean Smith and the Harvard Dental School:

> *We are trying hard to be worthy representatives of the Harvard Dental School. I would never think of disappointing you. It is my ambition to see dentistry respected and to have the Harvard Dental School assume such responsibility and creditability as it can.* [51]

"You can see from their faces," Dr. Kazanjian proudly reported in referring to the British medical officers, "the growing respect toward the dental profession."[52] Dr. Kazanjian's dental clinic in General Hospital No. 22 was an immediate and unqualified success and would remain so. However, the transition to treating jaw and facial wounds was more gradual and more complex.

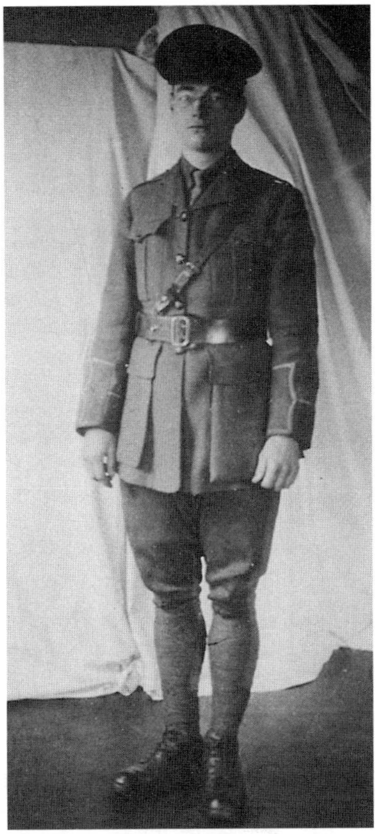

Dr. Ferdinand Brigham
The Harvard Medical Library
in the Francis A. Countway
Library of Medicine

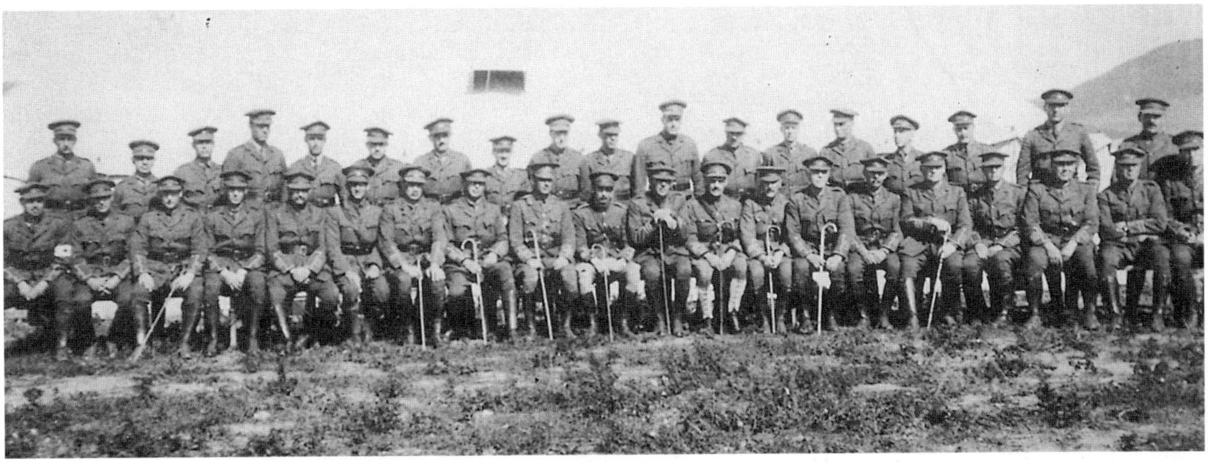

Group of officers with Dr. Kazanjian, back row, second from left
The Harvard Medical Library in the Francis A. Countway Library of Medicine

NOTES

1 Vincent Edward Grey of Fallodon, *Twenty-five Years, 1892-1916* (New York: Frederick A. Stokes, 1925), v. 2, p. 20. "The First World War was a tragic and unnecessary conflict," John Keegan wrote, and the Second World War was "the direct outcome of the first." John Keegan, *The First World War* (New York: Alfred A. Knopf, 1999), p. 3.

2 *Collected Poems of Wilfred Owen*, Edited by C. Day Lewis, (Norfolk, Conn.: New Directions. 1963), p. 129. Born in 1893, Owen served as a lieutenant in the Manchester Regiment. He was killed in France seven days before the Armistice. Owen and his fellow British officer and war poet, Siegfried Sassoon, wrote on the brutality and waste of war.

3 Richard Thoumin, ed., *The First World War,* translated by Martin Kieffer (New York: Putnam, 1963), Preface.

4 Francis A. March, *History of the World War* (Philadelphia: United Publishers, 1919), p. 247, states that 1,198 lives were lost and of these 124 were Americans. Among those lost was Alfred Gwynne Vanderbilt and the author, editor and publisher Elbert Hubbard and his wife. See also Francis J. Reynolds and Allen L. Churchill, eds., *World War Events* (New York: P. F. Collier and Sons, 1919), v. 1, p. 277.

5 Harvey Cushing, *The Life of Sir William Osler* (Oxford: Clarenden Press, 1925), v.2, p. 473; Richard Locke Hapgood, *History of the Harvard Dental School* (Peterboro, N. H.: Transcript Printing Co., 1930), p. 117. Ferdinand Brigham, "Harvard Goes to War," *Harvard Dental Alumni Bulletin* 24, no. 4 (1964): 100, indicated that the proposal came from Sir James Bryce and Sir William Osler in the first year of World War I. The *Harvard Alumni Bulletin* 17, no 37 (June 23, 1915): 692, gives the April 1915 date for Osler's request to Lowell.

6 David Cheever, "Experiences of the Harvard Unit with the British Expeditionary Force," *Transactions of the New Hampshire Medical Society*, May 16, 1916, p. 66. (Dr. Cheever served as Chief Surgeon of the Second Harvard Unit); internationally renowned neurosurgeon Harvey Cushing, who served in 1917 with Base Hospital No. 5, a Harvard Unit in Camiers, France, recorded his wartime exploits in his *From a Surgeon's Journal* (Boston: Little Brown, 1936), here p. 48; *Harvard Alumni Bulletin* 17, no. 32 (May 19, 1915): 600. Both President Lowell and former President Eliot vehemently opposed the war, and Lowell became a leading spirit of the League to Enforce Peace and later strongly supported the League of Nations.

7 *Encyclopaedia Britannica*, 11th ed. (1910-1911), v. 12, p. 592; Cheever, "Experiences," p. 67. Article XI of the Geneva Convention reads:

A recognized society of a neutral state can lend the services of its sanitary personnel to a belligerent only with the prior consent of its own government and the authority of such belligerent. The belligerent accepting such assistance is required to notify the enemy before making any use thereof.

Also F. N. L. Poynter, *Introductions to Exhibitions [of the Wellcome Institute of the History of Medicine,* London]: *Medicine and Surgery in the Great War, 1914-1918* (London: November 1968), p. 2. Dr. Poynter was Director of the Institute.

8 John F. Fulton, *Harvey Cushing, a Biography* (Springfield, Ill.: Thomas, 1941), v. 2, pp. 387-388; March, *World War*, p. 110. Ambulance was the usual name of a French military hospital.

9 "President Lowell's Report for 1914-15," *Harvard Alumni Bulletin* 18, no. 16 (January 19, 1916): Supplement, p. 16. A listing of the staff of the unit is contained in the appendix of this report. See also M. A. DeWolfe Howe, ed., *The Harvard Volunteers in Europe* (Cambridge, Mass.: Harvard University Press, 1916), pp. 32-54. This contains a description of the services of the American Ambulance hospital. A medical unit from Western Reserve University in Cleveland under Dr. George W. Crile had previously served in the American Ambulance hospital from January to April 1915.

10 Hapgood, *Harvard Dental School*, p. 141. There had been American dentists practicing in Paris since the early half of the nineteenth century. The most celebrated was Dr. Thomas W. Evans (1823-1897), who emigrated from Philadelphia to Paris

in 1847 and became the court dentist to Napoleon III and his wife Eugenie and for most of the royal families on the continent. See Gerald Carson, *The Dentist and the Empress* (Boston: Houghton, Mifflin, 1983), pp. 23-24. Also, W. S. Davenport, Jr., "The Pioneer American Dentists in France and Their Successors," *Revue d'Histoire de l'Art Dentaire* 3, no 7 (October 1965): 99-116. This paper is a speech delivered on the seventy-fifth anniversary of the American Dental Club of Paris (1890-1965). In addition to biographical material, it contains a chart illustrating the successors to the earliest American dentists in France. Also Cushing, *Surgeon's Journal*, p. 15 (entry for April 3, 1915).

11 Barbara W. Tuchman, *The Guns of August* (New York: Ballantine, 1962), p. 119; Brigham, "Harvard Goes to War," pp. 100-101; "Allied Battle Front is 1,656 miles long," The *New York Times*, April 12, 1915, p. 1, col. 7.

12 A. C. Champollion (Andre Cheronnet-Champollion), "Life and Death in the Trenches" and "We live like swine . . . " in Howe, *Harvard Volunteers*, p. 17. Champollion was killed at age thirty-five on March 23, 1915, by a bullet in the head. An edition of his 1914-1915 letters was privately printed in New York by the Cheltenham Press in 1915.

13 Some 20,000 British soldiers died on the first day of the Battle of the Somme on July 1, 1916.

14 "President Lowell's Report for 1914-15," p. 17. Also *Harvard Alumni Bulletin* 17:30 (May 5, 1915): 543, and 17:37 (June 23, 1915): 692. Dr. Samuel A. Hopkins, M.D., Columbia, D.D.S. New York College of Dentistry, 1882, had been Professor of the Theory and Practice of Dentistry at Tufts College Dental School (1903-1906) and Instructor of Dental Pathology at Harvard (1906-1909). He authored a book, *The Care of the Teeth*, published in 1902.

15 John M. Converse, "Plastic Surgery: The Twentieth Century. The Period of Growth 1914-1939," *Surgical Clinics of North America* 47, no.2 (April 1967): 261-278 (Quote comes from p. 263); Henry Morganthau, *Ambassador Morganthau's Story* (Garden City, N.Y.: Doubleday Page, 1919), p. 249 (caption to photograph, "The Dardanelles as it was March 16, 1915"); Thoumin, *First World War*, pp. 155-171, "The Dardanelles."

16 *The New York Times*, April 2, 1915, p. 2, col. 6; April 7, 1915, p. 2, col. 4; April 9, 1915, p. 1, col. 5; April 26, 1915, p. 3, col. 2.

17 Dr. John W. Cooke was a graduate of the Harvard Dental School in 1918 and served in Europe as a dental officer in the American Army. He practiced in Boston and taught at Harvard Dental School. His paper, "Kazanjian and Harvard," *Harvard Dental Alumni Bulletin* 3, no. 2 (January 1943), provided much valuable information (see especially p. 26). V. H. Kazanjian, Unpublished paper read before the Harvard Dental Alumni Association, June 18, 1919, in the Varaztad Kazanjian Archive in The Francis A. Countway Library of Medicine, folder AM-163, and "Remembrance of Things Past," *Plastic and Reconstructive Surgery* 35, no. 1 (1965): 8; Hapgood, *Harvard Dental School*, p. 118. Dr. Ferdinand Brigham's Unpublished manuscript on the Dental Unit of the First Harvard Unit is in the author's private collection.

18 *Boston Sunday Globe*, June 6, 1915, p. 11, cols. 3-6; Brigham, Unpublished manuscript on the Dental Unit of the First Harvard Unit.

19 Brigham, Unpublished manuscript.

20 Robert S. Catheron, Unpublished account included as a part of Dr. Brigham's longer manuscript on the Dental Unit of the First Harvard Unit during World War I; Address by Lieutenant-Colonel Herbert H. White at a reception in honor of the members who served with the Harvard Unit No. 22, Boston, Massachusetts, February 14, 1919, p. 2. The latter contains valuable information on the background, preparation, and administration of the Unit. V. H. Kazanjian Archives in The Francis A. Countway Library of Medicine, Folder C-446.

21 Catheron, Unpublished account; Kazanjian, Unpublished paper, June 18, 1919.

22 *Boston Transcript*, June 19, 1915, Part One, p. 14, col. 2; Postcards from Drs. Brigham and Cushman mailed to Dean Smith at noon on June 26, 1915, from Hoboken, N.J. (Kazanjian Archive, World War I Material, Section IV.)

23 Brigham, Unpublished manuscript. Also, list of cabin passengers, *Noordam*, June 26, 1915, where four dentists were listed: Drs. Kazanjian, Brigham, Cushman and Hopkins (Kazanjian Archive, World War I Material, Section IV); *Daniel Bartholomew Reardon (1877-1961), A*

Brief Biography (no publisher, no date, but probably 1963 or 1964), p. 13. His son, Judge Paul C. Reardon, was its presumed author. Dr. Reardon was one of the surgeons with the First Unit accompanying Dr. Kazanjian.

24 Brigham, Unpublished manuscript, p. 101; Hapgood, *Harvard Dental School,* p. 119.

25 Letter from Dr. Hugh Cabot to Herbert H. White, undated, only two pages survive, but probably written in 1916. Kazanjian Archive, Folder C-56. The letter states that "the Cushing outfit" insists that they are the Harvard Unit ". . . the question has been settled long ago by the War Office and #22 General Hospital appears upon the Army Register as the Harvard Unit." Apparently, President Lowell had originally designated Dr. Cushing's unit as "the official Harvard Unit."

26 A leather belt for a dress uniform supported by a light strap passing over the right shoulder.

27 A covering for the leg from ankle to knee consisting of a narrow cloth wrapped around the leg.

28 Hapgood, *Harvard Dental School*, p. 119. In the Harvard Unit there were two lieutenant colonels, six majors, and the remainder were either captains or lieutenants. Kazanjian, "Remembrance of Things Past," p. 8. Dr. Reardon's diary records that on July 8, 1915, they toured King George Military Hospital, which was originally a stationery factory that had been transformed into a military hospital. "Serves many wounded soldiers, who related many sad and sorrowful experiences. Told [p. 7] how Germans had spat in their faces and thrown hot coffee in faces when lying wounded." Daniel Bartholomew Reardon, "Diary," June 25, 1915 to Oct. 17, 1915. World War I, First Harvard Medical Unit—British Expeditionary Force, Camiers, France. Transcription by British Imperial War Museum. Courtesy of Mrs. Paul C. Reardon, Hingham, Massachusetts.

29 Hapgood, *Harvard Dental School*, pp. 118-119; Reardon, *Brief Biography*, p. 13. Letter from V. H. Kazanjian to Dean E. H. Smith, August 3, 1915. There are two versions of this letter in the Countway Library. Version no. 1 (the shorter) is in Kazanjian's handwriting and was mailed to Dean Smith. Version no. 2 is the original draft from which version 1 was prepared. The draft is also preserved in the library in two forms. One is in Dr. Kazanjian's handwriting and the other is a typescript copy marked "arrival in Camiers by V. H. K." and "copied from the original draft of letter by H. K. Sargeant." These version differ slightly. Kazanjian Archive, folders C-392 and WW-1269.

30 Robert S. Catheron, "The Work of the Dental Section of the Harvard Surgical Unit," paper delivered to the Harvard Dental Alumni sometime between May 1916 and August 1917. Kazanjian Archive, folder WW-1269. Also, Hapgood, *Harvard Dental School*, pp. 119-120.

31 *The Story of U. S. Army Base Hospital No. 5* (Cambridge, Mass.: Harvard University Press, 1919), p. 39. The reference to "soggy field" is on p. 4. Base Hospital No. 5 was located next to General Hospital No. 20.

32 Hapgood, *Harvard Dental School*, p. 120; Catheron, "Dental Section"; Kazanjian to Dean Smith, August 3, 1915; Letter from Kazanjian to Dean Smith, undated but written in answer to Dean Smith's letter to Kazanjian dated October 22, 1915, Kazanjian Archive, folder C-392.

33 Brigham, Unpublished manuscript.

34 Catheron, "Dental Section;" Brigham, "Harvard Goes to War," p. 102; George H. Makins, "The Development of British Surgery in the Hospitals of the Lines of Communication in France," *British Medical Journal* (June 16. 1917): 789. Makins wrote that "tented units under the climatic conditions of France have proved to possess one virtue, that of mobility." The author was a consulting surgeon to the British armies in France.

35 Brigham, Unpublished manuscript and "Harvard Goes to War," p. 102.

36 Reardon, *Brief Biography*, p. 14.

37 Quoted in a newspaper article, "American Dentists' Great Work in France," of which a clipping is preserved in the Kazanjian Archive, folder M-24. The only date on the newspaper clipping is "Sept-Oct. 1915." An exhaustive search of the microfilms of newspapers in the Boston Public Library failed to identify exact newspaper and date. Dr. Cushman's home was in Claremont, New Hampshire.

38 Letter from Hugh Cabot to Herbert A. White, undated, only p. 2 survives, but probably 1916. Fd c-56

39 Brigham, Unpublished manuscript. "On clear days when the wind was right," Dr. Catheron reported, "we could hear the cannonading from the hills behind the hospital" ("Dental Section").

40 Catheron, "Dental Section"; Brigham, "Harvard Goes to War," p. 102; also, Elliot C. Cutler, "The Organization, Function and Operation of an Evacuation Hospital," *Military Surgeon* 146, no. 1 (January 1920): 9-23.

41 Kazanjian to Dean Smith, August 3, 1915; Thoumin, *First World War*, p. 179; Cushing, *Sir William Osler*, v. 2, p. 489. H MS c51, Kazanjian Archive, folder c-392.

42 Kazanjian to Dean Smith, August 3, 1915.

43 [London] *Daily Telegram*, July 6, 1915. A Dental Aid Society was formed to help meet the dental needs of the men in service, "a Herculean task." Kazanjian Archive, folder M-24.

44 *Letters from Roger I. Lee, Lt. Col., U. S. Army Medical Corps, 1917-1918* (Brookline, Mass.: Privately printed, 1962), p. 20; Frank H. Cushman, "The Harvard Volunteers in Europe," in Howe, *Harvard Volunteers*, p. 182.

45 Cushman, "Volunteers in Europe"; Coningsby Dawson, "The Glory of the Trenches, the Road to Blighty," *Good Housekeeping* (January 1918): 17-18. Dawson, an honors graduate at Oxford in 1905, fought as an officer in the Canadian Field Artillery in France, where he was wounded. He wrote several books and poems about his experiences in the Great War.

46 Hapgood, *Harvard Dental School*, p. 170; *British Dental Journal* 36 (August 2, 1915): 713, 717, 767-768, 963; Letter from R. A. Cohen, Warwickshire, England, to the author, March 14, 1996, in the author's possession. *British Dental Journal* 37, no. 11 (June 1, 1916): 428, reports that Captain Leonard Renshaw, a dental student, was killed in action on May 13, 1916.

47 David Richards, "Dentistry in England in the 1840's: the First Indications of a Movement Toward Professionalization," *Medical History* 12 (1968): 151; Cushman, "Volunteers in Europe," p. 182; J. Taylor, *History of Dentistry* (Philadelphia: Lea and Febiger, 1922), p. 21. The U. S. Dental Corps of the Army was established in 1911 and the Navy Dental Corps was created in 1912. Cf. Milton B. Asbell, *Dentistry, A Historical Perspective* (Bryn Mawr, Pa.: Dorrance, 1988), p. 206. Also, Catheron, "Dental Section"; G. Villain, "The Physiological Treatment of Fractures and Dislocations," *The Lancet* 1 (June 24, 1916): 1267.

48 "Report of the Dental Department, Harvard Surgical Unit, General Hospital #22, July 1 - Oct. 1 [1915]," Kazanjian Archive, World War I Materials, Section IV; Catheron, "Dental Section"; Letter from Dr. Frank H. Cushman to Dean E. H. Smith, September 17, 1915, Kazanjian Archive, folder C-392; V. H. Kazanjian, "The Dentist and the Army," *The Mirror* (Harvard Dental School) (1917): 45-49.

49 "American Dentist's Great Work in France"; *The New York Times*, August 4, 1916, p. 4, col. 4; Brigham, Unpublished manuscript.

50 Brigham, Unpublished manuscript; Circular Memorandum No. 12, signed by Geo. Howell for the Director General Medical Services, British Forces in the Field, Étaples 11/8/15, Kazanjian Archive, folder C-818

51 Letters from Kazanjian to Dean Smith, August 3, 1915; undated but written in answer to Dean Smith's letter to Kazanjian dated October 2, 1915; July 31, 1915, Kazanjian Archive, folder C-392.

52 Letter from V. H. Kazanjian to Dr. William H. Potter, August 23, 1915, Kazanjian Archive, folder C-340

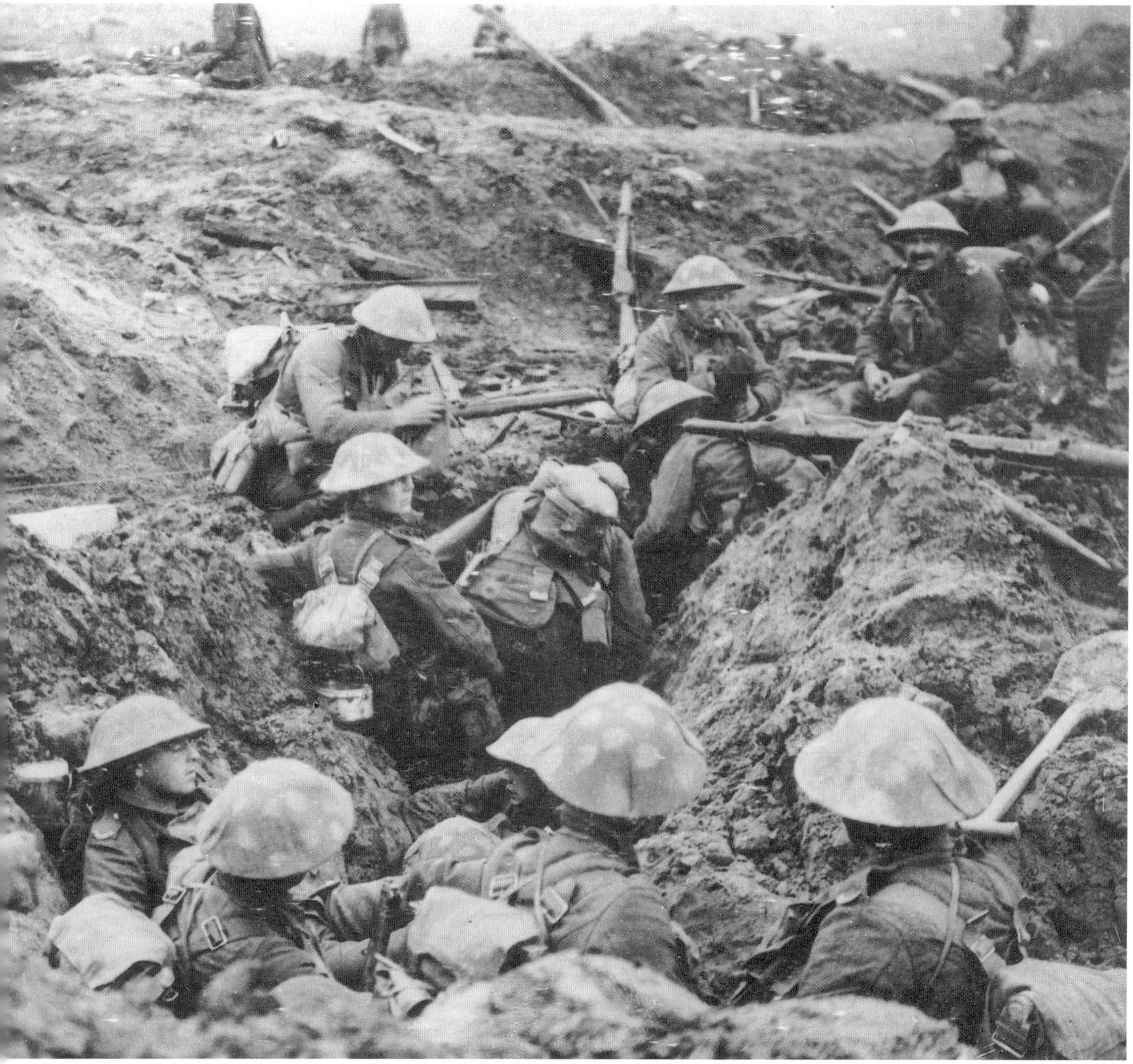

Battle of Menin Road Ridge; Q.5969, Courtesy of the Imperial War Museum, London

CHAPTER FIVE

No Man's Land

"A modern battlefield is the abomination of abominations. Imagine a vast stretch of dead country, pitted with shell-holes as though it had been mutilated with smallpox. There's not a leaf or a blade of grass in sight. Every house has either been leveled or is in ruins. No bird sings. Nothing stirs. The only live sound is at night — the scurry of rats. You enter a kind of ditch, called a trench, it leads to another and another in an unjoyful maze. From the sides feet stick out, and arms and faces — dead of the previous encounters." Thus wrote one combatant.[1]

Fought mostly in open trenches and in close combat, World War I produced a horrifying number of highly destructive and disfiguring wounds to the face. "No wounds of the European war have been quite so shocking," *The New York Times* reported, "as those of the human face. Shrapnel is the worst devastation. Noses are blown off, cheek bones crushed, upper jaws caved in, and lower jaws shot away." These injuries resulted when a soldier raised his head above the parapet of the trenches and offered a ready target to a bullet fired by the ever-present enemy. A volley of machine gun fire was invariably fatal. Most wounds were caused by rifle fire, shrapnel, grenades, or heavy munitions. Projectiles bursting on a soldier's steel helmet often struck the wearer's unprotected neck. An explosion of shells in the trenches could tear away part of the soldier's face.[2] One seasoned soldier wrote this poem as a warning to his comrades in arms:

Keep your head well down Chummy
Keep your head well down
When in the trenches
Keep your nut well down.
Bullets are a-flying
Nasty bits of lead
It's all up with you matey
If you stop one with your head.
Grills you through the temple
Comes out through your crown.
If you want to see your "Blighty"
Keep your head well down.[3]

"Hand grenades appeared to absolutely explode the tissues, bursting them open, destroying the hard tissues and forcing them into other regions, such as the tongue and pharynx," one study concluded.

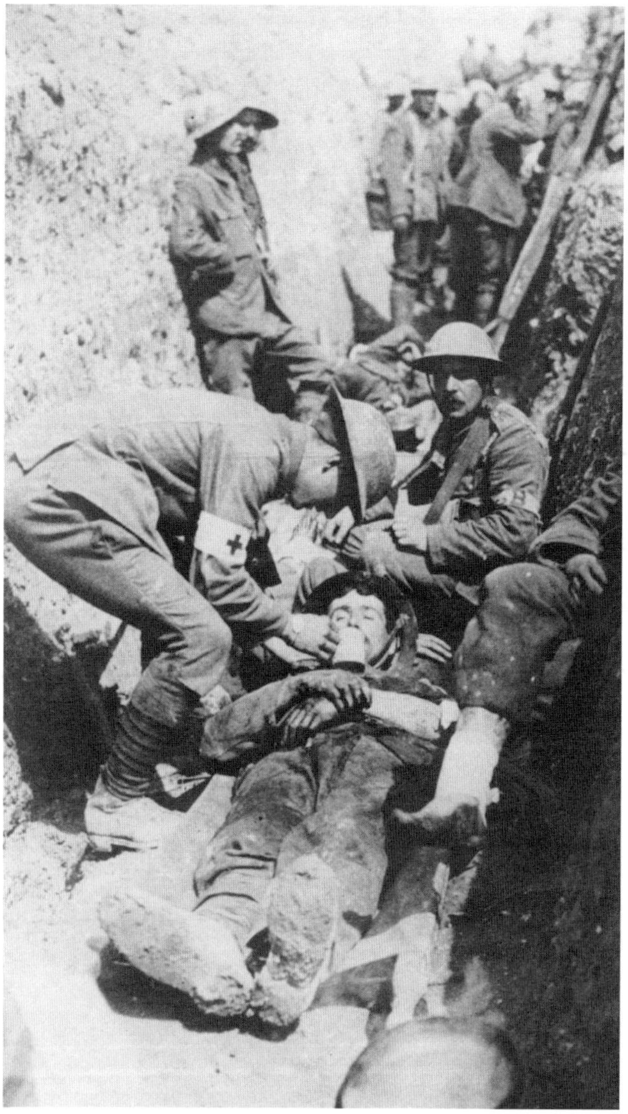

Battle of Menin Road Ridge; Q.5968, Courtesy of the Imperial War Museum, London

TABLE OF MISSILES CAUSING WOUNDS[4]

Rifle ball	128
Shrapnel ball	31
Shell	133
Shell fragment and rifle ball	5
Shell fragment and shrapnel	1
Doubtful	5
Bomb fragments	9
Hand grenade	3
Barbed wire	1
Mine explosion	1
Revolver ball	1
Total	318

Scarcely anyone was prepared to treat the avalanche of broken faces that dramatically increased in numbers as the war became more intense.

Shortly after his arrival in France, Dr. Kazanjian paid a call on Colonel William Carr, Deputy Director of Medical Services of the district with headquarters in nearby Étaples. "What is being done in the case of fractured jaws and mouth wounds?" Dr. Kazanjian inquired. Colonel Carr responded that men with such wounds were being returned to England, even though specialized treatment facilities were non-existent there. Indeed, there was at the time no recognized specialty of plastic surgery. "Harassed general surgeons at the base hospital were treating facial wounds by drawing the severed tissue together, stitching them up, and trusting to nature to do the rest. Men often were sent back to their units with permanently distorted features, depressing the morale of their fellows." Prior to World War I, the treatment of maxillofacial injuries, particularly gunshot wounds, was a minor preoccupation of surgery. "There was a considerable number of 'oral surgeons' . . . who, as a result of their dental training, took a special interest in surgical diseases of the mouth and jaws." There were no books written purely on the subject of traditional plastic surgery.[5]

"I am in a sense disappointed," Dr. Kazanjian wrote on August 3, 1915. "I have not seen any fracture jaw cases that we have heard so much of and I do not think there will be very many here in this hospital. The conditions here are entirely different from the American Ambulance Hospital in Paris. There, men like Drs. Potter, Hayes and Davenport put the foundation of the works and demonstrated their ability and established the clinic so that all the cases of that nature go to the American Ambulance Hospital. In English hospitals they do not do that; fracture jaws are scattered in different hospitals."[6]

"I have seen some of the crudest treatment done by English surgeons on fractured jaws," Dr. Kazanjian wrote to Dr. Potter on August 23, 1915. "I shall be back in school as soon as I can." Dismayed at his early setbacks, he wrote, "I shall start home perhaps at about the middle of October," when the contract of the First Unit was to expire. General surgeons set broken jaws, "but as a rule just badly enough that the teeth are not in exact alignment," Dr. Harvey Cushing declared. "Napoleon's army marched on its belly, Joffre's holds on with its teeth, and only experts can make 50 percent of lacerated faces and jaws capable of army crusts."[7]

Dr. Kazanjian's "disappointment" and his lack of involvement with jaw fractures was short-lived. As he had done once before in Boston when he treated patients with jaw fractures, Kazanjian took upon himself the mantle of concern for the untreated and disfigured. In the Harvard Unit, he could have chosen to render routine dental care alone and have been respected for it. After all, he was neither a physician nor a surgeon, but rather a prosthodontist. He extended himself, because, as he later said: "Nobody knew what to do with them."[8]

According to the recollections of Dr. Brigham, "It was bound to happen. One of the surgical wards had admitted two cases with gaping facial wounds and fractured jaws and I guess the surgeons called Kazanjian automatically. He took it all in his stride so easily, and the details of the treatment were organized so smoothly and quietly that I hardly recall those methods of treatment." Brigham became Kazanjian's surgical assistant and so remained during the entire war. Within two weeks, from August 9 to August 23, Dr. Kazanjian saw four cases.[9]

Dr. Kazanjian had the special ability to combine dental prosthetic appliances with plastic and reconstructive surgery for the treatment of facial and jaw wounds. In his performance of his professional duties, he crossed the thin line between the disciplines of dentistry and plastic surgery into a no-man's land which only a few had bridged. The dentist in the unit had embarked "upon an expedition which was at that time of indefinite and doubtful value . . . . The opportunities and the sphere of action had to be . . . created."[10]

During the Civil War Dr. James B. Bean (1834-1870) treated the fractured jaws of the Confederate soldiers by constructing interdental splints. He was so successful that a special ward was equipped for him in a Georgia hospital. At the same time, Dr. Thomas B. Gunning (1813-1889) of New York was treating jaw fractures in the Union Army with a splint named for him. The splints perfected by both Bean and Gunning were very similar, though developed independently of one another. Thereafter, Dr. Norman W. Kingsley (1829-1913) of New York, who is remembered as "The Father of Modern Orthodontia (Orthodonics)," invented an interdental splint made of vul-

DR. NORMAN W. KINGSLEY AND HIS SPLINT

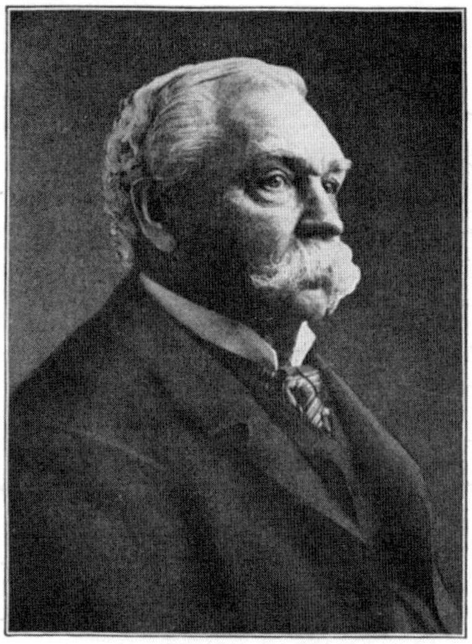

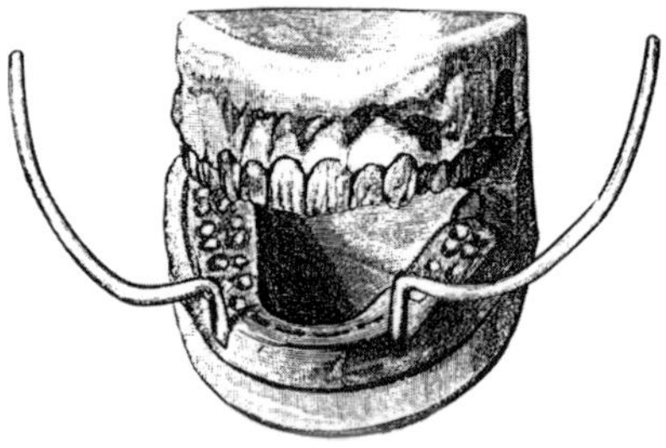

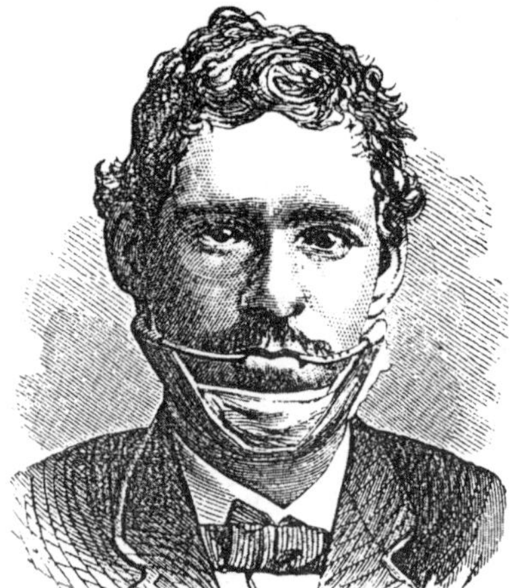

TOP: *Koch, v. 3, p. 543*
MIDDLE and BELOW: *Kingsley:* A Treatise on Oral Deformities, *(New York: Appleton, 1880) p. 401 and 404*

canite rubber for the reduction of mandibular fractures, which was widely used but which was cumbersome.[11]

"I would not care to go through another campaign," Dr. Bernard von Langenbeck, the great German surgeon, remarked following the Franco-Prussian War of 1870-1871, "without the help of skilled technicians to aid in the care of these jaw injuries." Early in World War I it was "the failure of the general surgeon and the dental surgeon to agree on the part which each should play in the treatment," Dr. Kazanjian noted, "and many cases of gunshot wounds of the face and jaws became grossly deformed as they passed to and fro."[12] Facial war wounds caused by projectiles often caused extensive shattering of underlying bones of the jaws and of the teeth. Using dental appliances attached to the teeth where possible, Dr. Kazanjian immobilized the bones in fractures of the jaws and fixed these fragments in harmony with the normal occlusion. He considered this to be the most important part of his treatment.

Dr. Kazanjian's prosthetic appliances were original and creative: no two were alike. He used them as a temporary framework to restore the lost parts of the jaw. To his appliances he often wired and suspended isolated fragments of bone and they showed "surprising regenerative powers." His appliances exerted forces to reposition the dislodged and shattered framework and allowed the external soft tissues of the face to be joined in a more esthetic position. He had developed "an extra-ordinary proficiency in constructing splints" and genuinely loved the work. Above all, "he showed a keen sense of organization that bordered upon genius."[13] He recalled the difficult years in "pulling wire" at the mill and the cases that he treated at the Dental School; he applied that special knowledge to these new circumstances.

"The treatment of facial injuries," Dr. Kazanjian asserted, "may be divided into two distinct phases or periods."

> *The first is the most critical for the patient and extends for about the first four weeks. It is characterized by exhaustion, blood loss, sepsis, pain and depression and with the possibility of "alarming complications" occurring such as bronchi-pneumonia, secondary hemorrhages and infection. In the second phase, the repair of the bony fragments begins with the construction of splints and prosthetic appliances. It is also a time when both minor and plastic surgical operations are performed for the correction of the facial deformity.*[14]

This was followed by a period of convalescence.

The first patient treated in the Department of Oral Surgery was Private J. H., who was admitted on August 10, 1915, with a compound fracture of the lower jaw. A bullet had entered on the right lower jaw and exited on the left side. His jaw operation consisted of "curette and extraction" and he was discharged on September 25, 1915.[15] It was the treatment of the second patient, far more complex, that demonstrated the scope of Dr. Kazanjian's skill. He was Private T. H., age twenty-three, of the 7th King's Royal Rifles, who was admitted in poor condition on August 17, 1915, with multiple fractures of both jaws, extensive wounds of the right cheek, and destruction of the anterior portion of the tongue. The following is Private T. H.'s description of his wounding and early treatment.

> *I was wounded at Hooge on the morning of July 30th during the action in which the Germans first used liquid fire [flamethrowers]. Six of us were engaged in erecting a barricade in our trench between the part occupied by us and a portion that had been captured that morning by the enemy, when a "whizz-bang" shell burst right on the top of the barricade. Two of us were placing sandbags on the construction, so that we were within a yard of the explosion. My companion was killed, while I had my jaws shattered. I was able, with assis-*

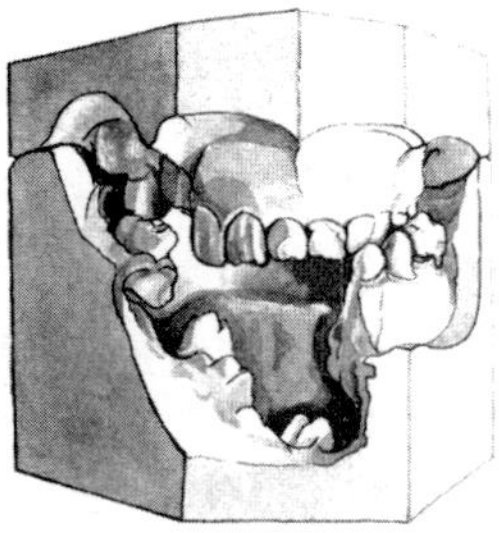

Model showing extensive displacement of the anterior fragments

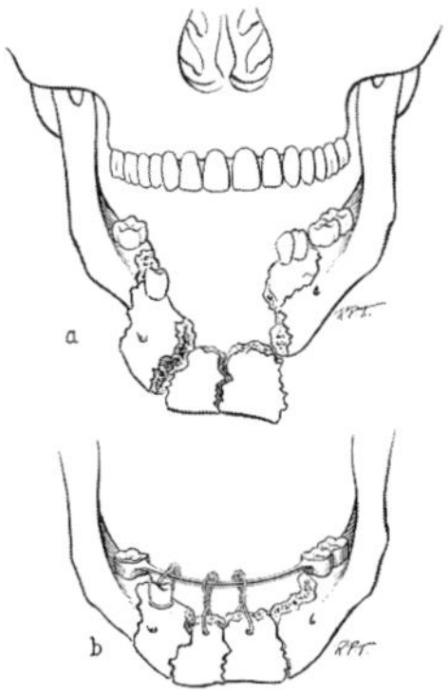

The fragments are raised to appropriate normal position

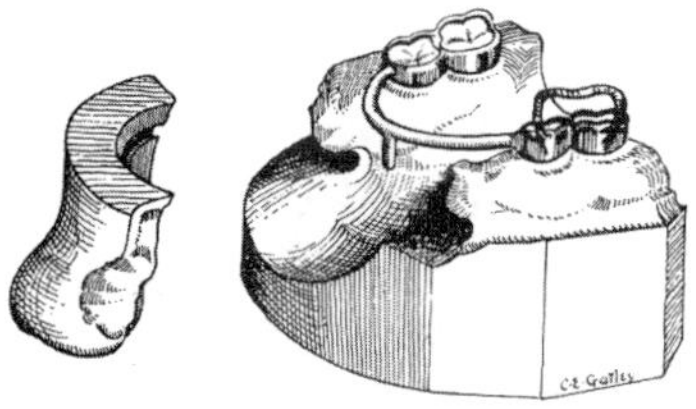

Band and arch splint with vulcanite appliance which supports soft tissue

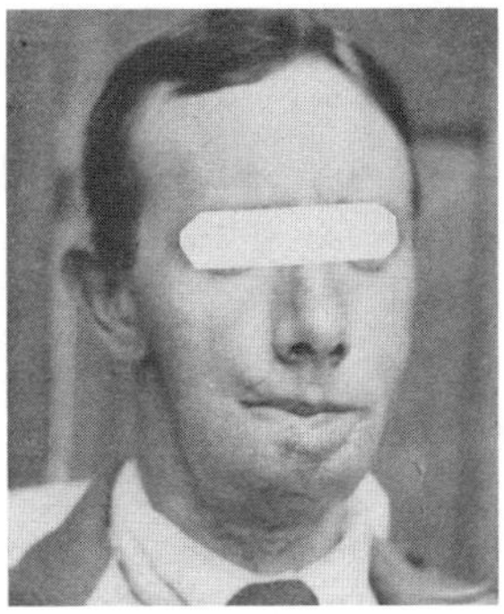

Following plastic reconstrucion.

V.H. Kazanjian, Immobilization of Wartime, Compound, Comminuted Fractures of the Mandible, Oral Surgery, *28:10 (Oct. 1942): 11*

tance, to walk to our dressing station, where my wound was dressed and the bleeding with some difficulty stanched. This was about 9 a.m. and I had to be in the trench until 4 o'clock the next morning, when I was removed to the R. A. M. Co. dressing station some distance in [the] rear. Here my wound was dressed afresh and I lay in the open until 10 p.m. when I was borne to Ypres and put aboard a motor ambulance which conveyed me to Toperinghe. At Toperinghe my wound was again dressed, and on the afternoon of August 1st I entrained for Étaples, arriving there on that night. My wound was then in a very foul state and was found to contain maggots, so that flies must have got to it while I was awaiting removal to Toperinghe. I was admitted into No. 26 General Hospital on the night of August 1st and left there on the afternoon of the 17th.

T. H. then related that for the first twelve days at hospital his wound was syringed with a fairly strong solution of hydrogen peroxide, and afterwards with a weaker solution of the same, and that the wound was treated with boric acid as well, but that the washings were done less often. His daily diet consisted of a couple of eggs in tea and a cup of beef tea. "My jaws were not bandaged at all until the last 3 days. Prior to that, the lower jaw was allowed to sag unsupported. No attempt was made to ascertain the exact extent of the fracture I had sustained, and I think it was the intention to close my wound somewhat before handing me over to the dental people."[16]

"They left the boy for seventeen days just dressing the wound," Dr. Kazanjian complained with a feeling of helpless exasperation. "Every one of my cases has a similar history."[17] The long delay from injury to admission had resulted in sepsis and extensive displacement of the bone fragments. Dr. Kazanjian's treatment, using bands, headgear, splints and dentures, lasted until February 5, 1916. It was his treatment of Private T. H. that firmly and finally established his reputation. He recorded it as follows:

There was a large wound on the right cheek which extended from the corner of the mouth nearly to the ear. The tongue was destroyed anteriorly as far as the frenum.

The Maxilla was fractured into three sections, and all the teeth, with the alveolar process, were destroyed except the third molars. These latter teeth, however, were unerupted. There were three fractures through the mandible: (1) anterior to the left bicuspid, (2) at the left angle, and (3) between the right bicuspids.

The patient was in critical condition upon admission because of lack of treatment. The wound was extremely foul, and the segments of the fractured maxillae were greatly displaced. The following means were employed to control the fractures: A Kingsley bar plate, with headgear, was fitted to the maxilla. A sectional band and arch splint were adjusted to the posterior teeth of the mandible. Inter-maxillary elastics were applied between hooks, attached to the upper and lower splints to control the fracture at the left angle.

On October 18 the jaws were cleaned of all useless roots and alveolar process, so that the only remaining teeth and roots were the upper third molars (exposed for purpose of splinting,) the roots of three upper incisors, the right lower third molar, and the left bicuspids. By this time the segments of the two jaws were in a satisfactory position so that it was possible to apply upper and lower bands and arch splints for the immobilization of the parts of each, while the use of intermaxillary ligation was continued.

On October 25 it was necessary to open externally an abscess which had developed at the left angle. Consolidation of the fracture progressed favorably, and on December 16 the splints were removed. An upper denture was made which was retained by Roach attachments on a bar attached to the roots of the incisors. The lower denture was retained by ordinary clasps on the remaining teeth. A plastic operation was performed to improve the right angle of the mouth. On January 7, 1916, adhesions to the lower ridge were cut. On January 22 the frenum of the tongue was cut to give added length to the tongue. The patient was evacuated to England on February 5, 1916, at which time the dentures were efficient and the fractures of the maxillae were uniting in a satisfactory manner.[18]

Confirmation of the treatment of these first two cases of jaw fractures appeared in the diary of Dr. Daniel B. Reardon, one of the surgeons of the hospital. Dr. Reardon witnessed and recorded the beginnings of "the remarkable work of Dr. Kazanjian . . . and his early miracles in plastic surgery" in his diary:

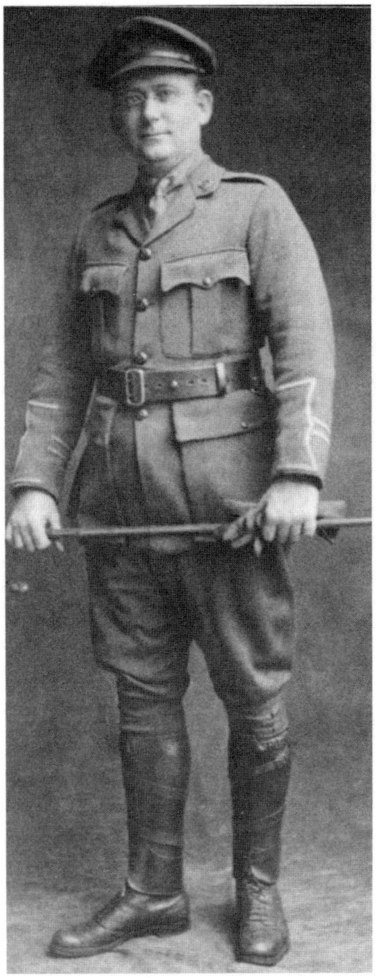

Dr. Daniel Bartholomew Reardon (1887-1961)
Photograph by Sue Rice Studios, Quincy, Mass.
Courtesy Mrs. Paul C. Reardon

Wednesday, August 18, 1915
22 General Hosp. British Exp. Force, Camiers, France

> *Breakfast at 8. Ward duties up to 10:30 A.M. Saw Dr. Kazanjian do 2 cases on multiple fracture of jaw which had been transferred from Hospital 26. They had been operated upon at 26 General Hosp. one for 17 days, other for 5 days. Both were caused by bullets. One entered left side of face & sent out right side of neck making large wound of eyes & fracturing lower jaw in 4 places. Took plaster cast, & held teeth together by wiring upper & lower teeth together. Later will apply splint. 2nd case was worse one because upper jaw was fractured in several places as well as lower jaw. This case was 17 days old & bone of upper jaw had partly united so it makes good apposition more difficult. Took cast and will try to make appliance to fit.*

Saturday, August 21, 1915
22 General Hosp. British Exp. Force, Camiers, France.

> *Dr. Kazanjian was still working on those 2 cases of badly wounded jaws today. Is gradually getting an apparatus made so as to bring the bones together & approximate the two jaws. It is a very clean piece of work.*[19]

Dr. Brigham complained that initially jaw centers were getting stale cases.

> *They were receiving facial cases only when the surgeons had failed, when the wound[s] were contracted and the remaining jaw seg-*

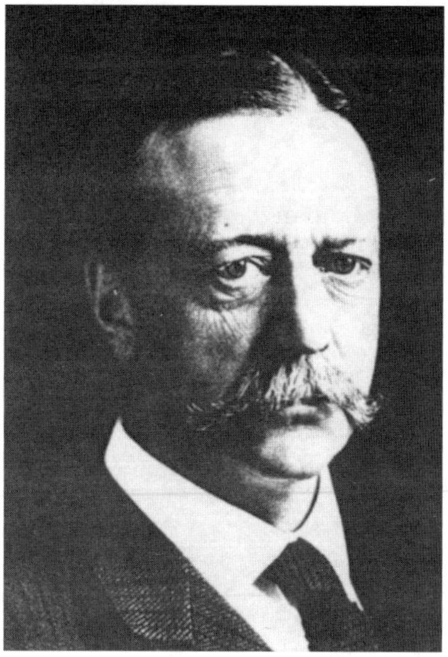

A. Lawrence Lowell, President
Harvard University
Photograph 1910
Courtesy Pusey Library,
Harvard University

ments displaced, when the poor soldier had been buffeted about from pillar to post, until he often healed with severe deformity . . . it was discouraging work . . . if a soldier who had a gunshot wound of the chin with the bone shattered and the flesh lacerated is left unattended, the soft tissues will draw together and heal in a knot, and the two parts of the jaw will be drawn inward and downward and will set in position. If a case could be treated within a few days of injury, the two halves of the jaw could be raised to normal biting position, then the tissues of the chin can be held in place and sewed properly. The surgeon was tempted to correct the soft tissue without first correcting the framework.[20]

With Dr. Kazanjian, the treatment of the external wound was secondary to that of the fractured jaws. Only later, when the fragments of the jaws were brought into correct relations and local sepsis was under control, would facial and plastic surgery be performed. The discharge of saliva through these wounds resulted in "wide-spread and persistent sepsis," most often foul and fetid. The control of infection was "the chief factor in delayed union or reformation of the jawbones." The removal of a foreign body such as the root of a tooth or bone spicule resulted in rapid "bone consolidation." According to the dictum of the English dental surgeon Dr. Kelsey Fry, the sun must never set "on undrained pus." Now Dr. Kazanjian was receiving about two new cases a day. The survival of soldiers with wounds above the shoulders was poor. A bullet wound a millimeter one way or another, particularly in the neck and brain, made the difference between life and death. Ninety percent of jaw cases were classified as "dangerously wounded, requiring grave responsibility" of the staff in their treatment.[21]

Early in September 1915, Dr Kazanjian demonstrated three cases to a clinic of medical men from the vicinity of Dannes-Camiers, and this "excited more interest than any of the others there. His surgical work has been something entirely out of the ordinary." Dr. Daniel B. Reardon, in his diary entry for September 1, 1915, recorded that he attended the first:

> *Medical meeting of "Étaples District Medical Society" at St. John's Ambulance Corps Hosp. at Étaples. Meeting was presided over by its president, Col. Carr A. D. M. S. at Étaples. About 135 doctors attended, coming from various hospitals. Papers were read and discussed.*[22]

By mid-September 1915, Dr. Kazanjian was in Paris, meeting with Dr. George B. Hayes at the American Ambulance Hospital Dental

Department. He was told that the department had treated more than 1,250 fractured jaw cases since its inception. There were five dental chairs in constant use, as well as a large laboratory where several highly skilled dental mechanics worked. "As an axiom," Kazanjian recorded in his notes, "the aim of the treatment of fractured jaws is to try to restore the tissue to normal occlusion and to hold them there."[23]

Six of the senior physicians of the First Harvard Unit now petitioned Harvard University President A. Lawrence Lowell, requesting that Dr. Kazanjian be granted permission to remain in France and that his position on the Dental School faculty not be in jeopardy. President Lowell quickly cabled his assent on September 24, 1915. "If Dr. Kazanjian thinks best and desires to stay, Harvard will gladly extend his leave of absence." In addition, the British War Office officially requested that Dr. Kazanjian extend his stay. "If I was not invited to do something," he remarked over fifty years later, "I did not do it." Dr. Kazanjian was completely "unqualified" as a surgeon and as such "he had no official right to perform operations." His skill as a dentist and his knowledge, "combined with a natural talent and a passionate interest in his cases, soon convinced the qualified doctors and surgeons of the unit that he was the best man for the job. Kazanjian developed his technique to such a degree that he could not be spared."[24]

What may have further influenced President Lowell to act favorably with regard to extending Dr. Kazanjian's service was a commendation that Sir William Osler wrote to him after a visit to the Harvard Unit in France: "The Dental men have been a revelation & I saw several cases of terrible mutilation of the face on the high road to repair." Sir William had visited the wards of General Hospital No. 22 on September 8-15, 1915. [25]

By October 1, 1915, Dr. Kazanjian's clinic had treated twenty-two compound fractured jaws. All cases were "complicated with wounds of various extent on the face, involving eyes, nose, ears, throat, etc., and many were very septic when first seen. The strength of many of the patients was also seriously impaired by the loss of blood and wounds in other parts of the body."There was a dramatic and far-reaching change in Dr. Kazanjian's status after October 1, 1915. "Lots of things have happened," Dr. Brigham excitedly reported to his father on that day. "There is a great deal of influence being used to keep us three here." There were more patients than at any previous time. "We naturally call our cases `fractured jaws' but . . . there usually goes with this condition a mutilation of the face, nose, head, throat, etc. which can easily result in a bad deformity for life." A high ranking British medical officer "was very insistent that we remain," realizing "that if Dr. Kazanjian will stay, countless men can be saved from mutilation and even death." Dr. Brigham went on to observe: "Where some thought we dentists were going to trail along and be an ornament . . . Dr. Kazanjian made this end the best known over a large territory."[26]

Initially, Dr. Kazanjian agreed to extend his stay for three months, from November 5, 1915, "with the probability of remaining longer should my services be required," but on several conditions. First, there were to be provisions made for extensive equipment and facilities for the soldiers suffering from wounds of the face and jaw and provisions were to be made for them to be kept in the hospital for longer periods than the three weeks that had been allotted. Second, both Drs. Brigham and Cushman would be allowed to remain if they wished. "I consider their services necessary," Dr. Kazanjian stated. Third, his wife was to come and live in a nearby village.[27]

When it was assumed initially that Dr. Kazanjian would be returning to America permanently with the First Harvard Unit, the parents of one of his patients had attempted to seek their son's discharge in order to send him to Boston to be treated privately by Dr. Kazanjian. Only one of his patients requested transfer to England before treatment was completed during the summer and winter of 1915. Soon after he arrived in England, the soldier asked to be transferred. Until he was healed and restored, a facially wounded soldier would not want to be seen by his friends or family. The fortitude and sheer "pluck" of the wounded Tommies was unparalleled. Young lads with broken jaws and faces half gone would respond "In the pink, thank you, sir" or "Champion, thank you sir," when addressed. It "did much to make the work easier" for the staff. "The British Tommy never complains. I repeat, never," Dr. Brigham observed. "He tells you, only if you ask."[28]

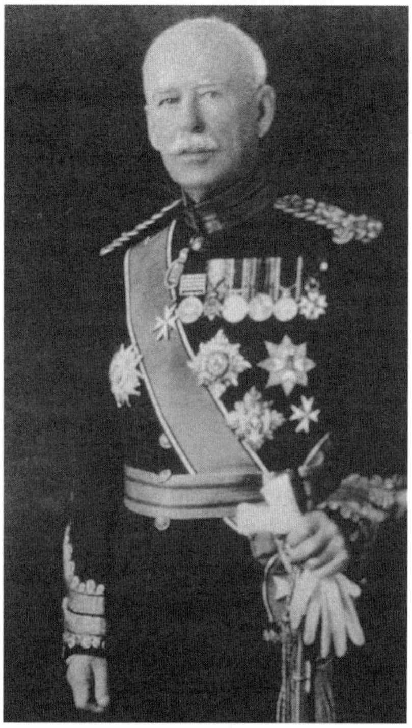

Lieut. General Sir Alfred Henry Keogh, M.D., Fr., C.D., Surgeon General, Late Director-General Army Medical Service Courtesy British Army Medical Services Museum, Keogh Barracks, Aldershot

The First Harvard Unit returned to America early in October 1915. As they left, Dr. Kazanjian admitted that he felt homesick. The only dentist of the original four who returned home was Dr. Samuel A. Hopkins. He was presented with a silver loving cup which was inscribed: "To Samuel A. Hopkins from his fellow members of the Harvard Unit in hearty appreciation of devoted services in the Royal Army Medical Corps in France 1915." A small number of officers with approximately half the nurses stayed behind and were billeted temporarily in hotels in Wimereux, a suburb of Boulogne.[29]

Columbia and Johns Hopkins universities did not fulfill their promises to send their surgical units to replace the First Harvard Unit. The period of three months seemed too short and the expenses involved too great to justify the effort. Expressing his disappointment that Johns Hopkins University would not be sending a unit, Osler wrote to the dean of that school: "When one has lived a completely comfortable life, to be wet and cold and muddy for weeks at a time, tests a fellow's mettle . . . get your boats ready—if we go under, you come next."[30]

It was up to Harvard to continue the project. A second Harvard unit was quickly organized under the direction of Dr. David Cheever with thirty new members of the medical staff and thirty-six nurses. They were scheduled to join and augment the members of the First Unit who had remained in France. The new dentists with the Second Unit were Drs. Charles F. MacDonald, John F. Dillon, and Robert S. Catheron, who replaced Samuel A. Hopkins. A portion of the funds raised to support the Unit came from a collection at the 1915 Harvard-Yale football game. The remainder of the funds was provided by Robert Beacon. The Second Harvard Unit was besieged with applicants. Dr. Wilfred T. Grenfell of Labrador fame was among the surgeons chosen.[31]

The Unit sailed out of New York harbor on November 17, 1915, on the steamship *Noordam* and arrived in England on November 27, where it was met by Lt. Col. Sir Allan Perry and Dr. Kazanjian. The Unit remained in England for ten days. When Dr. Catheron saw Dr. Kazanjian, he found a marked change in him; he had become a "personality." "One had only to see him to realize that he had been in contact with great events and had grown to meet them." Sir William Osler had written to Sir Alfred H. Keogh, Director General of Medical Services in England: "I think you should see Dr. Kazanjian of whom I spoke. He does the wonderful jaw and face work. Please give him a few minutes. He is over there meeting the new Harvard Unit."[32]

While in England on December 3, 1915, the Second Unit, with Dr. Kazanjian, visited Oxford where a large military hospital was located. The host for the day was Sir William Osler, resplendent in his uniform of a colonel of His Majesty's Forces. Luncheon was served with great formality at Christ Church College with "64 places—all the Imperial old silver and gold vases, tankards, etc., on the tables, with chrysanthemum, oak color to harmonize with the wood." Attending the luncheon was a Colonel Walker of the Royal Army Medical Corps, who described in glowing terms the treatment rendered to patients with fractured jaws by an American dentist. Dr. Kazanjian said not a word nor "flickered an eyelash." Finally Sir William Osler intervened and informed the astounded Colonel Walker, "You are now talking to that man."[33] Incidents such as this were to occur again and again.

The unit was also given a luncheon at the Savoy by the Harvard Club of London. Lord Bryce was present and spoke. Dr. Kazanjian personally thanked the British statesman for the great service which he had rendered to the Armenians in Turkey.

Scarcely two months earlier, on October 6, 1915, in a speech before Britain's House of Lords, Bryce had given the first full parliamentary revelation of the recent massacres of the Armenians. Bryce spoke of the massacres as premeditated, not spontaneous outbursts of fanaticism. The orders, he said, had come from Constantinople. The figure he gave of all those killed in this "uniform and contrived" manner was "around 800,000."[34]

Lady Osler expressed her concern for the health of the members of the newly arrived Second Unit. "It is simply horrible, the weather over there and I am terrified about the men being cold," Lady Osler said. "I am providing them with sleeping socks to their knees . . .

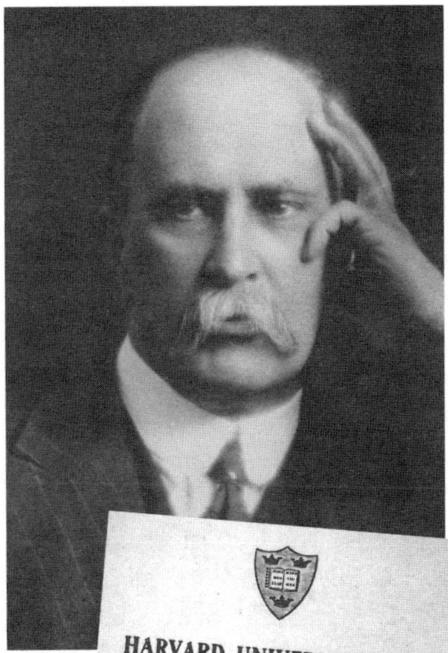

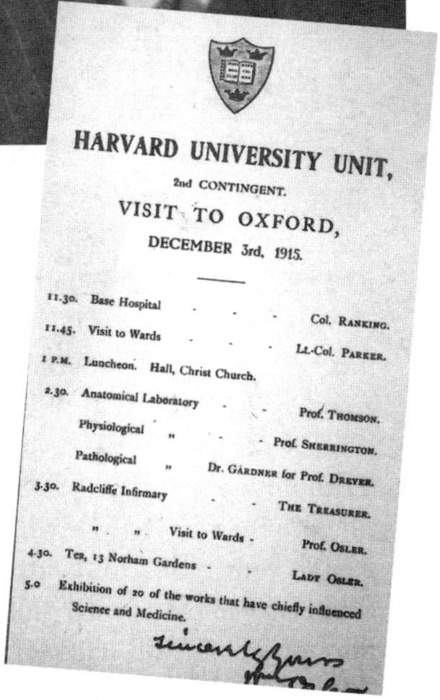

HARVARD UNIVERSITY UNIT,

2nd CONTINGENT.

VISIT TO OXFORD,

DECEMBER 3rd, 1915.

11.30.	Base Hospital - - -	Col. Ranking.
11.45.	Visit to Wards - - -	Lt.-Col. Parker.
1 P.M.	Luncheon. Hall, Christ Church.	
2.30.	Anatomical Laboratory - -	Prof. Thomson.
	Physiological " - -	Prof. Sherrington.
	Pathological "	Dr. Gardner for Prof. Dreyer.
3.30.	Radcliffe Infirmary - -	The Treasurer.
	" " Visit to Wards -	Prof. Osler.
4.30.	Tea, 13 Norham Gardens - -	Lady Osler.
5.0	Exhibition of 20 of the works that have chiefly influenced Science and Medicine.	

Above: *Sir William Osler, H MS c51, Fd. WW-1266*
Below: *Program of Harvard University Unit, 2nd Contingent, visit to Oxford, December 3, 1915 Dr. Kazanjian was present. The Harvard Medical Library in the Francis A. Countway Library of Medicine*

Socks are the most needed of all things, and khaki mufflers." It was reported that "Camiers had become a sea of mud" and "It was black, putrid, and unwholesome, to sit, sleep or stand in." The Unit crossed the English Channel on December 9, 1915, and was informed that General Hospital No. 22 had been temporarily moved from Dannes-Camiers, its summer quarters, to its winter quarters in Wimereux near Boulogne, in two large empty hotels. This move helped ameliorate some of the severe winter conditions that had concerned Lady Osler.[35]

With the coming of spring, the members of the Second Unit, together with those officers from the First Unit who remained in Wimereux, were settled back in Dannes-Camiers in General Hospital No. 22. Dr. Cushman served with this unit "with great energy and zeal" until February 1916, when he returned to America.

Dr. Kazanjian's jaw unit did not join them in Wimereux, but was assigned to an adjacent hospital in Dannes-Camiers, General Hospital No. 20, which was totally British. They were partially severed from the Harvard Unit. In essence, a hospital within a hospital was created for Dr. Kazanjian. The British commanding officer of the entire General Hospital No. 20 was Lt. Col. H. F. Shea, who was rated "one of the most efficient in the Corps." He was a "good surgeon, every inch an officer, almost Spartan in self-discipline . . . . His own tent looked like a friar's cell."[36]

Colonel William Carr, Deputy Director of Medical Services in charge of all the hospitals in the area of Camiers, issued a short, terse and all-inclusive order: In the future, all jaw cases in the area were to be treated by Dr. Kazanjian and his staff at General Hospital No.20. Recognizing his invaluable service to the British, Carr ordered, "Give that man, Kazanjian, anything he wants." Thus Kazanjian was provided with unlimited supplies and staff. Dr. Kazanjian acknowledged Col. Carr's "enthusiastic support and encouragement . . . and invaluable services . . . he was one of the first officers in the R.A.M.C. in France to recognize the importance of dental work in general, and the treatment of face and jaw injuries." The British assigned about a hundred beds to Dr. Kazanjian's jaw and facial unit. The unit was composed of five wards, each measuring sixty by twenty-four feet, with its own mess, laboratories, X-ray rooms, and operating rooms. This was to be the permanent home of the Unit until 1919.[37]

In a masterful stroke, Dr. Kazanjian placed himself and his unit under the direct supervision of Captain (later Colonel) Harold Burrows, Chief of the Surgical Section of General Hospital No. 20. Kazanjian considered him to be "one of the brilliant young surgeons of the British Army." Brigham described Burrows thus:

> *He had all the qualities, handsome, efficient, one of Britain's most respected general surgeons, keen in research, and resourceful in technique. The teamwork was ideal. Kazanjian provided the dental and mechanical skill while Burrows contributed the experience of a general surgeon. He was later promoted to the post of Chief Consultant of the British Expeditionary Force. Neither would shrink from any surgical sane responsibility and innovation, yet neither would over- step and attempt work illadvisedly.*[38]

Drs. Kazanjian and Burrows collaborated on two articles on gunshot wounds of the face, which appeared in the British Journal of Surgery in 1917 and 1918.[39]

Once the arrangements had been completed for Dr. Kazanjian to stay in France, there remained many unsolved problems, including his dental office and his patients back in Boston. He turned to Dean Smith, cabling him on October 25, 1915: "Leave care of practice to your judgment. Try arrange with Dr. Stone."

His dental patients were referred to Dr. Harry A. Stone at his old address at 157 Newbury Street

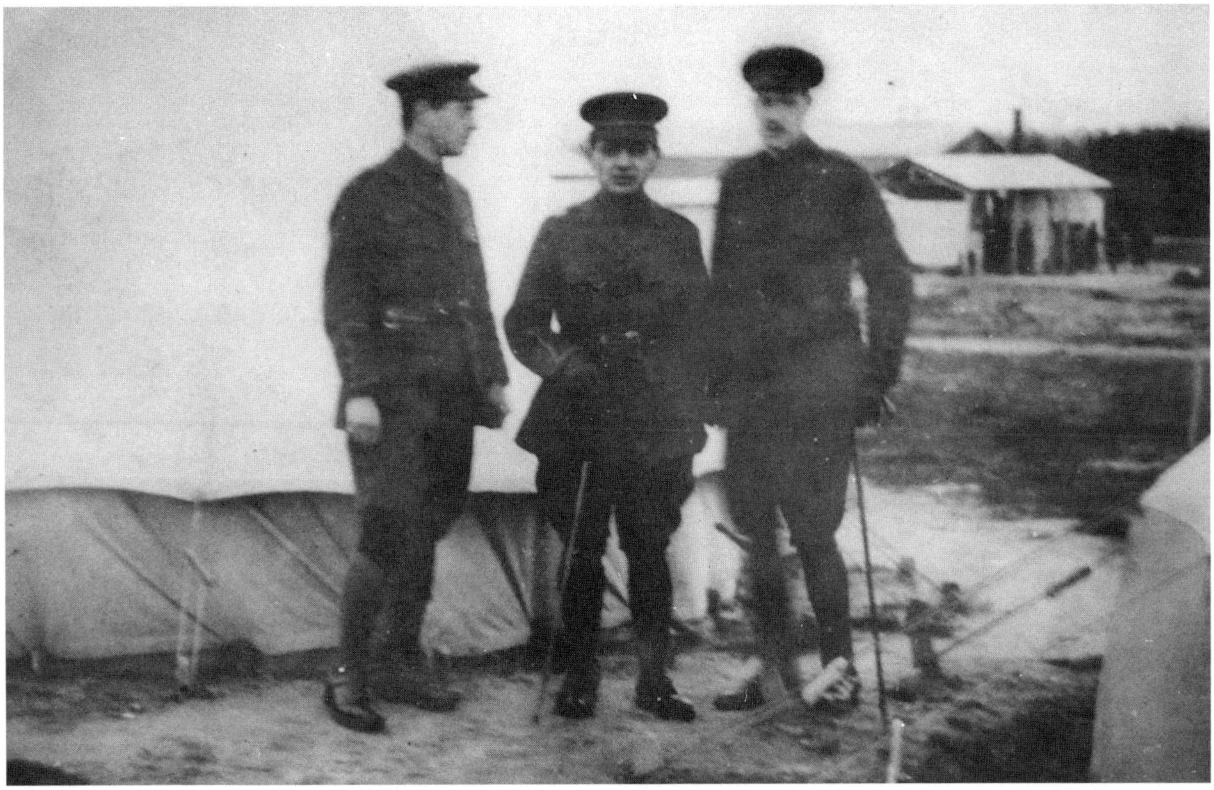

Dr. Kazanjian and two other officers in Dannes-Camiers,
The Harvard Medical Library in the Francis A. Countway Library of Medicine

in Boston. Apparently few of his patients were seen by Dr. Stone. "I guess I have scared off what of your practice did stay," Stone wrote afterwards.[40]

Dr. Kazanjian's humility became legendary. The description in The History of the Harvard Dental School characterized this best:

> *Yet, throughout it all, this Harvard dentist retained a modest simplicity and unassuming manner that gained him instant and spontaneous popularity. A short, black-haired, soft-spoken man with kindly eyes, he went quietly about his business and performed marvels upon the soldiers. His stature and appearance made him almost insignificant, yet in his presence, one felt there existed within him a vitality, a force, a genius, a keenness of perception that gave him extraordinary powers of accomplishment. It is small wonder that the stricken British soldiers, suffering untold agonies from splintered jaws and mangled faces, believed implicitly in his ability to help them.*[41]

A nurse who visited the hospital observed that when Dr. Kazanjian entered the ward, his patients would kiss his hand as a gesture of gratitude and respect.[42]

Dr. Kazanjian was able to set aside rules and regulations in an army that greatly valued such qualities. Yet he kept on the best of terms with the British officers. On off hours, the staff played field hockey. "All sorts of sports were indulged in," Dr. Daniel B. Reardon recorded. There was a

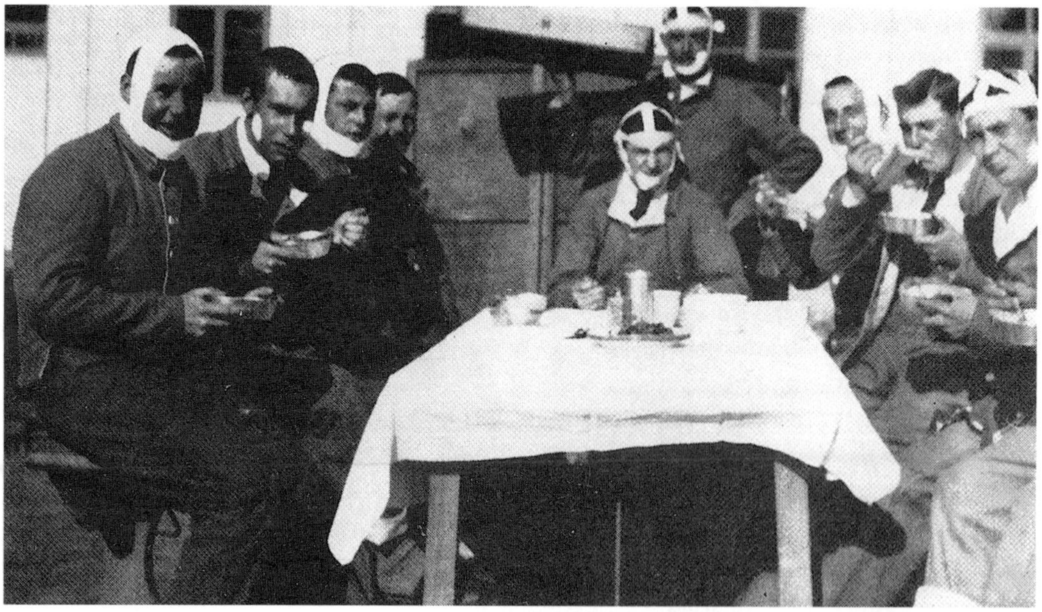

A group of patients at General Hospital No. 20
The Harvard Medical Library in the Francis A. Countway Library of Medicine

"keen rivalry between men of different camps." He mentions games of baseball, cricket, and tug of war. "The Camiers Y.M.C.A. provided many divertissements," Dr. Harvey Cushing recorded. One week's program was as follows:

> Tuesday—the 19th Ordnance Depot Concert Party;
>
> Wednesday—Lecture by J. Holland Rose on "The Crisis of 1914;"
>
> Thursday—Dramatic Performance: "Waterloo" and "Phipps;"
>
> Friday—Lecture by Prof. Perkins, "The Story of Baghdad."[43]

Dr. David Cheever, Chief Surgeon of the Second Harvard Unit, wrote that the experiences of the Unit expressed "the true feeling of sympathy and understanding, which exists between most Americans and most Englishmen." He also made it a point to report on "the splendid work which he [Kazanjian] and his associates are doing in the repair of destructive injuries of the jaws."[44]

With his "feet in the mud," Dr. Kazanjian was performing miracles of healing.[45]

NOTES

1 Coningsby Dawson, *Carry On, Letters of War-Time* (New York: John Lane, 1917), p. 50.

2 *The New York Times*, August 4, 1916, p. 4, col. 4, and January 16, 1916, Magazine Section, p. 6-7, col. 1-6; Ferdinand Brigham, "Harvard Goes to War," *Harvard Dental Alumni Bulletin* 24, no. 4 (1964): 103; Beth Haiken, "Plastic Surgery and American Beauty at 1921," *Bulletin of the History of Medicine* 68 (1994): 442.

3 John C. Phillips, "Tales and Poems of Patients in 22 General Hospital" (British), taken from books kept by nurses of the Harvard Surgical Units of 1915-16 (Sister Cunningham's booklet, p. 1). H MS c51

4 W. H. Gilmour, "Notes on a Visit to the Military Hospitals at the Base in France and Some Hospitals in Paris," *British Dental Journal* 37, no. 15 (August 1916): 562. E. C. Curtis, "Harvard Men in Hospital Work," *Harvard Graduates Magazine* 24 (September 1915), presents a statistical table (p. 229) of the kinds of missiles most likely to cause wounds. The wounded studied were 318 patients who were admitted to the American Ambulance Hospital.

5 Richard Locke Hapgood, *History of the Harvard Dental School* (Peterboro, N.H.: Transcript Printing Co., 1930), p. 120. Étaples, including Dannes-Camiers, became the largest hospital center for the British troops in France; see W. G. Macpherson, *Medical Services General History* (London: His Majesty's Stationery Office 1923), v. 2, p. 357. Also, Reginald Pound, *Harley Street* (London: Michael Joseph, 1967), p. 74; V. H. Kazanjian, "Remembrance of Things Past," *Plastic and Reconstructive Surgery* 35, no. 1 (1965): 10; John W. Converse, "Plastic Surgery: The Twentieth Century. The Period of Growth, 1914-1939," *Surgical Clinics of North America* 47, no. 2 (April 1967): 263. The scant number of books published before World War I relating to plastic, facial and jaw surgery, listed below, were for the most part in Dr. Kazanjian's personal library. James E. Garretson, *A System of Oral Surgery* (Philadelphia: Lippincott, 1873); Gordon Buck, *Contributions to Reparative Surgery* (New York: Appleton, 1876); Francis Mason, *On the Surgery of the Face* (London: Churchill, 1878); Norman W. Kingsley, *A Treatise on Oral Deformities as a Branch of Mechanical Surgery* (New York: Appleton, 1880); John S. Marshall, *A Manual of the Injuries and Surgical Diseases of the Face, Mouth and Jaws,* 2d ed. (Philadelphia: S. S. White, 1902); Frederick S. Kolle, *Plastic and Cosmetic Surgery* (New York: Appleton, 1911); John B. Roberts, *Surgery of Deformities of the Face Including Cleft Palate* (New York: William Wood, 1912); Vilray P. Blair, *Surgery and Diseases of the Mouth and Jaws* (St. Louis: Mosby, 1912). John S. Davis's important and pioneering book, *Plastic Surgery, Its Principles and Practice* (Philadelphia: Blakiston), appeared in 1919. See also John S. Davis, "Plastic Surgery in World War I and World War II," *Annals of Surgery* 123, no. 4 (April 1946): 610-621.

6 Letter from V. H. Kazanjian to Dean E. H. Smith, August 3, 1915, version no. 2, Kazanjian Archive, folders C-392 and WW-1269.

7 Letter from V. H. Kazanjian to William H. Potter, August 23, 1915, Kazanjian Archive, folder C-340. The idea of "crudeness" in the performance of operations of the jaw and face was observed about fifty years earlier by Dr. James E. Garretson, who "realized the crudeness that was characteristic of the early operations performed on the head, face and jaws." Garretson (1828-1895) founded the first hospital of oral surgery in Philadelphia in 1879. See Harold I. Faggart, "Dr. James E. Garretson and the First Hospital of Oral Surgery," *Bulletin of the History of Medicine* 17 (1945): 362. Also, Harvey Cushing, "Concerning Operations for the Cranio-Cerebral Wounds of Modern Warfare," *The Military Surgeon* 38: no. 6 (June 1916): 605. Cushing was referring to General and later Field Marshall Joseph Jacques-Césaire Joffre, French Commander-in-Chief. He discusses the work of Dr. Hayes and his colleagues at the American Ambulance in Paris, where 20 percent of wounds were fractured jaws.

8 Hapgood, *Harvard Dental School*, p. 120.

9 Ferdinand Brigham, Unpublished manuscript on the Dental Unit of the First Harvard Unit; John M. Converse and V. H. Kazanjian, *Kazanjian and Converse's Surgical Treatment of Facial Injuries* (Baltimore: Williams & Wilkins, 1973), 3rd ed., v. 1, p. viii.

10 Vilray P. Blair, "The Aims of the Sub-section of Plastic and Oral Surgery," *Gynecology and Obstetrics* 25, no. 6 (December 1917): 730 (Section on Symposium of War Surgery). Major Blair observed that "the surgeon is not technically trained to splint these cases [and] the dentist . . . is not trained to care for the wounded tissue. The majority are pursuing their separate ways." The concept of No Man's Land between surgery and dentistry, which only a few had bridged, is from Dr. Blair. For more information of Vilray Blair see Chapter 6. Also Ferdinand Brigham, "Dentistry in the Harvard Surgical Unit," *The Mirror* (Harvard Dental School) (1919): 51-53.

11 John M. Hyson, Jr. and Gardner P. H. Foley, "James Baxter Bean: The First Military Maxillofacial Hospital," and "Thomas Brian Gunning and His Splint for Jaw Fractures," *Maryland State Dental Association Journal* 40, no. 2 (Spring 1997): 77-81 and no. 1 (Winter 1997): 35-38. For a biographical sketch of Dr. Norman W. Kingsley, see Burton Lee Thorpe, "History of Dental Surgery," in Charles E. Koch, ed., *Biographies of Pioneer American Dentists and Their Successors* (Chicago: National Art Publishing Co., 1910), v. 3, pp. 542-559. For an illustrated history of interdental splints, see Norman W. Kingsley, *A Treatise on Oral Deformities as a Branch of Mechanical Surgery* (New York: Appleton, 1880), Chapter 17, pp 384-411, which includes an extensive description of the Kingsley Splint that was used and improved upon by Dr. Kazanjian.

12 Blair, "Aims of the Sub-section." Also, Robert M. Goldwyn, "Bernard von Langenbeck, His Life and Legacy," Chapter in Frank McDowell, *The Source Book of Plastic Surgery*, pp. 453-459. Bernard von Langenbeck (1810-1887) was the Surgeon-General of the German Army and Professor of Surgery at the University of Berlin. Dr. Goldwyn termed him "the productive nucleus of German Surgery in the mid-nineteenth century." V. H. Kazanjian, "Observations on War Surgery of the Face and Jaws," address delivered at the annual meeting of the New Jersey Dental Society, Atlantic City, July 16-19, 1919. Printed in *Dental Cosmos* 62 (1920): 283-294

13 Kazanjian, "Remembrance of Things Past," p. 12. Hapgood, *Harvard Dental School*, p. 126.

14 V. H. Kazanjian, "Early Treatment of Gunshot Wounds of the Face and Jaws," *Surgery* 15, no. 1 (June 1944): 22.

15 "Case #1, Private J. H.," Kazanjian Archive, Section IV, World War I Materials, folder WW-20, File on J. H.

16 "Case #2, Private T. H.," Kazanjian Archive, Section IV, World War I Materials, folder WW-20, file on T. H. A village about three miles east of Ypres, Hooge, in Flanders, was the site of major battles from May to July 30, 1915, when it became particularly furious. A planned Allied offensive was halted when the Germans used poison gas for the first time.

17 Letter from V. H. Kazanjian to William H. Potter, August 23, 1915.

18 Case #2, Private T. H.; Kazanjian, "Observations on War Surgery."

19 Daniel B. Reardon, "Diary," June 25, 1915, to October 17, 1915, p. 34, transcription by British Imperial War Museum. Courtesy of Mrs. Paul C. Reardon, Hingham, Mass. Dr. Reardon recorded in his diary entry for September 9, 1915: "I went down to Canadian No. 1 hospital with Dr. Kazanjian this afternoon to see fractured jaw cases with him." It did not take long for Dr. Kazanjian's reputation for skill to spread beyond the confines of General Hospital No. 22.

20 Brigham, Unpublished manuscript. Also A. D. Macalister, "The Queen's Hospital, Sidcup; The Foundation of British Oral Surgery," Mendies Campbell Lecture of the Royal College of Surgeons of England 1987, unpublished copy in the author's private collection. Macalister, who was Dean of the Dental Department of the Dental School at Dunedin, New Zealand, records the experience of Lt. Gen. Sir John Glubb, as a young officer in the Royal Engineers wounded during World War I and waiting for three months with his "wound pouring pus" until he received definitive treatment. John Glubb, *Into Battle: A Soldier's Diary of the Great War* (London: Book Club Associates, 1978).

21 Kazanjian, "Remembrance of Things Past," p. 11; Frank H. Cushman, "The Harvard Volunteers in Europe," in M. S. DeWolfe Howe, *Harvard Volunteers in Europe* (Cambridge, Mass.: Harvard University Press, 1916), p. 183; Vilray P. Blair, "The Maxillofacial Services of the American Army in the War," *Journal of the American Medical Association* 73, no. 5, (August 3, 1919): 325-327; Macalister, "The Queen's Hospital, Sidcup"; Brigham, "Harvard Goes to War," p. 103; V. H. Kazanjian, "Visit to American Ambulance

Hospital Dental Department, Sept. 14, 1915," Kazanjian Archive, World War I material, folder WW-1266; also, Brigham, Unpublished manuscript.

22 Letter from Dr. Frank H. Cushman to Dean Smith, September 17, 1915. Also, letter from V. H. Kazanjian to Dean Smith undated but written in answer to Dr. Smith's letter of October 22, 1915. "I read a paper before the Étaples Medical Society a few weeks ago which was received very favorably." Also, Reardon, "Diary."

23 V. H. Kazanjian, Notebook labeled "Sept. 14/15 Visit to American Ambulance Hospital Dental Department," Kazanjian Archive, World War I materials. The notebook contains descriptions and sketches of appliances that Kazanjian saw at the American Ambulance Hospital. For a detailed description and photographs of the work of the dental department of the American Ambulance, see George B. Hayes, "War Dental Surgery: Some Cases of Maxillo-Facial Injuries Treated in the Dental Section of American Ambulance at Neuilly (Paris), France," *Dental Cosmos* 58, no.3 (March 1916), I, pp. 249-258; II, pp. 389-401; III, pp. 511-523; IV, pp. 658-668; V, pp. 758-771; VI, pp. 1012-1028; VII pp. 1143-1163.

24 Hapgood, *Harvard Dental School*, pp. 122-123. The petition to President Lowell was sent with Dr. Kazanjian's approval. (Letter from V. H. Kazanjian to Dean Smith, undated but written in answer to Dean Smith's letter of Oct. 22, 1915.) Also, cablegram from A. Lawrence Lowell to Major Stookey, Twenty-Second General Hospital, France, Sept. 24, 1915, from the Harvard University Archives, Pusey Library, President Lowell's papers UA15. 160.7. Box 644; Kazanjian, "Remembrance of Things Past," p. 9; Taped interview of V. H. Kazanjian by Robin Anderson, 1971 (National Archives of Plastic Surgery in The Francis A. Countway Library of Medicine); Lyn Macdonald, *The Roses of No Man's Land* (London: Penguin Books, 1993), p. 153. Dr. Kazanjian was considered "unqualified" as far as the British system was concerned. He had not strictly met the educational and legal requirements of medical and surgical practice; he did not have the M. D. degree.

25 Harvey Cushing, *The Life of Sir William Osler*, (Oxford: Clarendon Press, 1925) v. 2, p. 490. Letter written before the end of September 1915. Also, *Daniel Bartholomew Reardon (1877-1961): A Brief Biography*, p. 14. Reardon "Diary", pp. 34-35.

26 Report of Dental Department, Harvard Surgical Unit, Gen. Hospital No. 22, July 21,-Oct. 1, 1915; also, Army Day Book 136, dental work beginning Aug. 8, 1915. Kazanjian Archive, folder C-333. Letter from Ferdinand Brigham to his father, Oct. 1, 1915, in Kazanjian Archive, folder C-42.

27 Letter from V. H. Kazanjian to Officer Commanding General Hospital No. 22, Nov. 5, 1915, Kazanjian Archive, folder C-333; Kazanjian, "Remembrance of Things Past," p. 9. These must not have been easy decisions to make. A cablegram was sent to Dean Smith from Drs. Kazanjian, Cushman, and Brigham on Oct. 3, 1915, reading: "Received cable. President Lowell permitting Kazanjian absence. Notify families. All waiting here for re-assignment. Our services very urgent." (translated from French).

28 Cushman, "Volunteers in Europe," p. 185; Hapgood, *Harvard Dental School*, pp. 123-124; Brigham, "Harvard Goes to War," p. 103.

29 Cushman, "Volunteers in Europe," pp. 184-185. Hapgood, *Harvard Dental School*, pp. 122-123, states that Dr. Nichols returned to America earlier on Sept. 14, 1915, and was temporarily replaced by Dr. William E. Faulkner. Also, letter from V. H. Kazanjian to Dean E. H. Smith, undated but written in answer to Dean Smith letter to Kazanjian dated Oct. 22, 1915; Robert S. Catheron, "The Work of the Dental Section of the Harvard Surgical Unit," Kazanjian Archive, folder WW-1269.

30 Harvard University, *Reports of the President and Treasurer of Harvard College, 1914-15* (Cambridge, Mass: Harvard University Press, 1916), p. 21; Cushing, *Sir William Osler*, v. 2, p. 503, footnote. Also, *Harvard Alumni Bulletin* 18 no. 3 (October 13, 1915): 42: "Thus Harvard is fortunately placed in the position of doing somewhat more than it promised."

31 The collection taken at the Harvard-Yale football game is reported in *Reports of the President and the Treasurer of Harvard College, 1914-1915*, p. 21; Hugh Cabot, "Harvard Surgical Unit with the British Expeditionary Force in France," *The Harvard Graduate Magazine* 25, no. 9 (1916-1917): 306; *Boston Sunday Herald*, Nov. 7, 1915, p. 4, col. 4-5.

32 David Cheever, "The Work of the Harvard Unit in France," *Harvard Alumni Bulletin* 18 no. 27 (April 5, 1916): 508; Robert S. Catheron, Unpublished

account included as part of Dr. Ferdinand Brigham's longer manuscript on the Dental Unit of the First Harvard Unit during World War I. Sir Alfred Henry Keogh (1857-1936), Director General of the Army Medical Service from October 1914 to 1918, administered medical services in England. For a biography of Keogh, see V. G. Plarr, *Plarr's Lives of the Fellows of the Royal College of England*, Supplement 1930-1951, by Dr D'Arcy Power and W. R. Lefanu (London: The Royal College, 1951), pp. 451-453. Also, Letter from Sir William Osler to Sir Alfred Keogh, Nov. 3, [1915], Kazanjian Archive, folder C-502. After observing Dr. Kazanjian's work, Sir William is reported to have said, "Why does a man like you marry?" Taped interview of V. H. Kazanjian by Robin Anderson, 1971.

33 Cheever, "Harvard Unit in France," p. 508; Cushing, *Sir William Osler*, v. 2, p. 504 (The quotation from a letter written by Lady Osler); Hapgood, *Harvard Dental School*, p. 128.

34 Catheron, Unpublished account included as a part of Dr. Ferdinand Brigham's longer manuscript on the Dental Unit of the First Harvard Unit during World War I. Christopher J. Walker, *Armenia: The Survival of a Nation* (London: Croom Helm, 1980), p. 231. Also,"800,000 Armenians counted destroyed," *The New York Times*, Oct. 7, 1915, p. 3, cols. 4-5: "The House of Lords is a very unemotional assembly, but it was thrilled in every fibre at the story of the horror . . . . There is not a case in history since the days of Tamerlane where a crime so hideous and on so gigantic a scale has been recorded."

35 Cushing, *Sir William Osler*, v. 2, p. 503 (Letter from Lady Osler, Dec. 3, 1915), pp. 502, 504; Cheever, "Harvard Unit in France," p. 508.

36 Hapgood, *Harvard Dental School*, pp. 123-125. Also, V. H. Kazanjian, unpublished paper read before the Harvard Dental Alumni Association, June 18, 1919, in the Kazanjian Archive, folder A-M 163. Cushman, "Volunteers in Europe," p. 186, reported that "between July 20 and December 1, over one thousand, two hundred cases of all kinds received treatment varying from a single visit to work covering daily attendance for several months." W. H. Gilmour, who visited 20th General Hospital soon after Dr. Kazanjian's arrival, commented "upon the ingenuity, he [Kazanjian] had displayed in the making and designing of the mechanical appliances" and marvelled at his results, "particularly in view of the really poor and inadequate equipment possessed by the Unit." W. H. Gilmour discussion of paper by V. H. Kazanjian, "Immediate Treatment of Gunshot Fracture of the Jaws," *British Dental Journal* 37:15 (1916): 332. See also, V. H. Kazanjian, "Immobilization of Wartime Compound Comminuted Fractures of the Mandible," *American Journal of Orthodontics and Oral Surgery*, 28, no. 10 (1942): 3; Brigham, Unpublished manuscript.

37 Brigham, Unpublished manuscript and "Harvard Goes to War," p. 103; V. H. Kazanjian, "Immediate Treatment of Gunshot Fractures of the Jaws": quote is from the hand-written draft in the Kazanjian Archive, folder-76, and is not included in the published article that appeared in the *British Dental Journal* 37 (1916): War Supplement, 297-336; Hapgood, *Harvard Dental School*, p. 124.

38 Kazanjian, "Remembrance of Things Past," p. 10, and Unpublished paper read before the Harvard Dental Alumni Association, June 18, 1919; Brigham, Unpublished manuscript.

39 V. H. Kazanjian and Harold Burrows, "The Treatment of Hemorrhage Caused by Gunshot Wounds of the Face and Jaws," *British Journal of Surgery* 5 (1917): War Supplement, 126, and "The Treatment of Gunshot Wounds of the Face Accompanied by Extensive Destruction of the Lower Lip and Mandible," *British Journal of Surgery* 6 (1918): 74.

40 Cablegram from V. H. Kazanjian to Dean Eugene Smith, Oct. 25, 1915, folder C-390; and letter from Dr. Harry A. Stone, to V. H. Kazanjian, June 29, 1916, folder C-410, in the Kazanjian Archive.

41 Hapgood, *Harvard Dental School*, p. 127.

42 Personal interview with Harry S. Cherken, Jr., July 11, 1996, King of Prussia, Pennsylvania. This had been reported to him by his grandmother who had been a nurse in France.

43 Hapgood, *Harvard Dental School*, p. 127; Reardon, "Diary" entries for Aug. 3, 5, 7, 13, and 18, 1915; Harvey Cushing, *From a Surgeon's Journal* (Boston: Little Brown, 1936), p. 157, covering the period of July 1917.

44 Cheever, "Harvard Unit in France," p. 511.

45 This concept of "feet in the mud" was suggested to me by Madeline Mullen of the staff of the V. H. Kazanjian Archive in The Francis A. Countway Library of Medicine during one of our many conferences, 1995-96.

CHAPTER SIX

Miracle Man of the Western Front

Word of Dr. Kazanjian's skill flew with wings along the entire battlefield. He became "probably the best known individual surgeon in the Allied Armies." His story, both personal and surgical, constituted "a veritable romance." An English writer characterized him as "the miracle man of the Western Front" and he "attracted the attention of the world." On January 1, 1916, his work was acknowledged in a dispatch from Field Marshall Sir John French, Commander-In-Chief of the British Army in France. On November 7, 1917, and April 7, 1918, he was mentioned in two additional dispatches from Field Marshall Sir Douglas Haig, "for gallant and distinguished service in France, both of which were signed by Winston Churchill."[1]

When Lieutenant Coningsby Dawson visited Dr. Kazanjian's jaw clinic, he observed: "There was a man who performed miracles. He was a naturalized American citizen, but was an Armenian by birth. He gave people new faces." Dawson graphically described a patient:

> *His face was entirely swathed in bandages with gaps left for his breathing and his eyes. He had been like that for two years, and looked like a leper. When he spoke he made hollow noises. His nose and lower jaw had been torn away by an exploding shell. Little by little, with infinite skill, by the grafting of bone and flesh, his face was being built up. Could any surgery be more merciful?*[2]

One of the best-known British war correspondents, H. F. Prevost Battersby, wrote an article, "Surgery's Miracle at the Western Front," which dramatized "the daring skill of the surgeon being used to make life once more of its old value to men whose hideous injuries made them beg to be destroyed." Of all the wonderful surgical achievements of the war none "moves us as does the reconstruction of a face, a third of which had disappeared." The surgeon "revels in restoring to the image of its Maker shapes that exceed in horror the devilish grotesqueries of the medieval masons."[3]

"How you came over to France—unknown, unsung, and really not yourself fully convinced of your mission, and influenced the British, particularly," a surgeon, Dr. Moses S. Strock, observed, "will always remain a miracle to me." The surgeon asserted that "the British . . . are . . . your greatest admirers," adding "to say to an Englishman, 'I had the good fortune to have been one of Kazanjian's assistants' is to break down all reserve." Dr. Kazanjian was very well liked by Europeans. "The general opinion here is that you should stay in Europe after the war," Dr. Catheron suggested in 1916. "A great many have said so." Kazanjian's friend, M. Vartan Malcom, as early as October 1915, had the "feeling that the rest of your life you will probably spend either in Paris or in London where you will be much better known . . . than in Boston."[4]

Back in America, on October 19, 1915, the *Boston Post* wrote of Dr. Kazanjian as performing "some most wonderful operations on the faces of

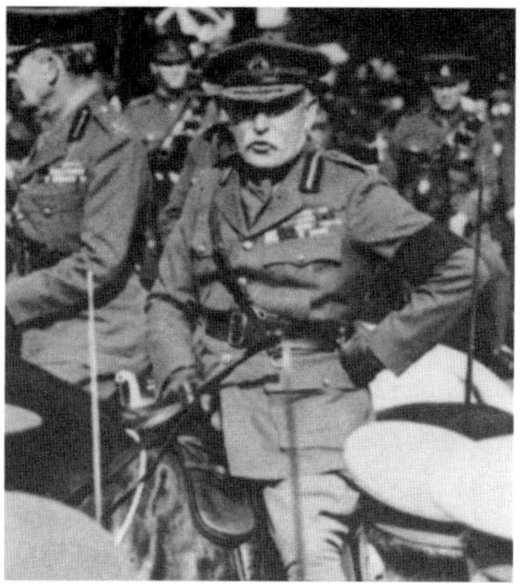

Field Marshall Sir John French, Commander-in-Chief of the British Army in France until December, 1915
Courtesy of the Imperial War Museum, London
Q.70032

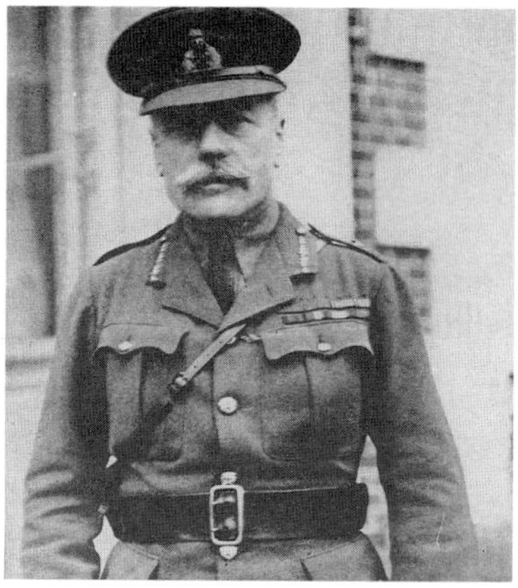

Field Marshall Sir Douglas Haig, Commander-in-Chief of the British Army in France beginning in December, 1915
Courtesy of the Imperial War Museum, London.
Q.3254

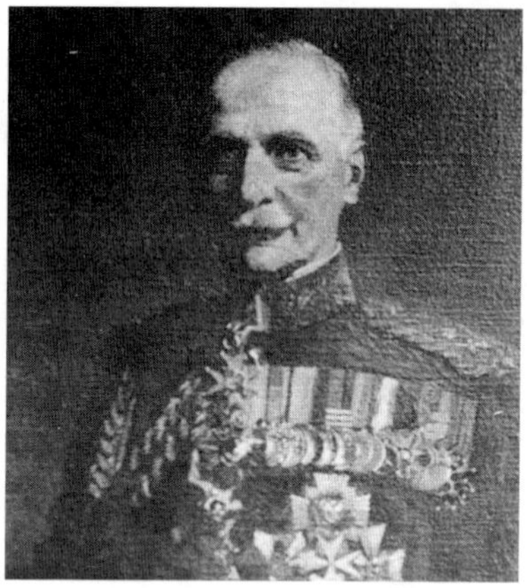

Lieut-General Sir A. T. Sloggett, K.C.B., K.C.M.G., K.C.V.D., F.R.C.S., K.V. Surgeon General, Director General of Military Services to the British Armies in France
Courtesy British Army Medical Services Museum, Keogh Barracks, Aldershot

men who have had their heads torn . . . his work can never be forgotten." His name was misspelled in this early newspaper account. American journalists were not, as yet, familiar with the scope of his work. However, change was not long in coming. On November 21, 1915, the *Boston Sunday Globe* featured Dr. Kazanjian with his photograph in an article, "Dentists Are Making History . . . Wonders of Surgery They Perform Are Beyond Anything Europe Had Ever Seen."

> *Just how valuable the dentists were to prove was not guessed. And just how great a step in advance they were to take was not dreamed. They turned out to be the best life-savers and pain removers, almost, among the lot of scientists.*[5]

In the summer of 1916, Dr. Carl W. Waldron was sent to Dr. Kazanjian's clinic in France by the Surgeon General of the Canadian Expeditionary Force. "It was my first meeting with Varaztad," he reminisced in 1955, "and here began our close friendship which has continued for more than thirty-eight years." Many of the techniques that were introduced by Dr. Kazanjian "are today standard procedures."[6]

Dr. Kazanjian's jaw clinic became a showplace, with many visitors, as there was no complete center like it anywhere, either among the Allies or the enemy. Not only did British surgeons come to spend from two to three months observing Dr. Kazanjian's techniques, but also doctors from Allied and neutral countries. One American visiting surgeon who stayed two or three days was Dr. Vilray P. Blair, who later became head of the Section of Oral and Plastic Surgery in the United States Army and Chief Consultant in Maxillofacial Surgery with the American Expeditionary Force during World War I. Many notables came, among them the sister of King George; Field Marshall Haig, the Commander-in-Chief of the British Army; Princess Victoria of Schleswig-Holstein, accompanied by two ladies-in-waiting; and Lt. Gen. Sir Arthur Sloggett, Director General of Medical Services of the British Armies in France. Sir Harold Gillies visited in the early days of the war and Sir Charles Valadier's presence was frequent. The visit by Sir William Osler in September 1915 has been previously recorded.[7]

At the request of his superiors, Major W. D. Anderson, of the Royal Army Medical Corps, toured the various dental centers in France from March 29 to April 11, 1916. In the report of his visit to the 20th General Hospital, he wrote:

> *I saw Major Kazanjian here, and had a most thorough and interesting show of patients and appliances. It is not possible to speak too highly of the work that is being carried out here. Major Kazanjian is doing nothing else but surgery connected with jaws and is getting most excellent results. I was especially struck with his ingenious and comparatively simply made appliances. Such appliances being* [sic} *made in vulcanite and involving much less expense than precious metal apparatus. The face wounds are doing well under his care, and altogether the work is of a very high order.*
>
> *One point worth mentioning was the brightness of the patients, in many cases suffering from unsightly wounds. The brightness Major Kazanjian attributes to some extent to their being all together so that the seeing of men, perhaps even in a worse plight than themselves, helps to cheer them up, and thus do away with the morbid sensitiveness so often found in bad face injuries. I think his own kindly treatment has also something to do with this brightness.*[8]

Dr. Kazanjian inspected military hospitals along the front lines and spoke to the staffs. He was received with honor and respect. In his first appearance before a civilian group in Europe, Dr. Kazanjian spoke in April 1916 to the American Dental Society in Paris. In preparing for the paper on that occasion, he acknowledged "the valuable

DENTISTS ARE MAKING HISTORY

Americans Who Went to France With Harvard Unit Retained by British Authorities — Wonders of Surgery They Perform Are Beyond Anything Europe Had Ever Seen.

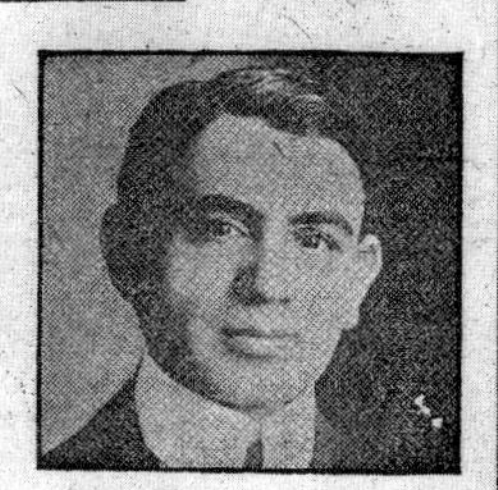

—VARAZTAD H. KAZANJIAN.

With the first Harvard unit that went to serve in a British base hospital in France, three dentists were included. With the second Harvard unit, which sailed this last week, went another three. Between the two events lies history.

The surgeons who composed the first unit said frankly that they did not expect to find much that would be new or instructive about war surgery.

It was recognized also that dentists were sure to be needed, partly because in trench fighting a large proportion of the wounds are likely to be head wounds, partly because the average English soldier, and more especially the cockney English soldier, is likely to have bad teeth.

Just how valuable the dentists were to prove was not guessed. And just how great a step in advance they were to take was not dreamed. They turned out to be the best life-savers and pain removers, almost, among the lot of scientists.

What the Specialist Does.

To begin with, a large proportion of wounds are head wounds, because the rest of the body is sheltered in a trench.

Now unless a head wound kills right away, the bullet is extremely apt to rake through the face, shattering the jaw, or cutting off the crowns of a row of teeth.

This is not all. The fragments of teeth or jawbone, under the impact of the modern high velocity rifle bullets, become themselves smaller bullets, and plow through the flesh of face or neck. They have to be followed up into the muscles of the cheeks, or dug out of the complicated mechanism of the throat, or even traced with probes far down among the neck muscles.

The dentist and the oral surgeon have found a great deal to do. The "general" surgeon, given a case in which part of a man's jaw has been carried away, is likely to excise the ragged part, fit the man up with an artificial appliance of some sort to carry teeth, and let it go at that.

The specialist in oral surgery has discovered and invented dozens of ways to improve on the old methods. If a lower jaw is shattered beyond hope of repair, the modern surgeon dentist will dissect it out altogether; he will crown two upper back teeth, and the gold crowns will carry sockets. He will form an artificial jaw of gold, mount artificial teeth upon it, and furnish it with balls to fit into the sockets, and springs to help a patient open and close his mouth.

Plenty of Work in France.

The dentist in these major operations works in conjunction with the new school of "plastic surgery," and does things unheard of till within a few years.

Most people of mature years have had the unpleasant experience of having a tooth nerve exposed, and are aware that it is unendurably painful. Men are brought into the base hospitals in France with a whole range of teeth smashed by a bullet, and a whole row of nerves standing naked. Imagine the pain of such a wound!

The dentists of today have learned the two points at which novocain can be injected in a jaw, numbing the whole set of tooth nerves. In five minutes they take away a soldier's anguish, and then hook out the devilish little white filaments calmly, with never a twinge for the patient.

It goes without saying that in the huge armies thousands of men need the ordinary dental attention which any crowd of like size would need. So there is plenty of work for dentists in France.

When the Harvard unit was being assembled, it was determined to add three dentists to the roster. Dean Eugene H. Smith of the Harvard Dental School made the selections of the men to go from among the volunteers, choosing Dr V. H. Kazanjian, Dr Frank Holmes Cushman and Dr Fred Brigham.

Dr Kazanjian was an instructor in the Dental School, and the others were students just ready to graduate when the expedition started. In fact, as the start was made before Commencement, they have not yet seen their diplomas unless they were forwarded.

Best Man in the Country.

Dr Kazanjian is a remarkable man. He is an Armenian who came to this country already well educated, who put himself through the dental school and earned his living while doing so, who then started to study medicine also, and who was grabbed by Dean Smith as an instructor in prosthetics, for the dental school, and so set to specializing instead of going on with a general education.

He is now the head of the department of prosthetics—which means mechanical dentistry—in the school, and is really the chief technician of the school. He is, what is more, probably one of the best men in the country in his specialty, and so recognized.

The other men are students who are just starting their careers. Dr Cushman is a graduate of Dartmouth with the degree of Bachelor of Science; Dr Brigham took his Bachelor of Arts degree at Tufts.

Their work in the war attracted immediate attention from the British authorities, and as the time for breaking up and sending the first Harvard unit home approached, the War Office sent for the three American dentists.

Sir Lionel Perry, or somebody else in high authority, told the Americans that their work had been so valuable that the War Office wished if possible to retain them when the rest of the surgeons returned to America.

Hospital at Their Disposal.

"You can all get extended leave of absence, for the Winter, anyway," the offisials said. "And if you will stay, we will build you a hospital, equip it completely, and will make financial arrangements differing from those under which you came. In other words, while under the arrangements of volunteering you get only the pay of soldiers, we will pay you salaries to make it possible for you to stay on."

Arrangements with Harvard for Dr Kazanjian's leave were readily made, and the British proposition has been accepted. Meanwhile, another Harvard unit has organized and started.

It had been obvious from the very first that three dentists could not handle all the work that was brought to them. So three more are going in the second unit, and the American Dental Hospital will start with the very latest of equipment and a staff of six surgeons.

The men of the second unit are Dr Franklin McDonald, who was graduated from the dental School in 1910, and who has been practicing in Brooklyn, N Y; Dr R. S Catheron, who is an instructor in anesthesia in the dental school, and Dr John F. Dillon of the class of 1915 who thus joins his classmates.

Whether these three men will be able to stay on for extended service has not yet been determined.

Boston Sunday Globe, Nov. 21, 1915
The Harvard Medical Library in the Francis A. Countway Library of Medicine

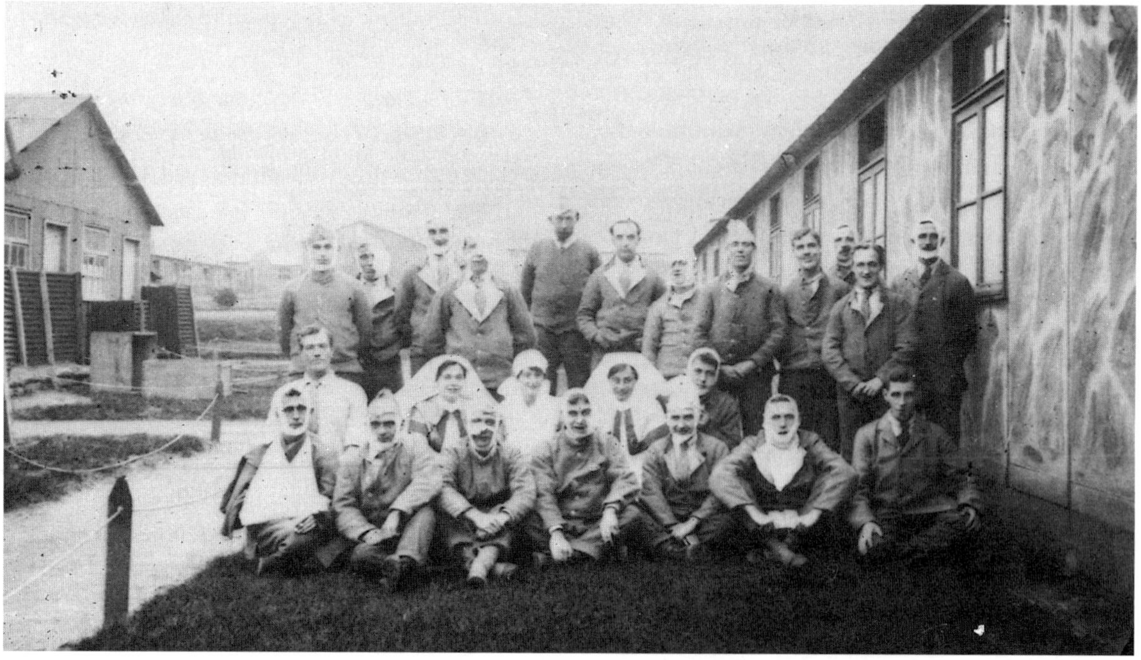

Patients and nurses in Dr. Kazanjian's clinic in Hospital No. 20
The Harvard Medical Library in the Francis A. Countway Library of Medicine

assistance of Catheron and Brigham in formulating, revising and illustrating it." The paper was well received by his colleagues and had "gained their support and good will." While in Paris, he again visited the American Ambulance Hospital in Neuilly-sur-Seine in the company of Dr. Catheron, who commented on "the splendid work they are doing."[9]

Dr. David Cheever completed his term as Chief of the Second Harvard Unit in March 1916 and was replaced by Dr. William E. Faulkner, who served as Chief until June 1916. Dr. Catheron's term of six months' service was up in May 1916, and he returned home. "His agreeable disposition gained him many friends," Dr. Kazanjian stated, "and long after he left the service [Catheron] was remembered by his British colleagues in the Unit." Catheron later recalled, "Outside of work hours, we walked to the nearby villages, the several miles of sand dunes between us and the channel . . . we talked of many things . . . and ate good food cooked at little cafes tucked away in tiny villages. We washed the good food down with St. Emilion or Graves Supérieures and thought the world not bad in spite of the war."[10]

The Third Harvard Unit, with Dr. Hugh Cabot as Chief, arrived in June 1916 for a six-month tour of duty. The dentists in the Third Unit were Dr. Harrison L. Parker, who arrived in May 1916, and Dr. Chauncy N. Lewis, who arrived in November 1916. Funds for the expenses of the Third Unit were obtained by a collection taken at the Harvard-Princeton football game in November 1916, which amounted to about $5,500. This sum was augmented by personal donations by Harvard graduates.[11]

The British Red Cross took a special interest in Dr. Kazanjian's clinic and allotted one thousand pounds (about $5,000) "to build and equip an additional ward which will be 90' by 22' and include 30 beds, two dental offices, a large laboratory, kitchen and nurses' room." It doubled the

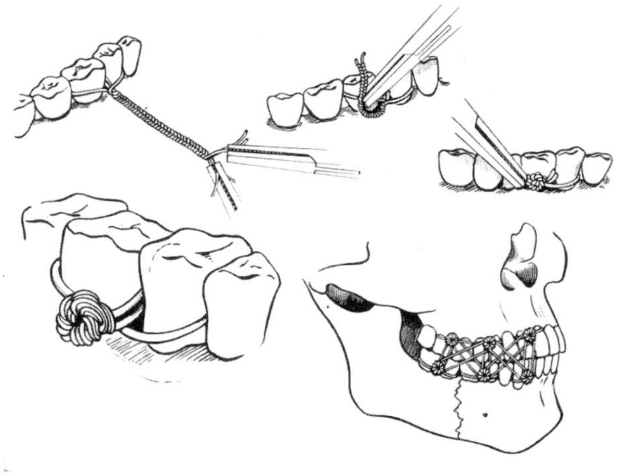

Kazanjian Button
Modified from P. D. Wilson,
Management of Fracture and Dislocations, *Lippincott (Philadelphia, 1938) p. 479, Illus. Robert H. Albertin*

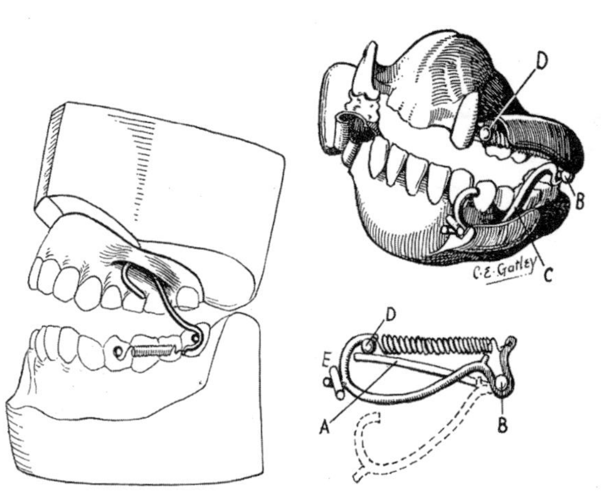

Illustrating the principles of the spring as a means of retention of the upper appliance
Kazanjian & Converse, 1st ed., 1949, p. 542

area of the clinic. All did not go easily, however, and "there were obstacles that had to be overcome." The greatest of these according to Dr. Kazanjian, was "the traditional disregard of the medical profession towards dentistry, which exists in the army as well as in civil life." He regretted to report to Dean Smith that "the present head of the Harvard Unit [Dr. Hugh Cabot] . . . is antagonistic, and not well disposed toward the dental department."[12]

An increase to six dentists in the Unit, which Dr. Kazanjian requested, meant that the number of medical men would be reduced to twenty-eight. Dentists would thus be "considered to be taking the places which others might have." It was argued that there were plenty of dentists from England who could "plug teeth," but what the War Office really wanted was "specialists in fractured jaws." It was Dr. Kazanjian's contention that there was a shortage of dentists. "In this district alone," he wrote, "there were . . . from five hundred to fifteen hundred soldiers . . . waiting for dental treatment . . . In view of this, why not support and encourage the dental department?"

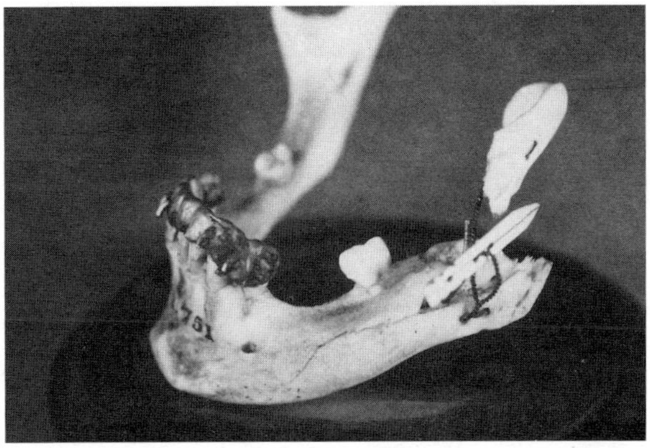

Anatomical Mandibular specimen, from a deceased patient illustrating the path of a projectile [right] and the cemented cast metal splint on the lower teeth
The Harvard Medical Library in the Francis A. Countway Library of Medicine
Photograph by Dr. Paul Davis

He pleaded that "our department wishes the support and not the antagonism of the medical men sent to France by the University." He appealed directly to President Lowell, but, deferring to his wishes, agreed to "try to utilize as many dentists as he sees fit to send."[13]

Lieutenant Kazanjian was promoted to Major Kazanjian in June 1916, skipping over the rank of captain. That same month, on June 15, he delivered a paper before the annual meeting of the British Dental Association on "Immediate Treatment of Gunshot Fracture of the Jaws." When the paper was published, it included his treatment plans and his classification of fractures.[14]

The daily routine in Dr. Kazanjian's unit began early, when the nurses, orderlies, and convalescing patients washed and fed the ill patients and removed bandages. Each wound was initially irrigated every two hours by a nurse with a syringe filled with a peroxide or a creosote-based solution. In a few days, the wound became less fetid. The tissues were swabbed with cotton pellets saturated with tincture of iodine. This was followed by Listerine or Dobell's solution. Drip irrigation with Carrel-Dakin's solution "worked wonders." Dr. Kazanjian then made his first rounds with the head nurse and assistants. Orders were given for special diets, minor surgery, splints, x-rays, medications, dressings, and special precautions, and consultations were arranged with other physicians.[15]

The dental staff then began their work. Impressions were taken, in bed if necessary, and minor surgical operations were performed under local anesthesia. More serious procedures were performed in the hospital operating rooms. It was late morning or afternoon when the appliances were actually fabricated with the help of the three dental mechanics (technicians). Each case required immobilization of the fractured segments of the jaw. If most of the teeth remained on both sides of the fracture, metal bands were made for the teeth. These were connected by a wire bar, and the entire appliance was cemented in place. These were the simplest types of appliances.

In those instances in which not enough teeth were present for anchorage, a vulcanite-rubber denture was fabricated that fixed the fractured portions of the jaw in place. A Barton bandage was placed, with great precision and perfection, in

CLASSIFICATION OF FRACTURES IN RELATION TO MECHANICAL FORCES GOVERNING THE CONSTRUCTION OF SLINTS [sic: splints]

I. Mandible....	1. Anterior to the last existing tooth 2. Posterior to the last existing tooth 3. Edentulous	(a) No loss of tissue (b) Comminution (c) Multiple fractures (d) Distinct loss of tissue
II. Maxilla......	1. Fracture of alveolar process and teeth 2. Partial fracture(s) with or without comminution and partial loss of bone 3. Complete fracture with or without loss of bone	
III. Mandible and maxilla	The foregoing conditions in combination	

From V. H. Kazanjian "Prosthetic Appliances in Surgical Treatment of Wounds of the Face and Jaws," The Dental Summary *39:12 (December 1919) chart: 923*

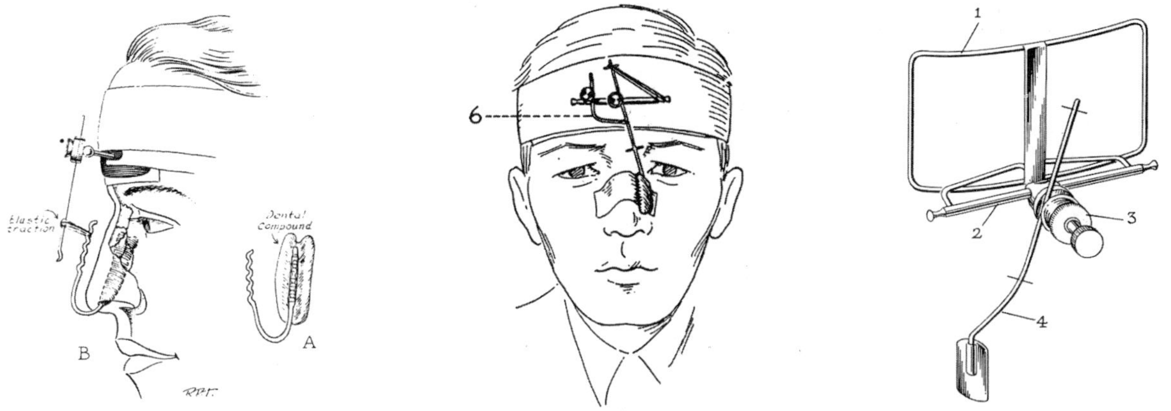

KAZANJIAN NASAL FRACTURE SPLINTS

LEFT: *V-splint for suspension of comminuted nasal bones* CENTER: *Splint anchored to forehead*
RIGHT: *Metal frame "This splint is designed to deliver the desired amount of continuous force against the lateral aspect of the nose at any selected point." Kazanjian & Converse,* The Surgical Treatment of Nasal Fractures, *(Baltimore: Williams & Wilkins 1949), pp. 176-78*

order to support the jaw and cover the facial wounds and forehead; it allowed the patient freedom to move about the ward. Very often more complex appliances were fabricated, using external support, such as plaster or vulcanite-rubber headgear over the forehead, to which splints or metal pads were attached, extending downward to support a fractured nose, for example, or to direct the wounded soft tissue into better position. Wires, like ropes, were anchored to the headgear, which also passed through the skin to gently direct a displaced fragment of bone into alignment. Where there was a gross amount of bone missing, Dr. Kazanjian replaced the lost bone with a mold made of vulcanite-rubber, over which the soft tissue of the face could later be surgically joined. If the temporomandibular joint was shattered, he fashioned a mechanical condyle.[16]

Hemorrhage was a constant complication and invariably occurred at night, when it "spoiled many well-earned hours of sleep for Dr. Kazanjian and his associates." In a survey of 400 patients treated at General Hospital No. 20, there were thirty-four cases of mild and serious hemorrhage. Of these, sixteen patients required surgical operations under general anesthesia. The remaining seventeen patients were successfully treated by packing, clamping or ligation of the blood vessel under local anesthesia. The majority of the hemorrhages occurred between the fourth and twelfth day following injury. To control secondary hemorrhages, particularly from the lingual artery, he invented the Kazanjian Clamp, one end of which exerted pressure in the mouth over the area of hemorrhage while the other end covered the corresponding area of the lower jaw extra-orally.[17] Other devices were also developed during this time. The Kazanjian Button was another brainchild. It was used during immobilization of the jaws with intermaxillary wiring with elastics.[18] The Kazanjian Nasal Fracture Splint "was designed to deliver the desired amount of continuous force against the lateral aspect of the nose at a selected point."[19]

Notwithstanding the presence of splints and appliances, which were often cumbersome, feeding was not a major problem. Dr. Kazanjian experimented in the kitchen and developed three separate diets: regular, minced, and liquid. For those who could not chew, rubber tubes of small caliber were inserted around the splint and either through the nose or the esophagus. "Teapot-type

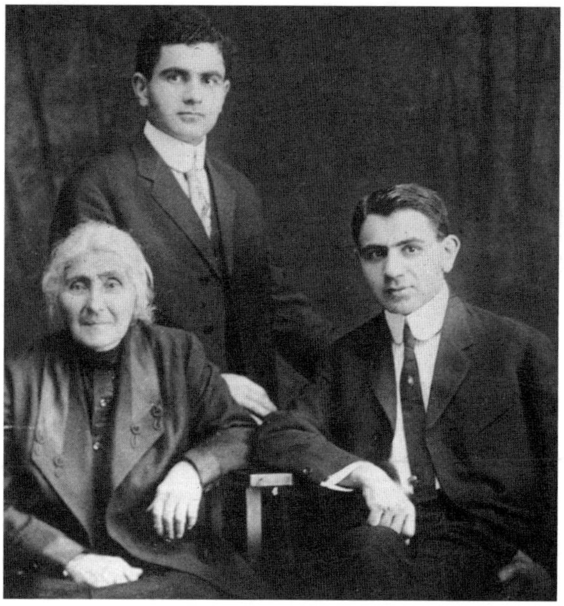

Anna, his mother, Yervant, his brother, and Varaztad Kazanjian. Mrs. Kazanjian died in 1918 while her son was in France.
Courtesy Melikian Studio

feeders" were filled with the liquid diet and the contents poured into the rubber tubes. The tubes were often left in place for several days.[20]

Dr. Kazanjian's wife, Sophie, arrived in Paris on November 18, 1915, but was unhappy there and moved to Dannes-Camier to be with her husband, at first living in a tent and later in a nearby village. She was the first wife in the war zone who was permitted to live with her husband. She endured "additional discomforts and sacrifice," but remained in France until 1919. "[My wife] became a very useful person," Kazanjian reported. "She helped the mothers and fathers of the sick boys at the base hospital." For them, she became a counselor and acted in the role of a social worker with the patients, apparently at the local Camiers Young Men's Christian Association. Mrs. Kazanjian made "life more of a joy at the base hospital." Her presence and support were a stimulus for Dr. Kazanjian to rise to even greater heights.[21]

Major Kazanjian's success and fame continued to grow as the war dragged on. His original three-month commitment for service stretched out to three-and-a-half years. He had prevailed in his technical differences with Valadier and Colyer —both will be discussed in the chapter that follows — and had found allies in Gillies, Fry, and James. "With a few exceptions," he wrote to Dean Smith, "I do the plastic operations on the patients in our department." The British authorities permitted him to perform maxillofacial surgery even though, according to their own standards, "he had no official right to perform operations" and "was completely unqualified as a surgeon," but "was the best man for the job, . . . and could not be spared." His superiors risked their reputations in allowing him to operate because his results were consistently superior. He made few, if any, serious errors in clinical judgment. He did not have "his hands slapped," but unlike the biblical admonition, the light of his candle was put "under a bushel." He was in an unconventional no-man's-land and was left alone and semi-ignored.[22]

There was a movement to separate the Harvard Dental Unit from the Harvard Surgical Unit. "Dr. Cabot would be delighted to be relieved of the dentists," Herbert H. White confided to Dean Smith. "Both Cabot and Nichols feel very strongly that Kazanjian is not a desirable person to represent the University as the head of anything."[23] This movement came to naught. Kazanjian continued as head of both units, and they were not separated. He continued to bring great honor to Harvard. Behind the scenes, Dean Smith must have stood his ground and remained loyal to his man.

President Lowell also supported him as the following letter, dated May 17, 1916, indicates:

> *It goes without saying that we need you very much here at the School, but at the same time we also want to do all we can to relieve the*

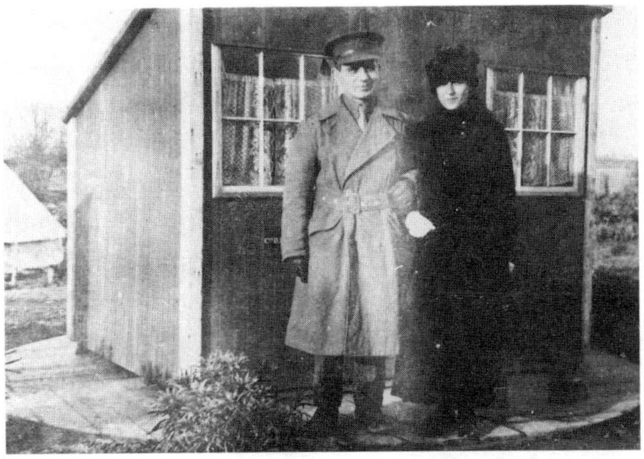

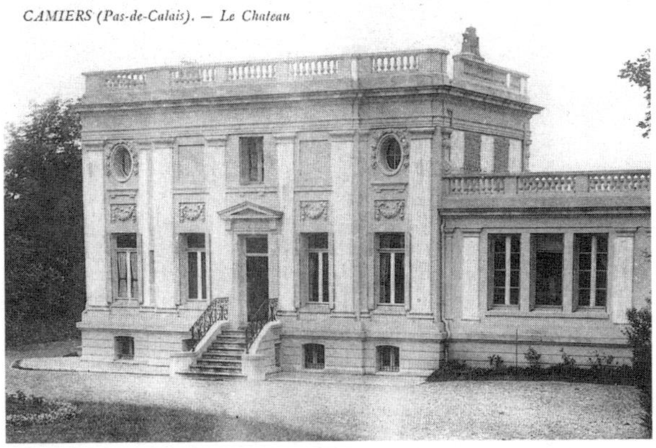

Left: Major and Mrs. Kazanjian in front of the "chicken coop" quarters in Hospital #20, which he occupied. Mrs. Kazanjian lived in the "Chateau" (right) in the nearby village of Camiers. It was the summer home of a gentleman before the war but served as quarters for the Scottish women volunteers.

The Harvard Medical Library in the Francis A. Countway Library of Medicine

> *conditions of the men who will suffer after the war from loss of their jaws; and if you think that your presence is important at the hospital, and cannot be thoroughly well supplied by someone else, by all means feel free to stay as long as that is the case.*[24]

A colleague at home, Dr. William H. Weston wrote: "You are courageous and a good sport to keep on with the work, when there is so much to call you back over here. You are needed in both places but probably we can do without your services better than some of the poor chaps who are trying to stop cannon balls with their faces."[25] To add to Dr. Kazanjian's dilemma, his family in Worcester was deeply concerned with his welfare and pressed him to return. "Don't you think you stayed there very long?" his ten-year-old nephew, Deron (Deran) Roopenian, pleaded in February 1917. "Dear Uncle in your last letter . . . you said that you looked older. We felt very bad for that. We think you did your duty . . . are you . . . going to come back?" His mother, Anna, died in 1918, which must have intensely saddened him. She had been the only parent that he had known since he was twelve years old and had been the anchor of the family.[26]

Dr. Kazanjian was aided greatly in his restorative work by the "Roses of No Man's Land," the valiant Army nurses, or sisters, as the British called them. The British designated them as V. A. D.'s (Voluntary Aid Detachment—female.) They were, for the most part, "gently nurtured girls" from comfortable Edwardian homes. To their patients they were "great ladies, medieval in their saintliness.". . . "the nearest approach to a sculptured Greek goddess . . . the divinity of womanhood . . . . Only her lips hold a touch of color; they have a childish trick of trembling when anyone's wound is hurting too much . . . . Men do not die in vain when they evoke such women." Gillies commended the nurses: "Bless their hearts, how quick their wits, how neat their knots! . . . the expert plastic sister . . . is often the deciding factor in success."[27] There's a Rose that grows in No Man's Land,

> *And it's wonderful to see.*
> *Tho' it's sprayed with tears,*
> *It will live for years.*
> *In my garden of memory.*[27]

The sisters, stationed in France, living in tents, "almost forgot what it feels like to be really warm." Their ankles were swollen and their feet ached and

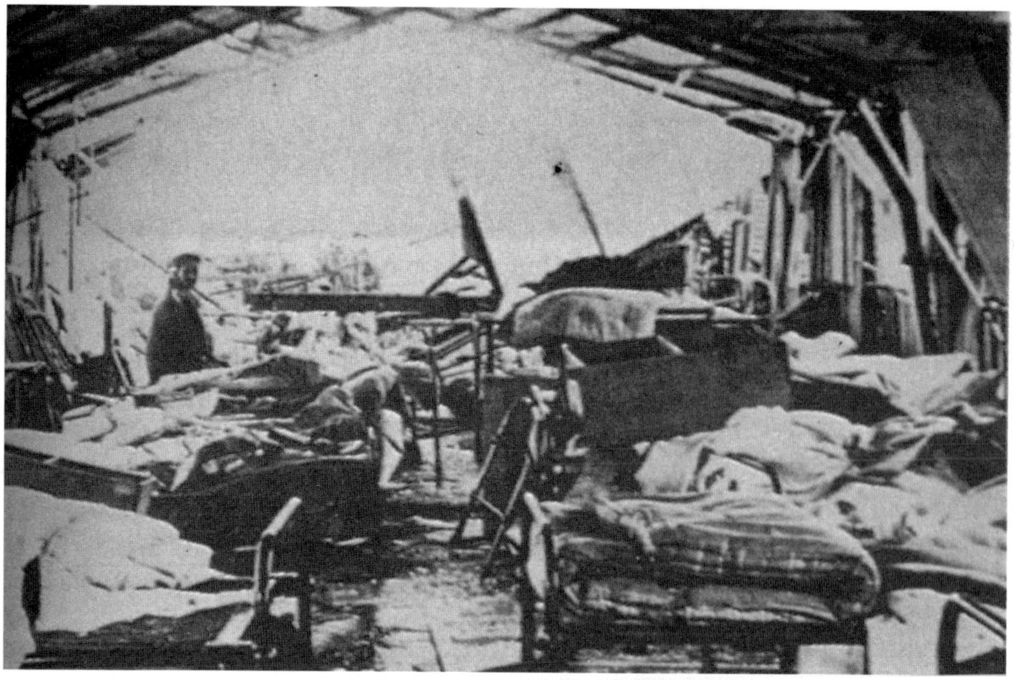

A bombed ward at No. 7 Canadian General Hospital in 1918
Macdonald The Roses of No Man's Land, *p. 176*

their hands were "reddened and rough."[28] Dr. Henry Potter described the life of nurses in Dannes-Camiers in a letter to his fiancee:

> *The nurses have to cut their own wood. It seems to me that they have a pretty hard time. They get up at six-thirty, breakfast at seven and get into the ward at seven-thirty. They are through at 6 pm. It certainly must take a good deal of nerve to stay on duty in a cold ward all day, with the thermometer usually around forty. Many have chilblains and several have ulcers on their fingers from the cold. There are always ten or twelve off sick.*[29]

Nurse Catherine Black treated facial wounds at Aldershot. These patients were "the most harrowing," she lamented. "Sadder even than the casualty clearing stations . . . for there death was swifter and even more merciful. . . . Hardest of all was the task of trying to rekindle the desire to live in men condemned to be week after week smothered in bandages . . . and all the while knowing themselves to be appallingly disfigured." Off-duty nurses were not allowed to be seen in the company of officers. It was a regulation impossible to enforce, notwithstanding the eagle eyes of the matron-nurses in charge. Junior officers "ogled the girls wherever they went" and contacts were made no matter at what peril. Ernest Hemingway portrayed Catherine Barkley as a nurse-heroine in *A Farewell to Arms,* his romantic novel set in a Red Cross hospital on the Italian front during World War I.[30]

An English nurse was one of the first martyrs of the war. Edith Cavell was matron of a hospital in Brussels, Belgium, when the city was occupied by the Germans. She was arrested and tried for having violated the German Military Penal Code in harboring Allied soldiers and assisting them to cross the Dutch border. Even the intervention of the American minister to Belgium, Brad Whitlock, could not save her, and she was sentenced to die. "She was deeply religious," Whitlock wrote, "with a conscience almost puritan, and was very stern with herself in what she conceived to be her duty." She was executed by a firing squad on October 11, 1915. "Even the Germans . . . knew that they had another . . . Lusitania, for which to answer before the bar of civilization." Later a statue was erected in her honor in London, and a mountain in Alberta, Canada was named for her.[31]

The winter of 1916-1917 in France was the coldest "in the memory of anyone living," Dr. Henry Potter wrote. "The wind is howling, the tents are flapping and blowing with a noise like a ship's sails when she comes up to the wind."[32] As a replacement for tents, chicken coops were imported.

The aftercare of Kazanjian's patients when they were evacuated to England was not always in keeping with his high standards. A V.A.D. nurse stationed at a hospital in Leeds, England, was horrified, while assisting the dental surgeons there, to see them rip off the doctor's "beautiful splints." The five or six patients involved "were progressing favorably, [but were] 'literally ruined' and . . . probably disfigured for life" as a consequence. She was forbidden to lodge a complaint against an officer, so she contacted her father, Major James M. Magee of the Canadian Army Dental Corps, who became incensed. "I urge you to have Dr. Cabot raise such a row over the maltreatment of your cases," Major Magee wrote to Major Kazanjian, "that the practice now being carried out in the Hospital above referred to may cease definitely." Similarly, Captain Leonard King, the dental surgeon who was with Gillies at Cambridge Hospital in Aldershot, England, cautioned Kazanjian in 1916, "It would be more than scandalous if your splendid work were being undone from lack of attention on this side." Leonard King also wrote: "Once again I am awful sorry and disappointed to tell you that not one of your patients has reached us since you were here."[33]

Recognizing that "it is a fearful thing to lead this great, peaceful people into war," President Woodrow Wilson on April 2, 1917, asked the United States Congress to declare that a state of war existed between the United States and Germany. "But the right is more precious than peace," he declared, "and we shall fight for the things which we have always carried nearest our hearts—for democracy." Following his message, Wilson was accorded the greatest ovation of his career. "Think of what it was they were applauding," he later said to his secretary. "My message of today was a message of death for our young men. How strange it seems to applaud that."[34] America officially entered the war "to make the world safe for democracy" on April 6, 1917. The most pressing needs of the Allies were for money and doctors. These arrived in ever increasing numbers.

The first hospital unit to embark with the American Expeditionary Force was the Peter Bent Brigham Unit, known as U. S. Army Base Hospital No. 5. Its director was Dr. Harvey Cushing, and its chief dental surgeon was Dr. William H. Potter, both of whom had served at the American Ambulance Hospital in Neuilly earlier in the war. The Unit sailed for France on May 11, 1917, less that five weeks after the declaration of war. It was housed in Dannes-Camiers next to General Hospital No. 20, where Dr. Kazanjian's facial unit was located.[35]

"Dr. Potter has been in this camp for some time, and I see him quite often," Kazanjian wrote to Dean Smith. "We have many pleasant conversations together, when, needless to say, we talk about our work and about the Dental School." Potter had been Kazanjian's teacher at Harvard Dental School and a man who "assumed great dignity, being one of the few with a Harvard A.B." He was now Lieutenant Potter, while his former student was Major Kazanjian. Brigham described Potter's

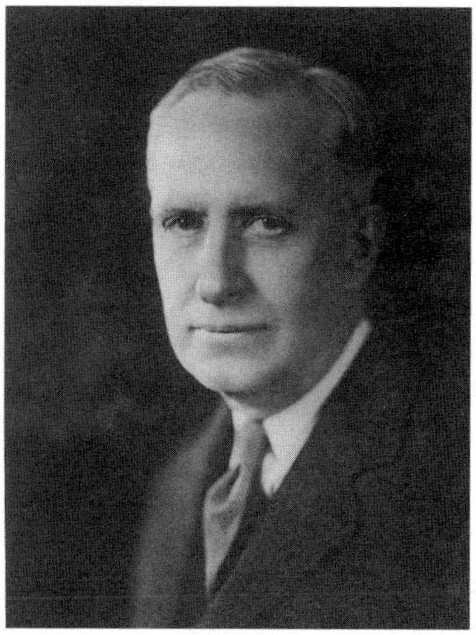

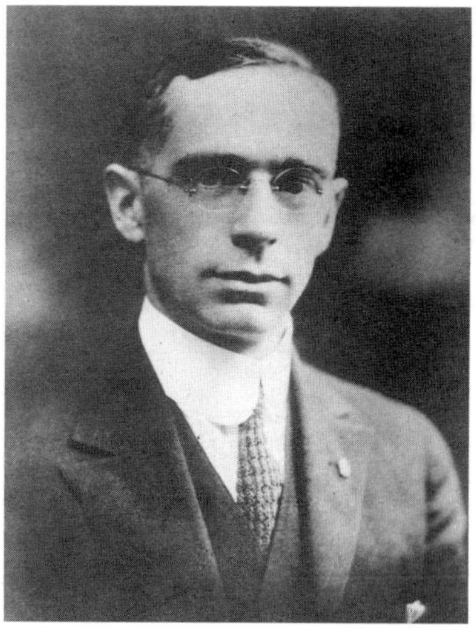

Left: Dr. Vilray P. Blair, The Harvard Medical Library in the Francis A. Countway Library of Medicine

Right: Dr. Robert H. Ivy, Photograph album of the American Association of Oral and Plastic Surgeons, November 1926, The Harvard Medical Library in the Francis A. Countway Library of Medicine

response as "outraged" and doing "everything to change this." Later when Potter was reassigned to teach maxillofacial surgery at the American Sanitary School at Langres, France and he needed teaching aids, he turned to Kazanjian."[36]

German air raids became a serious and frightening menace as the war intensified. "These raids," Major Kazanjian said, "were the most agonizing experience of the War." The hospitals were completely defenseless and vulnerable. A large cement factory and a machine gun corps base in the vicinity of the Dannes-Camiers hospitals were military targets.

Base Hospital No. 5 was "one of the first if not the first to suffer casualties." The evening of September 4, 1917, was "one hell of a night," according to Major Roger I. Lee. There were five direct hits on Base Hospital No. 5, resulting in the death of four men and the wounding of forty-three. "The only thing that saved the patients was that there were so few of them (730)," Major Lee observed, "otherwise the slaughter would have been tremendous." One medical officer "was literally blown to bits" by a bomb. Another medical officer was in his cot and miraculously survived, though wounded, with his tent peppered with over 400 holes.[37]

"Almost every clear night the raiders flew over, and we used to pray for rainy nights so that they would not be able to attack," Major Kazanjian recalled. "They threw the large group of hospitals in our vicinity, numbering more than thirty-five thousand beds, into complete disorganization . . . and on one occasion, a Canadian hospital was completely demolished with the loss of many lives." As a refuge from the air raids for the staff, trenches about six feet deep were dug, lined with wood and covered with sand bags. They were of no avail.[38] Dr. Ferdinand Brigham recalled the terror:

> *When the Germans bombed us by day, it was by a single plane flying . . . almost inaudible and invisible taking point blank shots at military objectives . . . . If we were bombed by night, the Boches (Germans) came in several squadrons of six, each remaining overhead for about a half hour. The planes dropped flares, chose their own altitude and bombed as they pleased.*[39]

As a consequence of the devastation caused by air raids, in the summer of 1918 there was a partial evacuation of hospital patients in the Camiers area. During this interval, a Harvard jaw center was organized at a Casualty Clearing Station in an advanced area. "I took one mechanic with me," Dr. Kazanjian wrote, "and was attached at different units 'up the line'." Only immediate and emergency treatment was provided.[40]

There were several men who completed a tour of duty with one of the earlier Harvard units of the British Expeditionary Force and later returned to France with the American Expeditionary Force. Prominent among these was Dr. Robert Catheron, who had served with Dr. Kazanjian from December 1915 to May 1916. He returned to France in the spring of 1918, was given an important post with the U.S. Army Dental Corps, and was promoted to Major. With America in the war, the question was raised of the future of Major Kazanjian's center at General Hospital No. 20, but both the British and the American authorities concurred that it would be ill-advised to abandon it or alter it. It was preeminently successful.[41]

The twenty-first annual session of the National Dental Association was held in New York City from October 22 to 26, 1917. The third General Session on October 24 was a symposium on "Dental Surgery and Restorative Prosthesis in the European War." Among the participants was Dr. Frank H. Cushman whose paper was "War Dental Restorative Prosthesis." "Dr. Cushman did finely," Dr. Laurence Baker, who attended, reported, "and when the slide of Major V. H. Kazanjian, in uniform, was thrown on the screen, the audience of over 6,000 went wild . . . it indicates the high regard America has for your brilliant work."[42]

"When we entered World War I," Dr. John S. Davis reported, "there was total ignorance of plastic surgery in the [American] Army." In the American Expeditionary Force, it was classed as "Faciomaxillary Surgery." Dr. Vilray P. Blair was appointed by Army Surgeon General Gorgas in 1917 to head the Sub-Section of Plastic and Oral Surgery and to be Chief Consultant in Maxillofacial Surgery with the A. E. F., with a commission as Major. Blair had in 1912 published a book, *Surgery and Diseases of the Mouth and Jaws,* which became the standard in the field and which firmly established his reputation. "I got to go to Washington where I spent a year trying to build up some framework of an organization," Blair wrote, "then spent nine months in France and England going from place to place trying to sell the stuff to the different hospitals, backed with orders signed by Pershing which swept away any difficulties I might otherwise have had."[43]

One of the hospitals in France which Major Blair visited was General Hospital No. 20 where he "stayed two or three days" observing Dr. Kazanjian's work. There was "a desperate need" to collect the knowledge and clinical experiences that the Allied surgeons had acquired earlier in the war. Dr. Robert Ivy reported that "very valuable information" was obtained from Kazanjian's reports.[44]

Blair wrote that "no surgical truth has received greater emphasis in this war than the necessity of correlating the skill and the knowledge of the general and the dental surgeons in the treatment of the combined injuries of the face and jaw injuries."[45]

Beginning in April 1918, a unit of about twenty surgeons and twenty dental surgeons was dispatched to the Chief Surgeon of the American Expeditionary Force for the purpose of observing the methods used in the treatment of facial and jaw injuries in the hospitals of the Allies. Prominent among these hospitals was Dr. Kazanjian's unit at General Hospital No. 20. In contrast to the Tommies with facial wounds that Dr. Kazanjian was treating, "secondary hemorrhage was a rare complication, largely because the

Corporal Fred N. Snowdon received an "extensive shell wound of the chin" July 16, 1916*

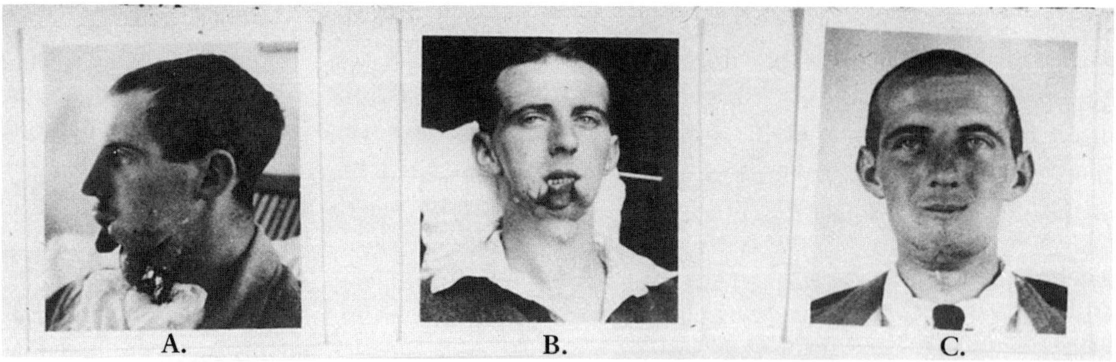

A. Great loss of the lower lip and the chin and entire body of the mandible missing. B. Dental splints to control the remaining ascending rami of the mandible and support of the lip and chin after operation. C. Plastic operation for the restoration of the lower lip and chin. Contour of the face is restored by artificial appliances.

Lydon, France
Halewhistle
Northld

Sept. 24, 1918

Dear Major Kazanjian

I have been such a long time in writing you that no doubt you will be thinking I have forgotten you. I am not likely to do that as the splendid results obtained by you on my face will always serve as a reminder. I am not really good at expressing myself but believe me when I say that both my people & myself are deeply grateful for what you have done & I will never forget the patience and interest shown by you when doing the work.

I was given my ticket immediately after landing at Sidcup & I started business the week I arrived home & as a result I have had very little spare time--work every day & looking up & visiting old friends after hours.

It would take too long to go through all that has been said about my face by professional men--dozens have examined it & all agree, & especially those at Sidcup, that it is a masterpiece. Major Ellis thinks bone-graft will be quite possible by what he calls the sectional system & so after the war I am to be recalled. In the meantime I am drawing a full pension. I am not at all keen on the grafting as the splints are working so well & I am having no trouble whatever with them. What do you think about it, if a failure, will it spoil the job at all. I am now eating much better than when at Camiers & "dribbling" is a thing of the past. I understand all the boys came to Blighty after the Bosche bombing stunt. You would miss them, all coming away together but no doubt by this time you will be full up again.

I hear occasionally from some of the boys- & all seem to be doing well

Are Capt. Brigham & Dr. Lewis still with you--if so give my kind regards to both.

I met L/Cpe a few weeks ago--he had two bone grafts done & both have been failures. I also saw Col. Shea last week in Blackpool & I see he is posted there for duty. If you are coming over to England soon you let me know. I will do my best to see you. Do you happen to know where had landed?

I hope you are not having to work so hard as in the old days. With kindest regards to Mrs. Kazanjian & yourself.

Yours v. sincerely

Fred Snowdon

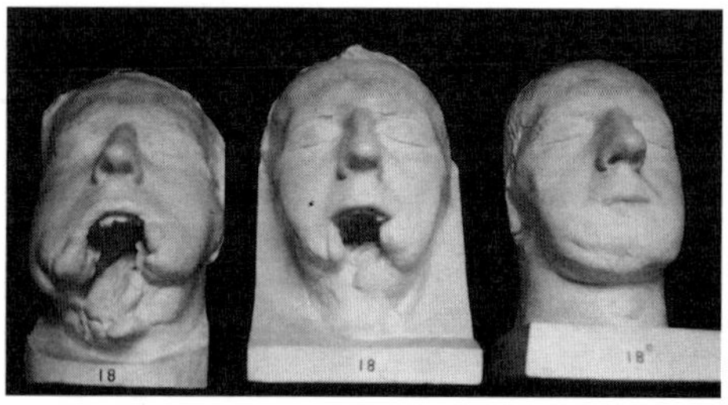

Plaster moulages of Snowden. Fd. WW 1219. Photograph by Dr. Paul Davis

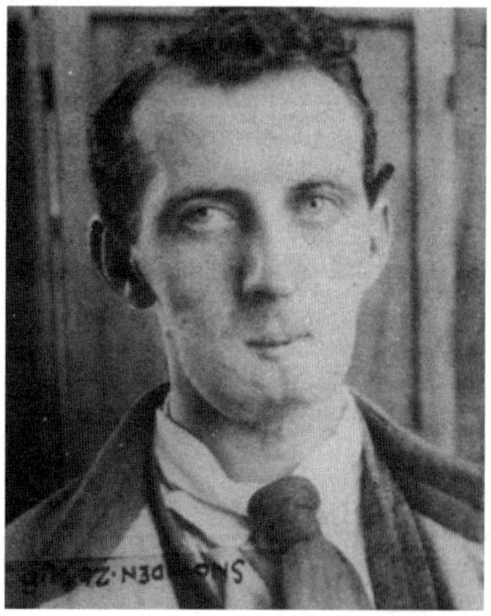

Snowden after treatment.

**The Harvard Medical Library in the Francis A. Countway Library of Medicine*

mouths of the American soldiers as a rule were free from sepsis." The treatment modality recommended by the U.S. Army Medical Corps essentially confirmed the methods adopted earlier by Dr. Kazanjian. "The jaw was first splinted . . . and the facial wound then repaired. . . . The reestablishment of correct occlusion took precedence over regard for apposition of fragments. . . . The cast-metal splint was more easily made and more satisfactory than the swaged-metal or vulcanite splint." Blair's team "treated thousands of soldiers with very complex reconstructive surgery" and Blair stood "out as a master of reconstructive surgery."[46]

The third edition of Blair's *Surgery and Diseases of the Mouth and Jaws,* considerably revised to meet the needs arising from World War I, appeared in 1917.[47] After the armistice, Dr. Blair organized several centers in the United States for the continuing care of these casualties and personally headed one at Jefferson Barracks, Missouri. In St. Louis as a civilian, Dr. Blair developed "one of the largest plastic surgery centers in the country and to train many of the top young American surgeons" who had a prominent influence in the establishment of plastic surgery as a medical specialty in this country. Among the most eminent were the three B's, Dr. James Barrett Brown and Dr. Louis T. Byars, with, of course, Dr. Blair, with Dr. Frank McDowell making up "The St. Louis Quadrumvirate."[48]

Dr. Robert H. Ivy was chosen as an assistant to Dr. Blair in organizing the Sub-Section of Plastic and Oral Surgery in 1917. It was a fortuitous choice, as Dr. Ivy had both dental and medical degrees and had a maxillofacial surgical background. "Whatever I may have achieved in later years," he admitted, "I owe chiefly to his [Dr Blair's] counsel and the opportunity for gaining experience he put in my way." There were several treatment centers for maxillofacial cases that the U. S. Army operated in France. One of these was in Paris, another in Bordeaux and a third was Base Hospital No. 115 at Vichy where Dr. Ivy served as consultant.[49]

Following the armistice, Dr. Ivy served in the office of the Surgeon General in Washington and was chief of the maxillofacial service at the Walter Reed General Hospital. He was discharged as a Lieutenant Colonel in 1919. It was in that year that the American Medical Association sponsored a meeting of the Section on Stomatology where the program consisted of papers by maxillofacial surgeons returned from the war. "It was here that I first met Kazanjian . . . and others who became lifelong friends." Dr. Ivy reported. The experiences and techniques that had been utilized during the war were recorded by Colonel Ivy, and Major D. Eby who wrote the section on standard practice of maxillofacial surgery for the United States Army Medical Department, which was published in 1924.[50]

"We probably had about 2300 cases of face and jaw injuries in the war, most of them occurring between July 14, and November 11, 1918," Dr. Blair related. "Only about 600 of these men returned to this country [United States] as patients, the remainder being discharged over there. It was chiefly due to the number of skilled dentists we had available that this result was possible. The work of Dr. Kazanjian was known to all of the Allies and I was very proud that he came from an American school."[51]

By the fall of 1918, the German war machine was utterly exhausted. The Armistice was signed on November 11, 1918, in a railroad car on a siding in the forest of Compiègne. Hostilities ceased at 11 a.m.

NOTES

1 Richard Locke Hapgood, *History of the Harvard Dental School* (Peterboro, N.H.: Transcript Printing Co., 1930), pp. 126-127. He was also called "The Wizard of the Western Front" in *The Mirror* (Harvard Dental School, 1919): 65. Eugene H. Smith, "The Harvard Dental School," *The Harvard Graduates' Magazine* 28 (September 1919): 48, extolled him, saying, "You are certainly a wizard," Dr. Elliott P. Joslin, famous for his knowledge and treatment of diabetes, wrote: "How grateful you should be that the Lord gave you the privilege of making over of unfortunate children!" Letter from Joslin to V. H. Kazanjian, May 19, 1938, V. H. Kazanjian Archive in The Francis A. Countway Library of Medicine, folder C-221. Also *The* [London] *Times*, "List of Recommendations," clipping, Harvard Dental School Archive, E17 Al.17, Box 53 under V. H. Kazanjian 1914, and copies of both citations, dated November 7, 1917, and April 7, 1918, in Kazanjian Archive, folder M-24. Also, *The* [London] *Times*, December 28, 1917.

2 Coningsby Dawson, "The Glory of the Trenches, The Road to Blighty," *Good Housekeeping* (January 1918), p. 20.

3 H. F. Prevost Battersby, "Surgery's Miracle at the Western Front," *British Dental Journal* 37 (January-June 1916): 427-428. Batterby's article originally appeared in the April 22, 1916, issue of the *Daily Graphic*.

4 Letter from Dr. Moses S. Strock to Dr. V. H. Kazanjian, May 27, 1943, folder C-415; letter from Robert S. Catheron to "Dear K," July 27, 1916, folder. C-65; and letter from M. Vartan Malcom to V. H. Kazanjian, October 22, 1915, folder C-278, V. H. Kazanjian Archive in The Francis A. Countway Library of Medicine. Strock was an oral surgeon stationed in England during World War II.

5 *Boston Post*, October 19, 1915, p. 12, col. 4; *Boston Sunday Globe*, November 21, 1915, p. 32, cols. 3 to 6.

6 Carl W. Waldron, "A Testimonial to Varaztad Kazanjian," *Journal of Oral Surgery* 13, no. 2 (April 1955): 96.

7 Hapgood, *Harvard Dental School*, p. 126; Taped interview of V. H. Kazanjian by Robin Anderson, 1971; Jerome P. Webster, "Vilray P. Blair: 1871-1915," chapter in Frank McDowell, *The Source Book of Plastic Surgery*, (Baltimore: Williams & Wilkins, 1977), p. 479; Robert S. Catheron, "The Work of the Dental Section of the Harvard Surgical Unit," Kazanjian Archive, folder WW-1269. Also, Daniel B. Reardon, "Diary" (Courtesy of Mrs Paul C. Reardon, Hingham, Mass.), entry for August 14, 1915. "Obituary: Lt. Gen. Sir Arthur Sloggett, *Journal of the Royal Army Medical Corps* 54, no. 1 (January 1930): 1-4. He was a highly decorated career medical officer. On one occasion, in 1898 at the Battle of Khartoum, he was shot through the chest and left for dead but survived. He was described as "a wise administrator," whose "savoir-faire, knowledge of the world and of men, enabled him to succeed where other men . . . would have failed." Letter from V. H. Kazanjian to Reginald Pound, May 1, 1962 or 1963, Kazanjian Archive, folder C-341. Ferdinand Brigham, Unpublished manuscript on the Dental Unit of the First Harvard Unit. Richard L. Golden and Charles G. Roland, eds, *Sir William Osler: An Annotated Bibliography with Illustrations*, Norman Bibliography Series, no. I (San Francisco, Calif.: Norman Publishing, 1988), p. 123, states that Sir William arrived in Camiers on September 8, 1915, and left on September 15. "He expressed himself in the highest terms of commendations upon the work which is being carried on by the various Departments. His visit here was one of encouragement and inspiration."

8 Extract from report by Major W. D. Anderson, of his visit to various dental centers in France, March 29 to April 11, 1916, dated June 9, 1916, in the author's possession.

9 Hapgood, *Harvard Dental School*, pp. 126-127. The Movement Orders granting Drs. Kazanjian and Catheron permission to proceed from Camiers to Paris is dated March 30. 1916, and is signed by Major Shea, O.C. 20th General Hospital, Kazanjian Archive, folder WW-1267. Also, letter from V. H. Kazanjian to Dean E. H. Smith, July 31, 1916, Kazanjian Archive, folder C-392, and Catheron, "Dental Section."

10 Hapgood, *Harvard Dental School*, p. 125; V. H. Kazanjian, unpublished paper read before the Harvard Dental Alumni Association, June 18, 1919, Kazanjian Archive, AM-163; Robert S. Catheron, unpublished account included as part of Dr. Ferdinand Brigham's longer manuscript on the Dental Unit of the First Harvard Unit during World War I.

11 Dr. Hugh Cabot served as Chief Surgeon until September 1916, and was succeeded by Dr. D. F. Jones in December 1916. At that time, Dr. C. M. Robinson was appointed Acting Chief. In the meantime, Dr. Cabot was again appointed Chief Surgeon and served as such for the duration of the war. Hugh Cabot, "Harvard Surgical Unit With the British Expeditionary Force in France," *The Harvard Graduate Magazine* 25, no. 9 (1916-1917): 306-307; Hapgood, *Harvard Dental School*, p. 125. On one occasion, it was learned, Dr. Kazanjian had spent 200 pounds of his own funds for supplies (*British Dental Journal*, (April 1, 1919): 247). Funds were also raised at the Harvard Dental School for a Kazanjian Fund. A list of contributors can be found in the Kazanjian Archive, folder WW-1266.

12 Letter from V. H. Kazanjian to Dean Smith, July 31, 1916, Kazanjian Archive, folder C-392.

13 Ibid.

14 Hapgood, *Harvard Dental School,* p. 126. Included in the Kazanjian Archive is a copy of his appointment as "Honorary Rank of Major" by order of King George, December 10, 1918, folder PAM 15. The date of his appointment in June 1916 is realistic. "Immediate Treatment of Gunshot Fracture of the Jaws" was published in the *British Dental Journal* 37 (1916): War Supplement, 297-336.

15 Dobell's solution was "an aqueous solution of sodium bicarbonate, borax, phenol and glycerine." W. A. Newman Dorland, *The American Illustrated Medical Dictionary* (Philadelphia: Saunders, 1932), p. 1180. Carrel-Dakin's treatment called for irrigation of the wound with a solution of chlorinated soda which had been modified with sodium bicarbonate (Dorland, p. 1353). *The New York Times*, Sunday Editorial Section, December 29, 1918, p. 4, cols. 1 to 6 quoted Sir Almroth Wright, writing in the *London Lancet*: "The Carrel-Dakin method of treating infected wounds is by far the most important contribution to surgical technique since the beginning of the war." See also Ferdinand Brigham, "Harvard Goes to War," *Harvard Dental Alumni Bulletin* 24, no. 4 (1964):103; V. H. Kazanjian report written for Sir George Makins, March 1917, Kazanjian Archive, folder C-277.

16 The Barton bandage, named for Dr. John Rhem Barton, American surgeon, 1794-1871, is a double figure of "8" bandage for fractures of the lower jaw. It helped reduce the downward and forward displacement of the mandible and held the upper and lower jaw in close proximity. V. H. Kazanjian, "Treatment of Maxillary Fractures," *The British Medical Journal* 1, (February 19, 1916): 266. An illustrated sketch of the Barton bandage and its application can be found in Seymour Barling and John T. Morrison, *A Manual of War Surgery* (London: Oxford University Press, 1919), p. 351, Figure 110. See also Brigham, Unpublished manuscript, and John M. Converse, "The Extraordinary Career of Doctor Varaztad Hovhannes Kazanjian, *Plastic and Reconstructive Surgery* 71, no. 1 (January 1982): 140. In 1941, George M. Dorrance and John W. Bransfield of Philadelphia compiled a comprehensive overview of articles and illustrations detailing just about everything known about jaw fractures at that time. Titled "The History of Treatment of Jaw Fractures" and edited by James B. Mann, it was produced through typescript on 506 leaves and reproduced in twelve copies through the photostat process, the only practical photographic process available at that time. Copies, each bound in two loose-leaf binders, were afterwards deposited in various medical libraries (the Surgeon General's Library in Washington, the College of Physicians of Philadelphia, etc.).

17 Catheron, "Dental Section"; V. H. Kazanjian, "Early Treatment of Gunshot Wounds of the Face and Jaws," *Surgery* 15, no. 1 (June 1944): 5. "It [the Kazanjian clamp] consisted of a piece of very heavy wire about eight or ten inches long, bent to a U shape, with a finger of modelling composition or vulcanite rubber on each end. One end is placed in the floor of the mouth and the other externally under the chin, between the hyoid bone and the lingual side of the mandible, and the tissues are pinched at the site of fracture by the use of elastic bands about the clamp." *The Lancet* 1, (June 24, 1916): 1273. Barling and Morrison, *A Manual of War Surgery,* pictures a

Kazanjian clamp on p. 341. It is illustrated also in V. H. Kazanjian, "Traitement Précoce des Blessures de la Machoire," Congrès Dentaire Interalliés, Paris, 10-11-12-13 (November 1916), *Comptes Rendus*, v. 1, p. 122. The Kazanjian lingual artery clamp is listed in the *Priced List of Medical Equipment*, Section X, Dental Appliances and Materials issued by the British War Office, October 29, 1941, p. 4, Kazanjian Archive, folder C-415.

18 Kazanjian and Converse, *The Surgical Treatment of Facial Injuries,* 2nd ed. (Baltimore: Williams & Wilkins, 1959), pp. 146-148, contains illustrations of the Kazanjian button. "A wire is passed around the neck of each tooth and twisted. The two twisted wires are then retwisted and cut about one inch from the teeth. The remaining ends of the wire are then reshaped into a small button." The button serves as an anchor for intermaxillary elastics.

19 V. H. Kazanjian and John M. Converse, *The Surgical Treatment of Facial Injuries* (Baltimore: Williams & Wilkins, 1949), pp. 176-78. The splint consists of an oblong-shaped metal frame; the lower surface is supplied with a round bar about one-fourth of an inch thick. The frame is embedded in dental compound spread over the forehead. The frame and compound are held in place securely with the aid of adhesive tape passed around the head. The horizontal bar of the splint is not covered with dental composition, but is left open for the attachment of a universal joint which can be passed freely along the bar and then held in place either to the right or the left of the median line. A vertical bar is attached to this joint, the lower end consisting of a flat base covered with soft dental compound, pressed against the side of the nose. Elastic bands are employed to exert pressure against the side of the nose; gentle pressure should be applied for the splint is used only to maintain the fractured bones in their correct position. Reproduced again in Kazanjian and Converse, *The Surgical Treatment of Facial Injuries*, 2nd ed., 1959, p. 237.

20 V. H. Kazanjian, "Treatment of Extensive Loss of the Mandible and Its Surrounding Tissues," *Journal of Oral Surgery* 1 no. 32 (January, 1943): 2.

21 M. Verazin, "A Famous Oral and Plastic Surgeon," *Hairenik Daily*, May 8, 1930 (in Armenian). See the notes from Dr. Ferdinand Brigham to Hélène Kazanjian Sargeant, 1974: "Nobody, but nobody . . . could have his wife overseas. Now come three historical exceptions. Sir George Makins, Chief R.A.M.C. Consultant, had his wife on visit. Dr. Dodd, [a Roentgenologist] with us in the Harvard Unit, had his wife serve as a nurse . . . Dr. K. agreed in Sept. 1915, to serve if his wife could be with him. The British Empire thought he was worth it." Dr. Brigham's notes are in the author's private collection. Letter from V. H. Kazanjian to Dean Smith, July 31, 1916; Taped interview with V. H. Kazanjian by Robin Anderson, 1971. Pass issued by Col. Carr, D.D. M. S. Étaples 7/15/17: "Mrs. V. H. Kazanjian has permission to visit the hospitals in this area." Kazanjian Archive, folder W-1267; Letter from V. H. Kazanjian to the American Consul, Lausanne, Switzerland, June 6, 1916. folder C-834. For information of the activities of the Y.M.C.A. during World War I, see Young Men's Christian Association, *Service With Fighting Men: An Account of the Work of the American Young Men's Christian Association in the World War* (New York: Association Press, 1924), 2 v. A copy of the article "Mends Faces of Wounded. Wife of Harvard Doctor Aids him in 'Miracle' work with British," *Boston Traveler*, January 4, 1918, p. 3, col. 6, is in the Kazanjian Archive, folder M-74.

22 Letter from V. H. Kazanjian to Dr. Smith, October 7, 1917, Kazanjian Archive, folder C-392; and Lyn Macdonald, *The Roses of No Man's Land,* (London: Penguin Books, 1993), p. 153. The Biblical reference is from Matthew 5:15 (King James version): "Neither do men light a candle, and put it under a bushel, but on a candlestick, and it giveth light unto all that are in the house."

23 Letter from Herbert H. White to Dean E. H. Smith, January 26, 1917, Kazanjian Archive, folder C-446. Also, letter from Dr. C. Franklin MacDonald to V. H. Kazanjian dated November 9, 1916. Kazanjian Archive, folder C-705. "Went to see Dr. Smith when up to Boston . . . Dr. Cabot had been in the day before and apparently was quite down off his `high horse' . . . something had happened evidently. " Also, Macdonald, *Roses*, p. 217: "Cabot is a tireless worker."

24 Letter from A. Lawrence Lowell to V. H. Kazanjian, May 17, 1916, Kazanjian Archive, folder C-676.

25 Letter from Dr. William H. Weston to "Dear Doctor Kazanjian, and Mrs. K. too," March 6,

1916, Kazanjian Archive, folder C-441. Dr. Weston shared Dr. Kazanjian's old office in Boston with Dr. Stone and paid $10 a month for half a day's use once a week.

26 Letter from Deron P. Roopenian to "Dear Uncle" dated February 1, 1917, Kazanjian Archive, folder C-357. Deron was the youngest son of his sister, Nouvart. The Roopenians lived at 117 Thomas Street in Worcester's "Little Armenia." According to a letter from Louise Roopenian to Virginia King Lane, dated August 11, 1972, in the author's private collection. Deron Roopenian was born in Worcester on April 23, 1906. Also, Hélène K. Sargeant, "Some Notes Concerning the Family of Varaztad H. Kazanjian," Kazanjian Archive. A record of the death of Annie H. Kazanjian is filed in the "Massachusetts Registry of Vital Records and Statistics" 1918, v. 1, p. 86, no 1112. She died on January 27, 1918, at 366 Center St., Boston, Mass., at the age of eighty. Letter from Betty Topjian, of Watertown, Mass., to the author, March 1, 1991.

27 "The Roses of No Man's Land" was a hit song of the period dedicated to the nurses: Macdonald, *Roses*, p. xi; Dawson, "The Glory of the Trenches," pp. 18, 20; Harold Gillies and Ralph Millard, Jr., *Principles and Art of Plastic Surgery,* (Baltimore: Williams & Wilkins, 1971), v. 1, p. xvi.

28 Macdonald, *Roses*, p. xi.

29 Quoted in Macdonald, *Roses*, p. 209.

30 Gillies and Millard, *Principles of Plastic Surgery*, pp. 8, 9; Macdonald, *Roses*, p. 200; Helen J. Lamb, *World War I, An American Nurse with the British Troops in France* (Provo, Utah: Stevenson's Genealogical Center, 1981) presents an account of the personal, social, and professional life of a nurse—a valuable memoir of the daily events. On Ernest Hemingway, *A Farewell to Arms* (New York: Scribner's, 1929), see Henry S. Villard, "A Prize Specimen of Wounded Hero," chapter in *The World Wars Remembered,* from the pages of *Yankee Magazine* (Dublin, NH: Yankee Magazine, 1979), pp. 90-101, and Henry S. Villard and James Negal, *Hemingway in Love and War* (Boston: Northeastern Univ. Press, 1989), who present the Lost Diary of Nurse Agnes von Kurowsky, her letters, and correspondence of Ernest Hemingway (she was the model after whom Hemingway patterned Catherine Barkley in his novel).

31 Brad Whitlock, "The Tragedy of Edith Cavell," in Francis J. Reynolds and Allen L. Churchill, *World's War Events* (New York: Collier, 1919), v. 1, p. 350, 364; *World Book Encyclopedia* (Chicago: Field Enterprises Educational Corp, 1973), v. 3, p. 246.

32 Macdonald, *Roses,* p. 195.

33 Letter from Major James M. Magee to Major V. H. Kazanjian, July 6, 1917, Kazanjian Archive, folder C-273, and letter from Leonard King to V. H. Kazanjian dated August 10, 1916, Kazanjian Archive, folder C-239.

34 Richard Thoumin, ed., *The First World War* (New York: Putnam, 1963), p. 353; S. L. A. Marshall, *World War I* (Boston: Houghton Mifflin, 1964), p. 281.

35 *The Story of U.S. Army Base Hospital No. 5* (Cambridge, Mass.: Harvard University Press, 1919). During mobilization, a proposal was made and plans were drawn to erect an encampment of the unit, including one typical ward, on the Boston Common. The plan was markedly opposed, and it was considered "as a desecration to the Common and a political dodge on the part of some rather than a patriotic movement." Harvey Cushing, *From A Surgeon's Journal* (Boston: Little Brown, 1936), contains maps, illustrations, letters, and orders of the unit. Other materials appear in Roger I. Lee, *Letters from Roger I. Lee, Lt. Col., U.S. Army Medical Corps 1917-18* (Brookline, Mass.: Privately printed, 1962). Lee served at Base Hospital No.5. His letters cover the period from May 11, 1917, to January 16, 1919. Also, Hapgood, *Harvard Dental School*, pp. 137-142. Dr. Potter served at Dannes-Camiers until November 3, 1917, when he was transferred to British General Hospital No. 13 at Boulogne until December 3, 1917, when he was again moved to the American Sanitary School at Langres, France. In 1918 he was reassigned back to Base Hospital No. 5, where he remained until the end of the war.

36 Letter from V. H. Kazanjian to Dean Smith, October 7, 1917; Brigham, Unpublished manuscript. Cushing, *Surgeon's Journal*, diary entry for June 25, 1918, refers to "William Potter, who is still a lieutenant and has worked unceasingly at his job here . . . . He's a patient soul—a veritable Job." Eventually Potter was promoted to the rank of lieutenant colonel. (Hapgood, *Harvard Dental School,* p. 142.)

37 Hapgood, *Harvard Dental School,* p. 129; Cushing, *Surgeon's Journal,* pp. 200-201; Lee, *Letters,* p. 70.

38 Hapgood, *Harvard Dental School,* p. 129. "It was rumored that the whole Étaples district was to be moved—33,000 hospital beds in the area," according to Cushing, *Surgeon's Journal*, p. 370, entry for June 3, 1918. Also, Lamb, *An American Nurse*, diary entry for June 16, 1918, p. 69.

39 Brigham, Unpublished manuscript.

40 V. H. Kazanjian, Unpublished paper read before the Harvard Dental Alumni Association, June 18, 1919.

41 Hapgood, *Harvard Dental School*, p. 144; Brigham, Unpublished manuscript.

42 National Dental Association 21st Session, October 22-26, 1917, *Program Booklet.* Courtesy American Dental Association Archives. Another speaker at that session was Dr. Alexis Carrell (1873-1944) of Paris, who spoke on "War Surgery." Letter from Laurence W. Baker to Major V. H. Kazanjian, November 24, 1917, is in the Kazanjian Archive, folder C-18.

43 John S. Davis, *Plastic Surgery, Its Principles and Practice* (Philadelphia: Blakiston, 1919), p. 610; Vilray P. Blair, "The Role of the Plastic Surgeon in the Care of War Injuries," *Annals of Surgery* 113, no. 5 (May 1941): 697. Jerome P. Webster, "Vilray Papin Blair, 1871-1955." writes that Blair was "one of the pioneers of plastic surgery in America . . . and almost single-handed, he was responsible for the formation of the American Board of Plastic Surgery." In addition to Webster's biographical sketch in McDowell, *The Source Book of Plastic Surgery*, another extensive statement on him is Robert H. Ivy's "Vilray Papin Blair," *British Journal of Plastic Surgery* 5, no. 4 (January 1953): 224-227.

44 Taped interview of V. H. Kazanjian by Robin Anderson, 1971; Francis X. Paletta, *History of the American Society of Plastic and Reconstructive Surgery* (Baltimore: Waverly, 1963), p. 68.

45 Quoted in Ivy, "Vilray Papin Blair," p. 226.

46 Vilray P. Blair, "The Maxillofacial Services of the American Army in the War," *Journal of the American Medical Association* 73, no. 5 (Aug. 3, 1919): 326. Robert H. Ivy and Joseph D. Eby, "Maxillofacial Surgery" in *Medical Department of the United States Army in the World War*, vol II, Surgery, Part 2 (Washington: Government Printing Office, 1924), pp. 398, 399, 401, 403; Webster, "Vilray Papin Blair," p. 10.

47 Vilray P. Blair, *Surgery and Diseases of the Mouth and Jaws, a Practical Treatise on the Surgery of the Diseases of the Mouth and Allied Structures . . . 3rd ed., Revised So As To Incorporate the Latest War Data Concerning Gunshot Injuries of the Face and Jaws* (St. Louis: C. V. Mosby, 1917).

48 Webster, "Vilray Papin Blair, 1871-1955," p. 476; Eric J. Steinicki, V. Leroy Young, Tom Francel and Peter Randall, "Vilray P. Blair, His Surgical Descendants and Their Roles in Plastic Surgical Development," *Plastic and Reconstructive Surgery* 103, no. 7 (June 1999): 1991; Bradford Cannon and Joseph E. Murray, "The Influence of the St. Louis Quadrumvirate of Plastic Surgery," *Plastic and Reconstructive Surgery* 94, no. 4 (April 1995): 1118.

49 For biographical material on Dr. Robert Henry Ivy (1881-1974), see Lydon A. Peer, "Robert H. Ivy, D.D.S., M.D., F.A. C.S., Sc. D.," *Plastic and Reconstructive Surgery* 4:30 (September 1954): 252-254; John M. Converse, "Robert H. Ivy, D.D.S., M.D.," *Plastic and Reconstructive Surgery* 51, no. 4 (April 1973): 411-412; Robert L. Harding, "Obituary, Robert Henry Ivy, 1881-1974," *Plastic and Reconstructive Surgery* 55, no. 1 (January 1975): 122-125; and Dr. Ivy's autobiography, *A Link With the Past* (Baltimore: Williams & Wilkins, 1962). See also, Davis, *Plastic Surgery,* p. 611.

50 Ivy and Eby, "Maxillofacial Surgery," p. 399.

51 V. P. Blair discussion of paper by V. H. Kazanjian, "Prosthetic Appliances in Surgical Treatment of Wounds of Face and Jaws," *The Dental Summary* 39, no. 12 (December 1919): 919-933. This was the paper which Kazanjian read in June 1919 before the Section on Stomatology of the American Medical Association. The maxillofacial cases returned to the United States for treatment were sent to General Hospital No. 11, at Cape May, N.J., to General Hospital No. 2, at Baltimore, to the Walter Reed Hospital, or to General Hospital No. 40, at St. Louis (Davis, *Plastic Surgery*, pp. 610-611).

CHAPTER SEVEN

The Development of Maxillofacial Surgery during World War I

It would be appropriate to pause here and consider in greater detail the development of maxillofacial surgery during World War I before continuing on with Varaztad Kazanjian's personal story, which formed but a single aspect of it—albeit an important one.

The war quickly settled into a four-year stalemate of trench warfare, in which artillery weapons of increasing efficiency and magnitude were employed. The use of such destructive innovations as the modern hand grenade, the trench mortar, and the flamethrower, resulted in an epidemic of trauma the likes of which the world had never seen before. Surgeons were challenged to cope with the human devastation this caused. This is especially true of the considerable number of survivors who had sustained horrible head and face injuries that left them in a condition that can only be described as grotesque.

This chapter, therefore, will consider some of the provisions made by the principal warring nations of Western Europe for the treatment and care of soldiers who had been severely wounded in the face and jaws, and to the dramatis personae who labored, as Varaztad Kazanjian did, to restore these victims to an acceptable condition so that they could return to civilian life. The lessons they learned would, in the years after the war, be employed by some of the homecoming surgeons and dentists to usher in a new era of plastic and reparative surgery that would, to some degree, repay humankind for the tragedy and suffering that war had inflicted.

In Germany, as early as August 1914, a hospital of 225 beds had been opened at Düsseldorf for the specific treatment of wounds of face and jaws, and by April 1915 similar institutions had been established in other parts of the German Empire. "The contributions of German-speaking surgeons [in Germany and Austria] to the field of *Kieferchirurgie*, surgery of the jaws, are outstanding," Wolfe and Berkowitz have written in their treatise on *The Plastic Surgery of the Facial Skeleton*, published in 1989. During World War I, the work done by August Lindemann at the Hospital for the Injuries of the Jaw at Düsseldorf, "set the standard for mandibular reconstruction." Lindemann was among the first to use "periosteal covered bone-grafts, usually from the tibia." In the post-war years, three important schools grew out of this war work, Wolfe and Berkowitz have noted, one in Vienna and two in Berlin.[1]

In contrast to their German adversaries, the British were less organized. The sequence in which the first British centers were established is somewhat clouded and lost in the mists of time, but the outline of a picture emerges. With the outbreak of World War I, Charles Valadier, a French-American dentist with a successful practice in Paris, offered his professional services first to the French, who did not accept him, and afterwards, through their Red Cross Society, to the British, who did, stationing him first in Abbeville and later at a field hospital at Boulogne. Valadier was

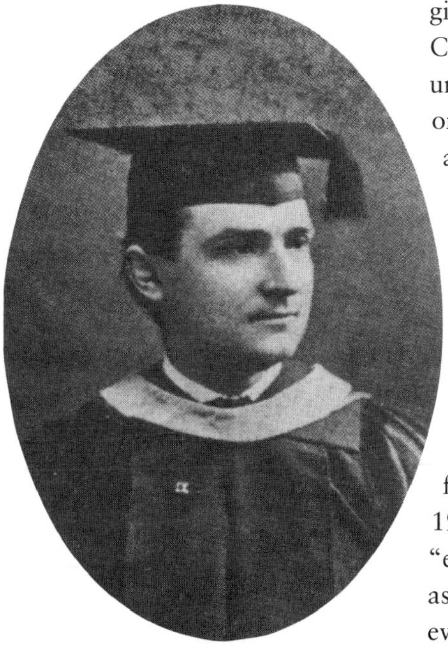

Auguste C. Valadier, (1873-1931)
From the 1901 class yearbook,
Philadelphia Dental College,
now Temple University
School of Dentistry
Reproduced from Robert H. Ivy,
"The Mysterious A. C. Valadier,"
Plastic and Reconstructive Surgery, *47:4 (April 1971), p, 367.*

given the honorary rank of lieutenant in the Royal Army Medical Corps on October 25, 1914, and afterwards organized a fifty-bed unit attached to the 83rd General Hospital at Wimereux. He not only provided a great deal of the equipment at his own expense, but a dental laboratory in which his technicians from Paris fabricated the prosthetic appliances used in the treatment of jaw fractures. He was left pretty much alone, but later the authorities, feeling that he should be assisted by a physician, assigned Dr. Harold Delf Gillies to his clinic. It should be noted that Valadier and Kazanjian had markedly divergent points of view on the treatment of war injuries.[2]

Valadier was joined in July 1916 by Captain H. Lawson Whale, "a rhinologist who became an enthusiastic plastic surgeon for the duration." The two published a comprehensive report in 1917 in which they advocated that all teeth should be preserved, "even old roots," and the facial "wounds should be closed as soon as possible; if necessary, before placing the jaw in position . . . however dirty the wound, it should be closed in a few days." A dental surgeon observed that Valadier's "cases continued with purulent discharge and sequestration." Valadier used boiled water for the cleansing of wounds, "avoiding antiseptics as much as possible." Valadier reported that he treated 1,010 cases of jaw injuries with only twenty-seven deaths.[3]

"When we went on a visit to Valadier," Dr. Ferdinand Brigham reported at a much later date, "we did not see much. He was content to pass his cases on to England. The cases we saw, and the few appliances he showed, looked very much like copies of what he [Valadier] had seen in our wards—and in the Val-de-Grace and the American Hospital in Paris." Brigham went on to describe Valadier as "pompous, using money, entertaining . . . an impresario, a pretender, a 'ham'." "Looking back, it is difficult to assess Valadier's ability as a surgeon," McAuley, a later biographer wrote, "but there seems little doubt about his ingenuity and clinical flare. . . . He was obviously a forceful, flamboyant character and may have been something of an empire builder." Another commentator, a dentist who saw him work, described Valadier as a "magnificent pioneer and did a lot for jaw work in the early days," claiming that his limitations were due to his "lack of orthodox surgical training."[4] It would appear, in the final analysis, that Valadier had neither the background nor the experience which Dr. Kazanjian had in treating jaw fractures or in the fabrication of appliances.

By 1918 Valadier, now a major, became less relevant and his

importance diminished. More of the surgical phase of treatment was performed by Captain Whale and later by Captain Frederick John Clemenison, another E.N.T. (ear, nose and throat) surgeon. Captain Leonard King, a dentist, fabricated the appliances as time passed on. Valadier's unit became more of a clearing center rather than a treatment facility, with cases being transferred to Gillies' Queen's Hospital, which was established in 1917 to specialize in the care of patients with facial wounds. With the Armistice, Valadier was ordered to terminate his operations and "the unit gradually ceased to function." Valadier won several honors for his military services. Most importantly, he received a knighthood from King George on March 16, 1920, after becoming a British citizen. He had friends and patients in high circles including Sir Arthur Sloggett and General Sir Douglas Haig. After the war, he practiced in Paris, where he "had an extremely successful dental practice" and served as president of the American Dental Club of Paris. He employed first-class assistants who did the majority of treatment, and "charged outrageous fees to outrageously rich patients." Valadier inherited a considerable fortune from his mother's estate and lived extravagantly. His downfall was his heavy gambling. He died penniless and in poor health on August 31, 1931. He is remembered chiefly "as one of those figures who make the fabric of history of medicine so fascinating."[5]

In publishing a report of his visit to the British military hospital in France in 1916, W. H. Gilmour quoted Valadier as asking, "What is the matter with you Britishers," and replied, "and the echo answers 'what'!" Gilmour expressed the concern that "whilst I am of the opinion that no one could give better service than they [the Americans] did, still one feels in principle that it was wrong." Actually, the British had already begun to address some of their problems, for a center for the treatment of facial injuries had been established in late 1915 by Harold Gillies in England at Aldershot. Gillies (1882-1960) was a New Zealander, born in Dunedin, the youngest of six sons. His father, an immigrant Scot, was a real estate agent, a noted amateur astronomer, and a member of the House of Representatives in the New Zealand Parliament. His great-uncle, Edward Lear, was a landscape painter and author of *The Book of Nonsense*.[6]

After graduating from Wanganui College, where he captained the cricket team, and later from Gonville and Cains College, Cambridge, where he excelled as an athlete both in rowing and in golf, Harold Gillies studied medicine at Saint Bartholomew's Hospital medical school in London. He graduated in 1908, with a fellowship in the Royal College of Medicine following in 1910. He won the Saint George's Grand Challenge Golf Cup in 1913. After a brief time as a general surgeon, he turned to otolaryngology and from 1910 to 1915 was an assistant to Sir Milsom Rees, "who was surgeon to the King's nose and throat."[7]

Early in 1915 "without undue remorse," Gillies "went off to France with the British Red Cross as general surgeon attached to the Army," where he was initially attached to Valadier's center for jaw injuries located near Boulogne, at the nearby town of Wimereux. "I was invited by Valadier," Gillies later recounted, "to accompany him to assist in his initial incision." Gillies' service with Valadier introduced him to "a new kind of wound." Although the British Army authorities would permit Valadier to operate only under the direction of a qualified surgeon, such as Gillies, "Gillies may have owed more to Valadier's experience . . . than he was disposed to admit." However, Gillies had no reservations acknowledging his indebtedness to "my American dental friend, Bobs Roberts [Dr. C. W. Roberts], . . . who had just returned from six months [of] jaw surgery in the American Hospital in Paris," for intro-

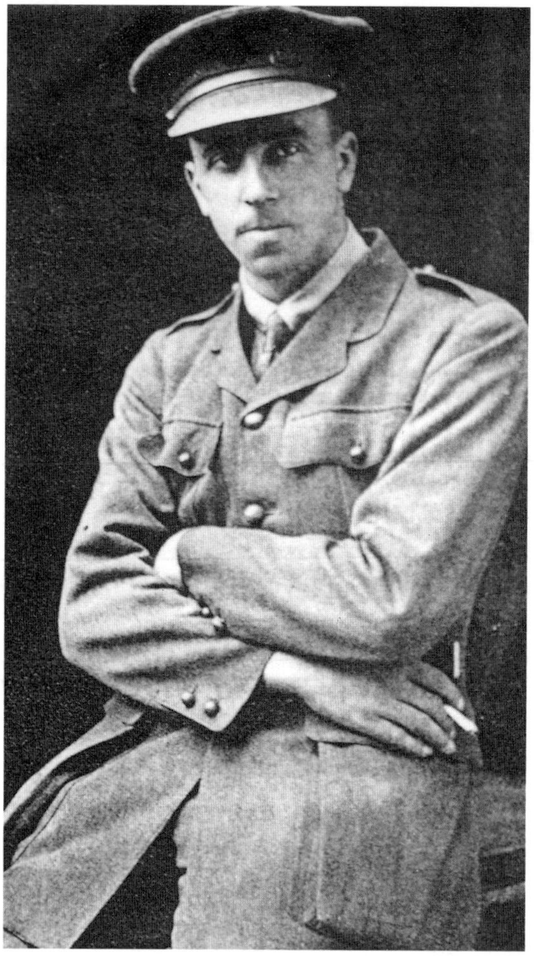

Sir Harold Delf Gillies (1882-1960) as a medical officer working with the Red Cross, 1915, Reginald Pound, Gillies: Surgeon Extraordinary, *(London: Michael Joseph, 1964.) p. 41*

ducing him to a book by Lindemann, which he had received from Germany, on "the good work they were doing on jaw fractures and wounds about the mouth. . . . Bobs presented this book to me with [the suggestion], 'Gillies, why don't you take up this work'?" The transformation from otolaryngology to the treatment of facial wounds by Gillies began in this manner. It was soon enhanced when, in June 1915, he had a leave and visited in Paris "the famous Morestin from Martinique [who] was rumored to be performing unbelievable feats of surgical reconstruction." Gillies was "captivated" as he observed Morestin operating and said, "I fell in love with the work on the spot."[8]

Gillies' enthusiasm was transmitted to his chiefs, Sir Anthony Bowlby and Sir John Rose Bradford, and through them to Sir Alfred Keogh, Director General of Army Medical Services. As a result, the center for the treatment of facial injuries was established by Gillies late in 1915 at Aldershot, southwest of London. On arrival there, Gillies "was allotted a young dental surgeon named A. L. Fraser, who very soon proved his worth. . . . He was followed by Captain [L. A.] King," with whom Gillies spent a "very happy year."[9]

The Aldershot center soon proved inadequate and was transferred to the Frognal Estate, the residence of the Earl of Sydney at Sidcup, Kent. The queen commanded that it be named for her; hence it was called Queen's Hospital. Initially it had 320 beds and was later augmented to 600. The hospital was very advanced in concept and design, with "spacious, single storied, well-lit wards . . . the wide verandas were available as open air wards . . . additional charm was offered by the beautiful grounds and surrounding countryside." It was described as being "years ahead of its time." It was also heavily funded. The move to Sidcup took place on August 18, 1917, and "was simultaneous with a flood of casualties." These stately and palatial surroundings contrasted sharply with the tent wards and huts in the field where Dr. Kazanjian was performing miracles "with his feet in the mud."[10]

A group of trained nurses was sent from the Cambridge Hospital at Aldershot to General Hospital No. 12 in France, a unit that was quartered under tents. Conditions were strikingly different between the two hospitals. "They were very smart and grand and very critical of our rough and ready ways," Nurse Kit Dodsworth recorded in her diary. "One of these new people was . . . horror-stricken to think that she would have to keep the linen in packing cases stood on end. 'In the Cambridge Hospital' she said, 'we had wonderful linen cupboards. I never imagined we should have to put up with this sort of thing.' . . . Nurse Dodsworth reported that she was a bit irritated and couldn't resist pointing out that we were after all on ACTIVE SERVICE."[11]

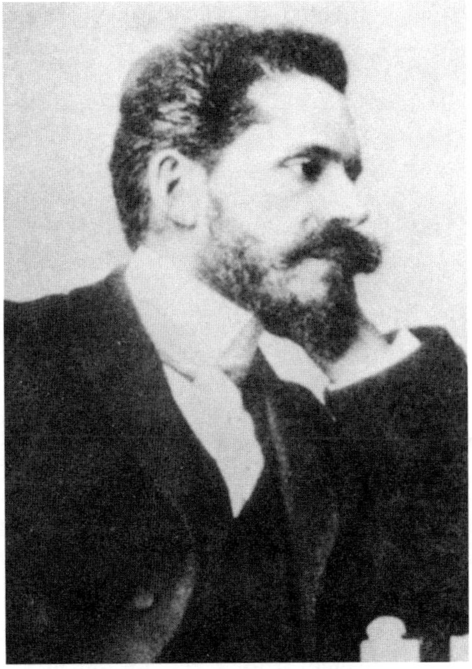

Hyppolylte Morestin (1869-1919), Courtesy National Library of Medicine, Bethesda, Md.

There was frequent and cordial interchange between Dr. Kazanjian and Gillies. "Sir Harold visited me in the early days of the First World War," Dr. Kazanjian reported. "As the years of the War continued, I visited Sir Harold frequently at Queen's Hospital at Sidcup, where many of my patients were who had been forwarded for further reconstructive surgery." Gillies acknowledged that he had received from Dr. Kazanjian "much kindly encouragement." He also observed that "cases coming from Kazanjian's Harvard Unit always showed excellent care. His work about the mouth and his use of weighted dentures produced such soft lips and ample chins that we would always gather around his cases on arrival to see exactly what he had done." According to John M. Converse, Gillies described "the remarkable condition of those patients received by him at Sidcup who had been treated by Kazanjian at Étaples before their evacuation to England." It is not surprising that Sir Harold invited Dr. Kazanjian to join him at his hospital in Sidcup. "I had been sent to France by Harvard," Dr. Kazanjian responded in declining, "and had responsibilities."[12]

Queen's Hospital "became the largest and most fruitful center of its kind in the world." It eventually treated over 11,000 cases. Sir Harold became "the only British surgeon attempting this type of work at the time." At Sidcup, the "famous dental surgeon, Sir William Kelsey Fry took Captain L. A. King's place." "I take the hard tissues," Fry proposed to Gillies. "You take the soft." This arrangement of shared responsibility remained in place during the war and thereafter. The staff also included Henry Tonks, who had been qualified as a surgeon and was a Fellow of the Royal College of Surgeons. Abandoning the practice of medicine, he became "one of the great artists of his day" and a professor of the Slade Art School. Gillies used Tonks's abundant talents in painting to draw portraits of patients with facial wounds, which were used to plan their treatment. One of Tonks's pastels is reproduced on a forepage of the first volume of Gillies and Millard's book.[13]

In 1920 Gillies published his classic text, *Plastic Surgery of the*

Face, a chronicle of his surgical experiences in World War I, with 424 pages and 844 illustrations and case histories. W. Kelsey Fry contributed a chapter titled, "The Prosthetic Problems of Plastic Surgery." Gillies acknowledged that, "in the early treatment of all wounds involving the oral cavity, the dental surgeon must be encouraged to take a large share of responsibility."[14]

Concerning bone-grafting to the mandible, Gillies reported that "in the early stages, the operation . . . was very much on trial . . . but a large number of cases of successful rib-grafts were obtained in 1916 and beginning of 1917." By 1920 he was able to announce "the operation for bone-grafting is uncomplicated." "Mr. Gillies' book," the *Lancet* reviewer wrote, "should go beyond the circle of his professional brethren and . . . might well be a patent factor in promoting peace among the nations." It was dedicated to Queen Mary.[15]

Gillies devised "the tube pedicle flap, [described by John S. Davis as probably the most important innovation in plastic surgery to come out of the war], the onlay eyelid graft, the palate push-back; he has conceived and executed a multitude of original thoughts and techniques." He formulated sixteen classical and enduring principles. "The father and mother of them is that *plastic surgery is a contest between blood supply and beauty*." These principles represented much more than surgery; they were a "philosophy of life." Gillies was described by Battle as "a born showman and extrovert" with "a penetrating sarcasm for the inefficient colleague." Throughout his life he maintained a "'Peter Pan' streak" and delighted in practical jokes. Those who worked with him "were inspired by his almost boyish enthusiasm for his work and by his superb craftsmanship."[16]

Gillies and Kazanjian maintained a respectful friendship throughout their lives. "How I would love to come, and discuss all the problems of our work with you," Gillies confessed to Kazanjian. Gillies acknowledged "the great regard I have always had for your work." Following Kazanjian's favorable review of the Gillies and Millard book in *The New England Journal of Medicine* (August 29, 1957), Sir Harold wrote, "So I thank you, dear friend, for all that has happened since the day that you arrived in Wimereux in 1915 right up to this lovely critique of my book." There were differences between them, not only in temperament, but in their relationship toward the students who came to them for training. Gillies charged them a fee while Kazanjian "gave freely of his time and talents, saying that he was complimented when anyone wanted to learn from him." Among the Allied surgeons who came to Sidcup to learn from Gillies were Ferris Smith from the United States, Carl Waldron and Fulton Risdon from Canada and Pickerill from Australia and New Zealand.[17]

Over the years, Kazanjian and Gillies exchanged visits, each to the other's country and home. On one of Gillies' early visits to Boston, Kazanjian took him to the traditional Harvard-Yale football game. Sir Harold was "the perfect guest" and cheered for Harvard, which, of course, was Kazanjian's school. "I never really knew," Kazanjian wondered, "if he actually preferred the Harvard team."

"I personally considered Sir Harold to be a resourceful surgeon, with original ideas which he was not hesitant in putting into practical use," Dr. Kazanjian stated. "He was thus responsible for many outstanding contributions to the advancement of plastic surgery."[18] Knighthood was conferred upon him in 1930 by King George V.

Three British dentists who were deeply involved in the treatment of jaw injuries during the war should be mentioned. Frank (J. F.) Colyer, William Kelsey Fry and William Warwick James. In July 1915, about a year after the beginning of the war, the Eastern Command of the British Army opened a special center for jaw cases at the Croydon War Hospital, located ten miles south of

London, where Frank Colyer (1866-1957) became the best known British exponent of jaw treatment. Colyer's treatment modality of jaw fractures differed markedly from the Kazanjian method, which emphasized the primacy of the restoration of the occlusion of the teeth. To Colyer, however, "the consolidation of the fracture" was "above all the result to be attained." He considered the maintenance of the arch and occlusion of the remaining teeth of no great importance." In common with Kazanjian, he strongly advocated removal of the teeth on either side of the fractures, as well as any necrotic bone, "in order to diminish sepsis and to lessen the risk of subsequent infection." He avoided the use of wire splints and ligature "which may irritate the gum."[19]

Colyer asserted that "Valadier's methods . . . were unsound." When Valadier's patients were evacuated to Croydon Hospital, Colyer sometimes found it necessary to remove splints and to extract questionable teeth. They became "bitter antagonists." Brigham described Colyer as "a dynamic person of inflexible opinions. . . . He expressed loud disapproval of most work except his own."[20]

Later, Colyer served at Sidcup with Gillies. "To . . . Sir Frank Colyer," Gillies wrote, "and to many other senior dental surgeons do I owe great technical and moral support." The son of a dental surgeon, Colyer studied dentistry at Leicester Square, where he was doubly qualified as a surgeon and dentist in 1889. He was knighted in recognition of his war work.[21]

William Kelsey Fry (1889-1963) was a regimental medical officer early in the war. Landing in France in October 1914, he served in the front lines with the Royal Welch Fusiliers. He was awarded the Military Cross for bravery, once in May 1915, and again in August 1916. "He was steadfastly courageous and his calm, happy temperament carried him through . . . apparently unaffected." On one occasion, he carried a wounded colonel across no-man's land and, in the process, received a bullet in his own arm.[22]

The direction of his life was forever changed after the needless loss of a young soldier's life.

> *A young lieutenant who had had his jaw blown apart . . . staggered back to the dugout soaked with blood. . . . Captain Fry made a quick examination, and then the two of them marched . . . toward the aid station. Fry walked in front so that the wounded officer could lean against him. . . to allow blood and bits of jaw to fall free of the airway. They arrived without mishap. . . The medical orderly was informed about the patient, and as the lieutenant's condition seemed quite good, Fry started back up the line. He had not gone fifty yards . . . when a message caught up with him that the lieutenant was dead. He had been laid on his back on a stretcher and had died immediately of respiratory obstruction. Fry had to wrap him in a blanket and bury him in the mud that very night.*[23]

It was after this unfortunate incident that Fry was drawn to the treatment of jaw injuries. He initiated a vigorous campaign about the importance of keeping the face down and the airway open in mouth and jaw wounds.[24]

Beginning in October 1916 and for the remainder of the war, Fry served as a dental surgeon, first at Aldershot and later at Queen's Hospital in Sidcup with Gillies. They "worked together in friendly cooperation and were responsible for many advancements in plastic surgery." At Sidcup both Gillies and Fry admittedly "learned a great deal from observing the treatment that some of the cases had received from . . . Kazanjian." Fry displayed a "remarkable combination of mechanical ingenuity and technical skill with surgical and medical acumen." To Gillies, Fry became his "very closest dental colleague . . . the combination of his mind and my surgery made for very considerable progress."[25]

Gillies observed that "no one could have been more critically co-operative than Kelsey Fry in the early days" and wrote of "his wisdom and charm in guiding us to adapt our work to fit the dental problem." The appliances for buccal inlays for bone graft cases, the sculpture and fixation of retaining molds for bird-chins, flat faces, and depressed noses were his special contribution. Fry was born in 1889 in Greenwich and went to school at Hurstpierpoint. He entered Guy's Hospital in 1908 and became qualified in both dentistry and medicine by 1913. He was knighted in 1951.[26]

William Warwick James (b.1874), the son of a shopkeeper, was apprenticed to a local dentist, in keeping with the custom of the time, but was so proficient that he soon was assisting in surgery rather than in the laboratory. Seeking formal education, he entered the Royal Dental Hospital of London in 1894 and later the Middlesex Hospital, thus becoming qualified in both dentistry and in medicine by 1905. In 1915, when he was forty-one years old, W. Warwick James began his service in France with the Anglo-French Red Cross at Yvetot in Normandy, where he met Valadier and Kazanjian. The latter's strong and constructive influence and friendship remained with him life-long. Thereafter, until 1919-20, James served with the Maxillo-Facial Unit at the Third London General Hospital at Wandsworth Common, "where he showed great skill in repairing extensive facial injuries and, along with a surgical colleague, performed many successful bone-grafts of the mandible."[27]

The Unit of the Third London Hospital was in place before the establishment of Gillies' Queen's Hospital at Sidcup. As a result "great initiative and perseverance were required [by James] to develop new methods in the treatment of the severe facial wound." James reported that it was not until he employed intermaxillary wiring for fractured jaws (Kazanjian's method) that the incidence of secondary hemorrhage and pneumonia "decreased rapidly." James was present when Major Kazanjian was invested as a Companion of the Order of Saint Michael and Saint George by King George V in 1919, and there is a photograph of Mr. and Mrs. James accompanying Major Kazanjian to the ceremony. For his own meritorious wartime services, James was made a member of the Order of the British Empire.[28]

In 1940, in cooperation with Ben W. Fickling, James published *Injuries of the Jaws and Face with Special Reference to War Casualties*, in which he acknowledged that he was "much influenced by the work of Major Kazanjian at the Twentieth General Hospital." The book was written at the outbreak of World War II in nine months and was an analysis of the case records that James had preserved from the end of World War I. "This work was much facilitated by his prodigious memory," since many records of that period had been destroyed. The cooperative relationship between Gillies, Fry, and James continued until after World War I, when they served on a British Army Advisory Standing Committee on facial and maxillary injuries, which formulated and executed principles of treatment. James maintained a life-long friendship with Major Kazanjian and never forgot "the help I received from you."[29]

In France, Dr. Hyppolyte Morestin operated successfully on many horrible face wounds at the Val-de-Grace Hospital during World War I. Born on the island of Martinique in the Antilles in 1869, of part-Negro extraction, the son of a physician (who died in 1902 when a volcano erupted in Martinique, killing 25,000 inhabitants), he was said to be "a quiet, moody and, unfortunately, a lonely man." Harold Gillies characterized Hyppolyte Morestin as "a strange and moody octoroon whose dagger-like sharpness was accentuated by his pointed mustache and tapered beard as well as the agility of his long, thin hands." About his visit at Paris in June 1915 Gillies wrote: "In the space of a single movement, he could reveal the gentleness of a kitten and the savagery of a tiger. . . . I stood spellbound as he removed half a face with a horrible cancer and then deftly turned a neck flap to restore not only the cheek but the side of the nose and lip, in one shot." After this sole visit in Paris, Dr. Morestin's door was closed, and there was no further contact between him and Gillies.[30]

Originally Morestin "disdained the services of the dental surgeon and claimed that he could 'do everything with his knife'," John Converse has written. In time and of necessity, his views changed. Truman Brophy related that, "Instead of producing chins for his patients, which could only be correctly formed by the use of a prosthesis, "he [Morestin] found the patients were severely deformed. . . . He therefore secured the co-operation of Dr. [Kelsey] Fry . . . and from that time on his results were better."[31]

Blair O. Rogers has written that Morestin was "born out of his time. . . . He was not the first man to attempt plastic surgery, but he was the first . . . to apply himself to every branch of it. . . . He realized that even in the simplest operation there had to be an aesthetic approach."[32] As soon as the patients' lives were out of danger, Hélène Baillaud, who was a nurse in Dr. Morestin's service, stated, "we began the task of restoring their appearance."

> *There was no question of leaving them with a hole in the middle of their face. After thirty or so operations, the great specialist, Doctor Morestin, remade the nose they lacked and gave them back their human appearance. He achieved this using the skin of their forehead and a fragment of cartilage from their rib cage. The surgeon's skill was truly great and we were full of admiration."*[33]

Following the end of World War I, Eleanor Roosevelt was in Paris, where she toured Val-de-Grace Hospital. "It was here that Morestin operates," she recalled, "and he has been so successful with the horrible face wounds." What she witnessed devastated and revolted her "even though one does not show it." She was in the company of her Aunt Dora (Doe), who was unaffected. To the sensitive and sympathetic Eleanor even the plaster casts were offensive, and she "could hardly bear to look at the men with the horrible face wounds."[34]

Dr. Hyppolyte Morestin died in France soon thereafter, in 1919, at age forty-nine, as a result of pulmonary complications during the global influenza epidemic in 1918-1919. His death left a tremendous "void in French plastic surgery." He "contributed so much" to his specialty, including 634 articles and discussions and "literally gave his life at much too young an age." He did one of the first modern western mammoplasties. As one of the founders of the specialty of Plastic Surgery, Morestin was to France what Sir Gillies was to England[35] and what Kazanjian was to America.[36] A search of the literature has failed to unearth any preserved communication between Morestin and Kazanjian.

Dr. Georges Villain, Professor of Prosthetic Dentistry of the University of Paris Dental School, was in charge of an ambulatory treatment center for French soldiers with jaw wounds that the school instituted in August 1914.[37] Born in Paris in 1881, he studied in England with an established dental practitioner as a preceptor and in the process acquired a precise knowledge of English. Thereafter he qualified as a Chirurgien Dentiste in the Faculty of Medicine in Paris in 1903. He furthered his education by entering the University of Pennsylvania, where he received the D.D.S. degree in 1906. Returning to Paris, he began a long teaching career at l'École Dentaire at the University of Paris. After serving in various capacities, he was appointed dean in 1926.

His belief was that "if a fractured jaw was to perform its normal function and not merely to be united in any portion, a state of muscular dynam-

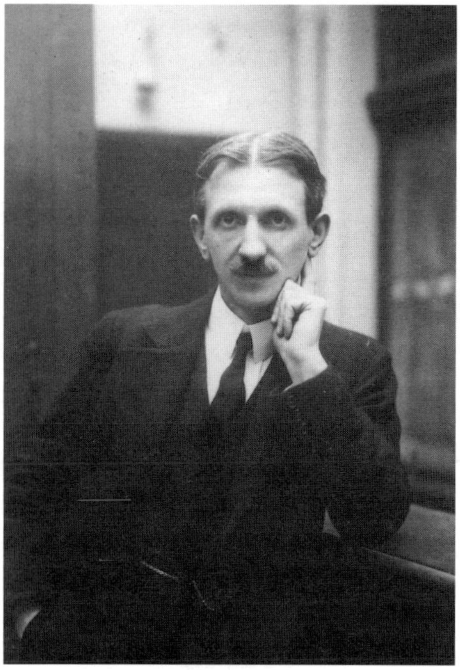

Georges Villain, (1881-1938)
Hospital Val-de-Grace, Paris,
Bibliothèque de l'École Dentaire de Paris (section de la Bibliothèque Interuniversitaire de Médecine)
Courtesy Pierre Gremeaux

ic equilibrium must be returned." He came away from the war with a strong belief in the universality of man. "The duties of man are wider than the limits of his family and of his native country," he maintained. "Human solidarity, which goes beyond the bounds limiting the individual nations, is the most sacred of these duties." This credo led him to assume a most active role in the Federation Dentaire Internationale, and in 1931 he was elected its president. He wore the Legion of Honor ribbon and was awarded honorary degrees from Laval University, Montreal, University of Pennsylvania, and Loyola University in Chicago. He died tragically as a result of an automobile accident at the age of fifty-seven. He was "a most important figure in French dentistry."[38]

Two American dentists who contributed significant services to France in the Great War were Dr. George B. Hayes and Dr. William Slocum Davenport. After receiving his D.D.S. degree from the University of Michigan in 1889, Dr. Hayes (1865-1957) practiced in Tacoma, Washington from 1890 to 1895, and then in Berlin, Germany from 1895 to 1897, in the court of Kaiser Wilhelm II; but disliking the Prussian sternness and rigidity of character, he moved to Paris, where he graduated from l'École Dentaire and began a practice in 1900. Upon the outbreak of war in 1914, Dr. Hayes volunteered his services as a dentist to the Medical Board of the American Hospital. This was the first instance of the appointment of a dental surgeon to the medical board of a military hospital.[39]

Dr. Hayes and Dr. William Davenport jointly operated the dental department at the American Hospital for the French for treatment of jaw fractures, a facility that was highly regarded by Kazanjian. Following his services at the American Hospital from 1914 to 1917, Hayes became director of the dental department of an American Red Cross military hospital in Paris from 1917 to 1919. For his wartime services, the French government made him a Chevalier of the Legion of Honor in 1918. He also received the American Distinguished Service medal. Dr. Hayes continued his dental practice in Paris until 1932, when he retired to La Jolla, California.[40]

Dr. Davenport came from a family of ministers; the Davenports of New Haven were among the founders of Yale University. Born in New York State in 1868, Dr. Davenport received the degree of D.D.S. from the University of Pennsylvania in 1890, subsequently joining his brother Isaac, who had established a practice in Paris. The Davenports represented a dental dynasty that was emulated in Europe, and they made the title "American Dentist" respected there.

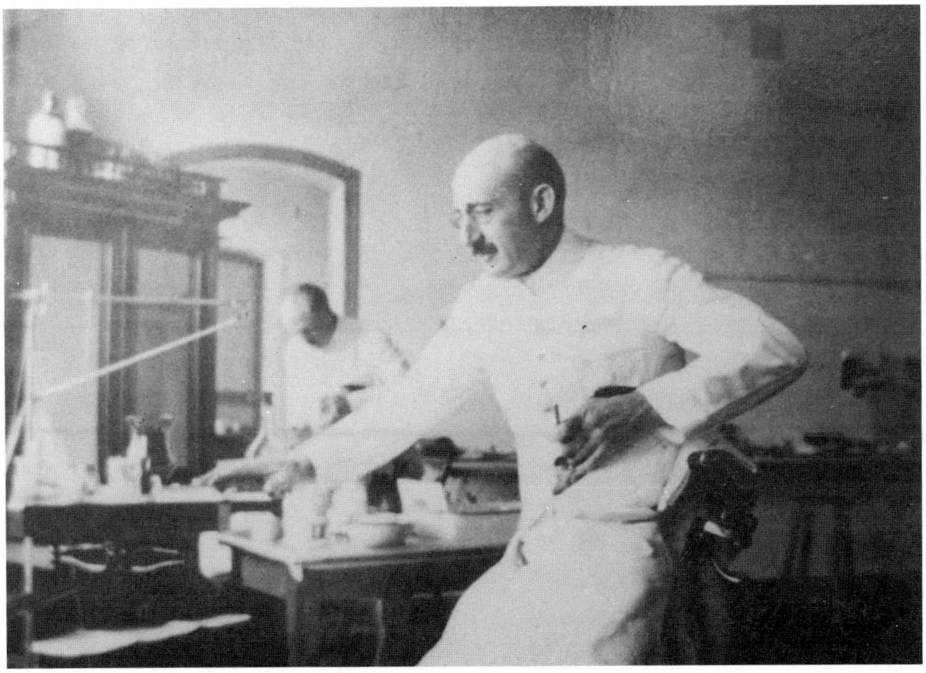

George B. Hayes (1865-1957)
Courtesy Dept. of Rare Books and Special Collections, University of Rochester

During World War I William Davenport devoted half of his time to service at the American Ambulance Hospital, and from 1917 to 1919, at the 63rd French Military Hospital. He was assistant chief of the dental department at each hospital. In a paper published in October 1916 he reported the invention of a bone graft from the rib following multiple fractures of the mandible.[41]He practiced for nearly fifty years and had a very select clientele, including the royal family of Belgium.

Two others, who were neither surgeons nor dentists, made significant contributions to the correction of face injuries in England and France during and after World War I. They were Captain Francis Derwent Wood and Anna Coleman Ladd, artists who fabricated external facial prostheses "that made a man's face as near as possible to what it had looked like before he was wounded."[42]

Not all faces could be successfully rehabilitated during and after World War I. "There were many others whose faces contained gaping holes, who had no lower jaws; these were the veterans whose faces could not be reconstructed," Dr. John M. Converse wrote. "They formed an organization of mutual aid, 'Les Gueules Cassées'— the broken faces."[43]

Francis Derwent Wood was a sculptor and an Associate of the Royal Academy. After the outbreak of the war, he was a nursing orderly in the Royal Army Medical Corps with the rank of private. His artistic talents in fabricating external facial prostheses eventually earned him a commission as a captain in 1916. At the Third London General Hospital he established the Masks for Facial Disfigurements Department, which the Tommies nicknamed the Tin Nose Shop. "My

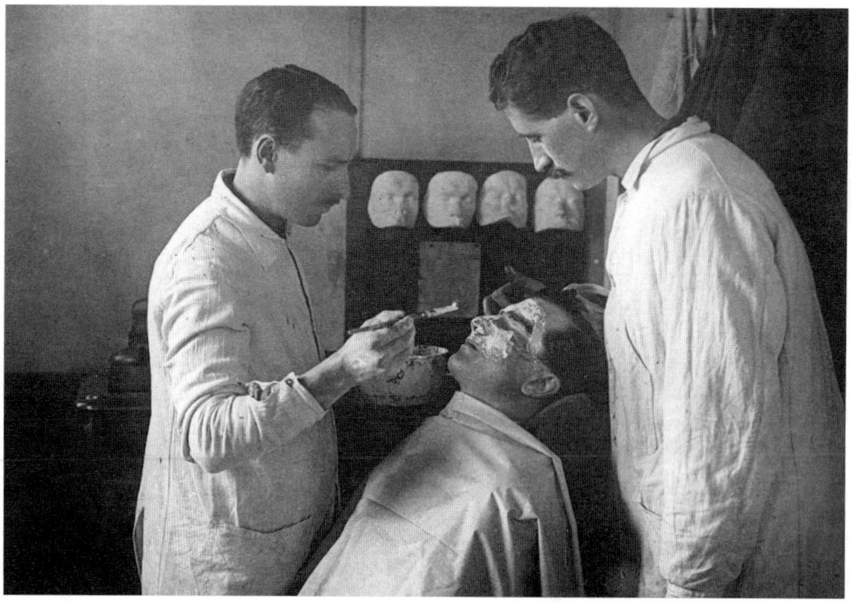

Capt. Francis Derwent Wood, R.A.M.C., and assistant,
Courtesy of the Imperial War Museum, London
Q.30452

work begins where the work of the surgeon is completed," Wood wrote. Wood reported that the cases that came to him were "so severe as to remove them beyond the range of even the most advanced plastic surgical operations."[44]

The basis of his treatment was the natural "restoration of features . . . originally ugly or beautiful." He worked from a pre-wound photograph. The size of the area affected did not concern him, but the materials did. He found that "only a rigid mask can be depended upon, both for hygiene and cosmetic reasons." He rejected soft substances "such as gelatin mixtures." The mask was made of an electrolyte plate of pure copper, with a thickness of 1/32 inch. "The necessary fitments of glass eye and attachments are fixed," he wrote, "and it is finally well covered with an electric deposit of silver." The mask was attached to the face usually with strong spectacles. It was pigmented to match the patient's coloring. Wood's masks were intended to make his patient's presence "no longer a source of melancholy to himself nor of sadness to his relatives and friends."[45]

There were 2,000 facially disfigured and mutilated soldiers (*mutilés de la face*) in France alone in 1918.[46] Some of them were the patrons of a cafe in Paris in the 1920s whom Ernest Hemingway described in his posthumously published sketches of his life in Paris in that era, *A Moveable Feast*:

> *There were other people too who lived in the quarter and came to the Lilas, and some of them wore Croix de Guerre ribbons in their lapels and others also had the yellow and green of the Médaille Militaire, and I watched how well they were overcoming the handicap of the loss of limbs, and saw the quality of their artificial eyes and the degree of skill with*

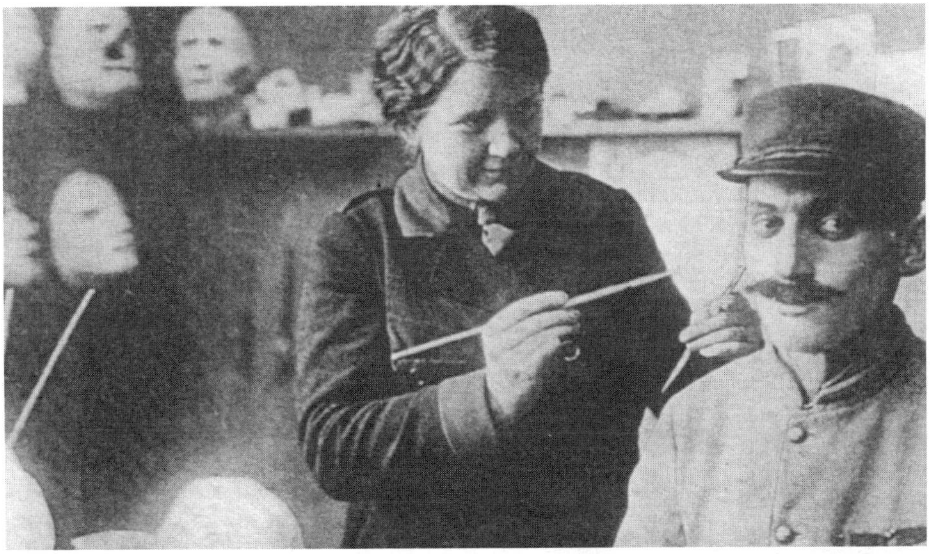

Anna Coleman Ladd, (1878-1959)
New Faces for Mutilated Soldiers, *Henry P. Davison* The American Red Cross In The Great War *(New York: MacMillan Company, 1919). American Red Cross Collection, the Hazel Braugh Records Center and Archives, Division of the Historical Resources Department of the American Red Cross*

which their faces had been reconstructed. There was always an almost iridescent shiny cast about the considerably reconstructed face, rather like that of a well packed ski run, and we respected these clients more than we did the savants *or the professors, although the latter might well have done their military service too without experiencing mutilation.*

In those days, we did not trust anyone who had not been in the war, ... [47]

Just as Captain Wood had done for the Tommies, an American socialite, Anna Coleman Ladd, dedicated herself to sculpturing masks for these mutilated French soldiers. It was Wood's article in the June 23, 1917 issue of *Lancet,* "Masks for Facial Wounds," which served as her guide. Born into a socially prominent Pennsylvania family in 1878, Anna Coleman lived with her family in Paris until she was twenty-one, receiving a classical education, and was tutored in the private tradition. She studied sculpture in Rome and began to receive commissions and exhibited her work in several important galleries and museums in America and abroad. In 1905 she married Dr. Maynard Ladd, a Harvard Medical School graduate who became chief of staff of the Children's Department of the Boston Dispensary. During the war he served in France in 1917 with the Children's Bureau of the American Red Cross. [48]

Anna Coleman Ladd devoted about a year of her life, beginning in November 1917, to the sculpting of portrait masks in Paris. This was done under the direction of the American Red Cross, but at her own request. She created ninety-seven masks, mostly for French soldiers who were facially wounded and disfigured. "My objective was not simply to provide a man with a mask to hide his awful mutilation," Ladd related, "but to

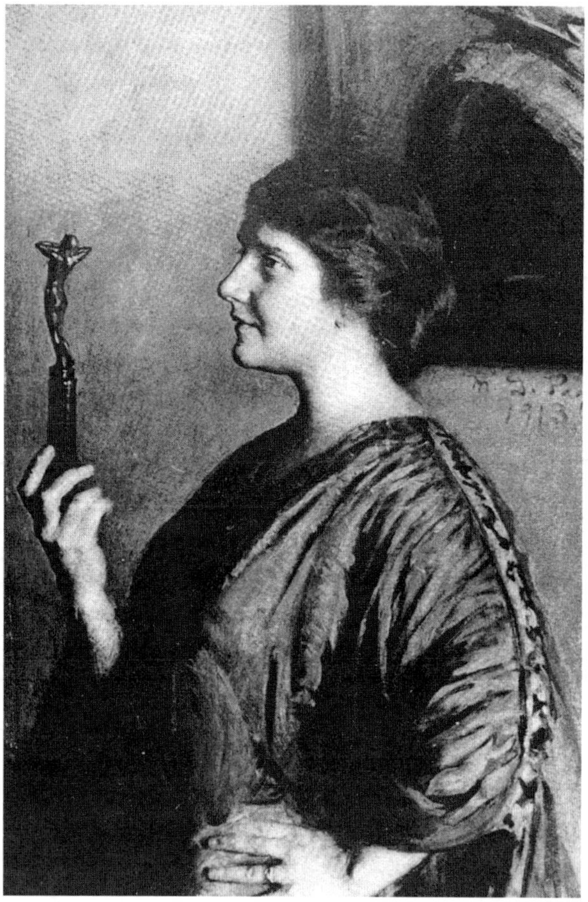

Mrs. Anna Coleman Ladd, (1878-1959) oil on canvas by Marie Danforth Page (American, 1869-1940), Skinner's, Auctioneers and Appraisers of Antiques and Fine Arts, Boston and Bolton, MA.

put in the mask part of the man himself--that is the man he had been before the tragedy." Ladd was aided by the French sculptor, Jane Poupelet (1874-1923), who voluntarily served as the co-director of the Studio of Portrait Masks in Paris. Apparently Ladd worked primarily in the field, visiting hospitals which specialized in the treatment of facial injuries, while Poupelet supervised the day-to-day operations of the studio, Mrs. Ladd accepted nothing for her services. She returned to the United States early in 1919 and was made a Chevalier of the Legion of Honor by the French government in 1931. She died in 1939 and is remembered as one who contributed "to the reconstruction of lives begun where the plastic surgeon left off."[49]

From the perspective of the American medical experience with masks, Vilray Blair reported that

> *The matter of making masks to camouflage these face injuries was investigated extensively by the Surgeon-General, and personnel trained for the work. A few were made for our soldiers by the Red Cross in Paris, and several here, by our own staff; but the men will not wear them, preferring plastic reconstruction. There is not, to my knowledge at present, a single mask in use by our soldiers, and Major Gillies of the British service tells me that the soldiers have the same preference.* [50]

NOTES

1 W. H. Dolamore, "The Treatment of Injuries of the Face and Jaws at Düsseldorf," *British Dental Journal* 38, no. 1 (January -June 1917): War Supplement, 1-31; S. Anthony Wolfe and Samuel Berkowitz, *Plastic Surgery of the Facial Skeleton* (Boston: Little Brown, 1989), pp. 10-11.

2 The best account of August Charles Valadier's yearly life and career is Robert H. Ivy's "The Mysterious A. C. Valadier," *Plastic and Reconstructive Surgery* 74, no. 4 (1971): 365-370. Charles Auguste (or Auguste Charles) Valadier was born in Paris in 1873, the son of American parents. He moved with his parents to America as a boy and entered the Philadelphia Dental College, now Temple University School of Dentistry, in 1898, graduating with the degree of Doctor of Dental Surgery in 1901. He passed the New York Board of Dental Registration examinations of May 2, 1902, and afterwards practiced as a dentist who advertised his services on Fifth Avenue in New York City. By 1910, following the death of his father, he was in Paris, where he was licensed as a dentist and established a successful dental practice. Sir Harold Gillies, in his and Ralph Millard, Jr.'s *Plastic and Reconstructive Surgery* (Boston: Little Brown, 1957) v.1, p. 6, describes him as then "a fat man . . . who had equipped his Rolls Royce with dental chair [and] drills . . . whose high brown riding boots carried a polish equal to the glitter of his spurs." Also, William P. Cruse, "Auguste Charles Valadier: A Pioneer in Maxillofacial Surgery," *Military Medicine* 152, no. 7 (July 1987): 338; and J. E. McAuley, "Charles Valadier: A Forgotten Pioneer in the Treatment of Jaw Injuries,"*Proceedings of Royal Society of Medicine, Section of the History of Medicine* 67 (August 1974): 787.

3 McAuley, "Forgotten Pioneer," pp. 786, 788; A. C. Valadier and H. Lawson Whale, "A Report on Oral and Plastic Surgery and on Prosthetic Appliances," *The British Journal of Surgery* 5, nos. 17-20 (July 1917 to April 1918): 151-170.

4 Brigham's observations are quoted in Ivy, "Valadier," p. 369, based on a 1970 interview; McAuley, "Forgotten Pioneer," p. 787; Letter from Dr. Leonard King to Dr. V. H. Kazanjian, August 10, 1916, V. H. Kazanjian Archive in The Francis A. Countway Library of Medicine, folder C-239. Also, A. C. Valadier and L. A. B. King, "A Few Appliances of Probable Interest to the Dental Surgeon," *La Restauration Maxillo-Faciale* 1 (January 1918): 511-517.

5 McAuley, "Forgotten Pioneer," pp. 785, 787, 788. Promoted to the rank of Honorary Major in 1916, Valadier was mentioned three times in dispatches during the war: he was appointed a Companion of St. Michael and St. George in June 1916; an Associate of St. John of Jerusalem in January 1917; and in 1919 he was made a Chevalier of the Legion of Honor by the French government. Valadier and Whale, "Report," pp. 160-168, lists twelve typical cases; initially Major Valadier does the operating either alone or with Captain Whale assisting, but from case eight to twelve, the roles are reversed, and it is Captain Whale who is operating with Major Valadier assisting. Also, Cruse, "Pioneer," p. 338; and Ivy, "Valadier," p. 369. Ferdinand Brigham's Unpublished manuscript on the Dental Unit of the First Harvard Unit states that Valadier claimed to have treated as dental patients "from the Prince of Wales and General Sir Douglas Haig down."

6 W. H. Gilmour, "Notes on a Visit to the Military Hospital at the Base in France and Some Hospitals in Paris," *British Dental Journal* 37, no. 51 (August 1, 1916): 566; Jerome P. Webster, "In Memoriam: Sir Harold Delf Gillies, 1887-1960," *Plastic and Reconstructive Surgery* 27, no. 1 (January 1961): 1-6.

7 H. D. Gillies and Ralph Millard, Jr., *The Principles and Art of Plastic Surgery* (Baltimore: Williams & Wilkins, 1971), v. 1, p. 6.

8 Gillies and Millard, *Principles of Plastic Surgery*, v. 1, pp. 6, 7; McAuley, "Forgotten Pioneer," p. 786; Reginald Pound, *Gillies: Surgeon Extraordinary* (London: Michael Joseph, 1964), p. 22. Dr. C. W. Roberts was born in Hannibal, Missouri, in 1877, graduated from Northwestern Dental School in 1899, and practiced dentistry in London beginning in 1908. He became a naturalized British subject. Early in 1915 he gave up his practice and served as dental surgeon at the American Hospital in Paris. He is discussed in G. H. Leatherman, "The American Dental Society of

London, An Historical Record (1908-1958)," paper read at a meeting of the Society of London on October 14, 1958, in the author's possession. See also George B. Hayes, "War Dental Surgery," *Dental Cosmos* 58, no. 3 (March 1916): 254.

9 Gillies and Millard, *Principles of Plastic Surgery*, v. 1, p. xviii.

10 A. D. Macalister, "The Queen's Hospital, Sidcup," 1987, manuscript, unpaged, in the author's possession. Gillies received funding for his hospital from the British Red Cross, the Order of St. John of Jerusalem, the British Red Cross of Australia, Canada and New Zealand, the National Relief Fund, the War Office, the Admiralty and a number of substantial donations by private individuals. Gillies and Millard, *Principles of Plastic Surgery*, v. 1, p. 31.

11 Lyn Macdonald, *The Roses of No Man's Land*, (London: Penguin Books, 1993), p. 109.

12 Letter from Varaztad H. Kazanjian to Reginald Pound, May 1, 1962 or 1963, in the Kazanjian Archive, folder C-341; H. D. Gillies, *Plastic Surgery of the Face* (London: Oxford University Press, 1920), Preface, p. x; Gillies and Millard, *Principles of Plastic Surgery*, v. 1, p. 22; Pam Hait, "History of the American Society of Plastic and Reconstructive Surgeons, Inc. 1931-1994," *Journal of Plastic and Reconstructive Surgery* 94, no. 4, (September 1994): 13A. Also, John M. Converse, "The Extraordinary Career of Dr. Varaztad Hovhannes Kazanjian," *Plastic and Reconstructive Surgery* 71, no. 1 (January 1982): 138.

13 Webster, "In Memoriam," p. 2; Gillies and Millard, *Principles of Plastic Surgery*, v. 1, pp. xvii, 11; Pound, *Surgeon Extraordinary*, p. 31. For a biography of Tonks, see *Plarr's Lives of the Fellows of the Royal College of Surgeons of England*, Supplement 1930-1951, by D'Arcy Power and William LeFanu, pp. 775-777.

14 W. Kelsey Fry, "The Prosthetic Problems of Plastic Surgery," in Gillies, *Plastic Surgery,* pp. 6, 193-208.

15 Gillies, *Plastic Surgery*, p. 177; Pound, *Surgeon Extraordinary,* p. 65.

16 Gillies performed his first tube pedicle on October 3, 1917, on a sailor who was badly burned during the Battle of Jutland in May 1916 (Gillies and Millard, *Principles of Plastic Surgery,* v. 1, pp. 34, 49-54, v. 2, Epilogue). John S. Davis writes in "Plastic Surgery in World War I and World War II," p. 611: "Probably the most useful plastic procedure developed during World War I was the tubed flap which was reported independently by Filatov, in 1916, in Russia, and Gillies, in 1917, in England." See Harold Gillies, "Experiences With Tubed Pedicle Flaps," *Surgery, Gynecology and Obstetrics* 60, no. 2 (February 15, 1935): 291-303. Gillies acknowledged that it was first described by Filatov in 1917 "but the idea occurred to me quite independently in the same year." Anthony R. Wallace, *The Progress of Plastic Surgery* (Oxford: Willem A. Meeuws, 1982), pp. 162-163, contains material on Vladimir P. Filatov (1875-1956), who was an ophthalmic surgeon in Odessa. Also, G. M. Fitzgibbon, "The Commandments of Gillies." *British Journal of Plastic Surgery* 21 no. 3 (July 1968): 226-239; Richard Battle, "Plastic Surgery in the Two World Wars and the Years Between," *Journal of the Royal Society of Medicine* 71 (November 1978): 844; T. P. K., "The Late Sir Harold Gillies," *British Journal of Plastic Surgery* 21, no. 3 (1960-1961): 193.

17 Letter from H. D. Gillies to V. H. Kazanjian, October 3, 1957, Kazanjian Archive, folder C-171; Hait, "History of the American Society" p. 13A; John Converse, *Reconstructive Plastic Surgery* (Philadelphia: Saunders, 1964), v. 1, p. 10.

18 Letter from Kazanjian to Reginald Pound, May 1, 1962 (or 1963).

19 Ferdinand Brigham, unpublished manuscript on the Dental Unit of the Harvard Surgical Unit; L. Impert and P. Regal, *Fracture of the Lower Jaw*, edited by J. F. Colyer (London: University of London Press, 1918); J. F. Colyer, "Injuries of the Mandible in Military Practice," *British Dental Journal* 38, no. 1 (January-June 1917): *War Supplement,* 57-97 (This paper was a study of the cases at the Croydon War Hospital); McAuley, "Forgotten Pioneer," p. 787; G. Villain, "The Physiological Treatment of Fractures and Dislocations," *Lancet* 1 (June 24, 1916): 1273-1274.

20 Cruse, "Pioneer," p. 340; Brigham, Unpublished manuscript.

21 Lillian Lindsay, "Obituary, Sir Frank Colyer," *British Dental Journal* 96, no. 8 (April 20, 1954):

197; Gillies and Millard, *Principles of Plastic Surgery*, v. 1, p. xvii. Gillies and Colyer had their differences. Gillies wrote (p. 39), "Competition was keen, for the game was on. Take, for instance, the scramble for the building of a buccal sulcus. It all started when Sir Frank Colyer began to scorn our lovely bone grafts to the jaw. He opposed restoring the oral arch at all, because he maintained that our bone grafts were in the substance of the cheek or the floor of the mouth and no dental prosthesis could be fitted over them." The problem was resolved with the placement of a skin-lined sulcus. "Dentures can now be fitted into it and over the bone graft. Complicated, yes, but quite obviously answer to our problem." Also, Lindsay, "Sir Frank Colyer" p. 197; "Sir Frank Colyer," *British Dental Journal* 114, no. 10 (May 21, 1963): 410.

22 Biography of Sir William Kelsey Fry in *Plarr's Lives of the Fellows of the Royal College of England*, Supplement 1930-1951, by Power and LeFanu, p. 141; D. Ralph Millard, Jr. *Cleft Craft, The Evolution of Its Surgery* (Boston: Little Brown, 1980), v. 3, pp. 413-414.

23 Gillies and Millard, *Principles of Plastic Surgery*, v. 1, p. 23.

24 Millard, *Cleft Craft*, v. 3, p. 413-414.

25 Millard, *Cleft Craft*; T. G. W. "Great Teachers of Surgery in the Past: Sir William Kelsey Fry (1889-1963)," *British Journal of Surgery* 53, no. 4 (April 1966): 318; M. A. R., Obituary: "Sir William Kelsey Fry," *British Dental Journal* 115, no. 1 (November 19, 1963): 422; Gillies and Millard, *Principles of Plastic Surgery*, v. 1, p. xvii.

26 Gillies and Millard, *Principles of Plastic Surgery*, v. 1, p. xvi; M.A.R., "Sir William Kelsey Fry," pp. 422-423.

27 B. W. F. (Ben W. Fickling), "Obituary: William Warwick James," *British Dental Journal* 119, no. 7 (October 5, 1965): 326; B. W. Fickling and J. Boyes, "No End to Talk About: Personal Recollections of the Late William Warwick James," *British Dental Journal* 138, no. 5 (March 4, 1975): 182; Z. C. (Zachary Cope), "In Memoriam: William Warwick James," *Annals of the Royal College of Surgeons of England* 37 no. 5 (November 1965): 318.

28 Fickling and Boyes, "No End to Talk About," pp. 182, 186. Photograph in the Kazanjian Archive, folder M-18.

29 W. Warwick James and B. W. Fickling, *Injuries of the Jaws and Face with Special Reference to War Casualties* (London: John Bale and Staples, 1940), p. vi; Unpublished address by B. W. Fickling at the memorial service for William Warwick James, England, the Middlesex Hospital Chapel, 11 November 1965, p. 2, in the Kazanjian Archive, folder C-146; B. W. F., "William Warwick James," p. 326; T. G. W., "Great Teachers of Surgery," p. 319; Letter from W. Warwick James to V. H. Kazanjian dated July 24, 1940, in the Kazanjian Archive, folder G-217. "So far the work in this War [World War II]," James wrote, "is in no way comparable with that of the last."

30 Blair O. Rogers "Hippolyte Morestin (1869-1919), Part 1: A Brief Biography," *Aesthetic Plastic Surgery* (1982): 142; Gillies and Millard, *Principles of Plastic Surgery*, v. 1, p. 7; John M. Converse, "Plastic Surgery: The Twentieth Century, the Period of Growth, 1914-1939," *Surgical Clinics of North America* 47, no. 2 (April 1967): 262.

31 Converse, "Plastic Surgery"; Truman W. Brophy, in Thomas L. Gilmer, "Fifty Years Observation of Oral Surgery," *Journal of the National Dental Association* 9, no. 7 (July 1922): 7.

32 Rogers, "Morestin," Part 1; p. 145.

33 Hélène Baillaud, "Mémoires d'une Infirmière du Val-de-Grace," 11 p. manuscript, Archive du Val-de-Grace, Carton 169, p. 7. Quoted in Claudine Mitchell, *Work and the Image* (London: Ashgate, 2001), Chapter "Facing Horror: Women's Work, Sculptural Practice and the Great War," p. 38.

34 Joseph P. Lash, *Eleanor and Franklin: The Story of Their Relationship, Based on Eleanor Roosevelt's Private Papers* (New York: W. W. Norton, 1971), p. 233.

35 Converse, "Plastic Surgery," pp. 146, 262; Personal interview with Dr. Robert M. Goldwyn on April 22, 2002, Boston, in the author's possession; Wallace, *Progress of Plastic Surgery*, p. 156. For obituaries of Morestin see J. L Faure, *La Presse Médicale*, February 20, 1919; Albert Mouchet, *Paris Médical* 32, no.1010 (1919): 92-93; and P. Leceme and H. Mondor "L'Oeuvre Chirurgicale de H. Morestin," *Journal de Chirurgie* 16 (1920): 1-8.

36 B. W. F. (Ben W. Fickling), "Obituary: V. H. Kazanjian," *British Dental Journal* 138, no. 2

(January 21, 1975): 73-74. "He [Kazanjian] virtually founded American Plastic Surgery as Sir Harold Gillies did in this country."

37 Angelo Chiavaro, "Organizzazione Metodi Di Cura," *Odontologia* (Rome, 1920), p. 47, provides a review of the French, American, and British jaw center in 1917; also Brophy in Gilmer, "Fifty Years Observation of Oral Surgery," p. 7.

38 Villain, "Physiological Treatment," *The Lancet* 1 (June 24, 1916): 1273; Obituary: "M. Georges Villain," *The Dental Magazine and Oral Topics* 55 (May 1938): 432; Obituary: "Dr. Georges Villain," *Journal of the American Dental Association* 25, no. 7 (July 1938): 1131-1133.

39 A comprehensive sketch of Dr. Hayes's life is found in Malvin E. Ring, "The Life and Work of Dr. George Byron Hayes, Pioneer Maxillofacial Surgeon," *Journal of the History of Dentistry* 4, no. 3 (November 1999): 105-109. See "Miracles of Surgery on Men Mutilated in War," *The New York Times Magazine*, January 16, 1916, pp. 6-7, for the support that William K. Vanderbilt and other Americans gave to the work of Drs. Hayes and Davenport.

40 *Journal of the National Dental Association* 5, no. 6 (June 1918): 631; Robinson Field, "A Few Remarks on the Role of the American Dentists in Paris During the Great War," *Dental Items of Interest* 45, no. 3 (March 1923): 213-214; Ring, "The Life and Work of Dr. George Byron Hayes," p. 109.

41 Jacques Foure, *American Dental Club, Paris: The First Hundred Years* (Paris Club, 1990), no p.; "Dr. William Slocum Davenport," *The Dental Magazine and Oral Topics* 55 (May 1938): 433-434. Also, W. S. Davenport,"Multiple Fracture of the Mandible and Lost Substance Restored by Bone-Graft," *Dental Cosmos* 58, no 10 (October 1916): 1135-1141. The bone graft operation was performed by Dr. R. B. Greenough of the Harvard Unit.

42 Francis D. Wood, "Masks for Facial Wounds," *The Lancet* 1 (June 23, 1917): 949.

43 Converse, "Plastic Surgery," p. 264.

44 Macdonald, *Roses*, pp. 155-156; Wood, "Masks."

45 Wood, "Masks," pp. 949, 951. Some Tommies rejected these masks, saying: "These blankety tin faces are no good to us. Can't you give us something that we can wash and shave and won't fall off in the street?" William S. Bainbridge, "Report on Medical and Surgical Developments of the War," *United States Naval Medical Bulletin* (1919): 88, contains a description of Wood's methods.

46 Grace S. Harper, "New Faces for Mutilated Soldiers," *Red Cross Magazine* 13 (November 1918): 44.

47 Ernest Hemingway, *A Moveable Feast, Sketches of the Author's Life in Paris in the Twenties* (New York: Scribner's, 1964), p. 82.

48 Brophy, in Gilmer, "Fifty Years Observation of Oral Surgery," p. 7. Also, P. Desfosses, "Nos Amis Les Américains," *Press Médicale* no. 30 (May 30, 1918): 345-346 (This article was one of the first to publicize Ladd's work); Claudine Mitchell, "Facing Horror: Women's Work, Sculptural Practice and the Great War," in Valerie Mainz and Griselda Pollock, *Work and The Image* (London: Ashgate, 2001), p. 39; Sharon Romm and Judith Zacher, "Anna Coleman Ladd: Maker of Masks for the Facially Mutilated," *Plastic and Reconstructive Surgery* 70, no. 1 (July 1982): 104-105. Also, *The Work of Anna Coleman Ladd* (Boston: Seaver-Howland Press, 1920), which contains photographs of her work.

49 Romm and Zacher, "Anna Coleman Ladd," p. 8; Mitchell, "Facing Horror," p. 41.

50 Vilray P. Blair, "The Maxillofacial Service of the American Army at War," *Journal of the American Medical Association* 73, no. 5 (Aug. 3, 1919): 327.

CHAPTER EIGHT

Glory and Anguish

Deemed indispensable, Major Kazanjian remained on active duty until January 8, 1919, when he relinquished his commission, and the Harvard Unit was mustered out of service and the hospital closed. He had served for about 1,300 days, during which time between 2,500 and 3,000 cases had been recorded, "of which 2,000 received extensive treatment." The foundation of modern plastic surgery had been laid in the battlefield hospitals of France, and this immigrant American dentist was its architect. Dr. Kazanjian "undoubtedly set the standard and formulated the principles of treatment," Dr. Robert Ivy acknowledged, "that were followed so successfully by others in World War I and even World War II."[1]

Dr. Frederick A. Washburn, who as a colonel had been the commander of Base Hospital No. 6 during World War I, the Massachusetts General Hospital unit, and who later served as director of the General from 1922 to 1934, paid the following tribute to Dr. Kazanjian: "In this work of reconstruction and plastic surgery, his skill was unrivalled." Throughout the entire period, July 17, 1915, to January 18, 1919, General Sir Charles Burtchaell, Director General of Medical Services, British Armies in France, reported "Major Kazanjian performed very important and successful work . . . and his duties were at all times characterized by zeal, energy, and ability."[2]

The Harvard Unit itself sailed home from Liverpool on the White Star liner S.S. *Megantic*, on January 20, 1919, but without Kazanjian, who was still needed in Europe. Before embarking, the members of the Unit were entertained at luncheon by Sir William Osler (who would die on December 29 that year), Lt. Gen. Thomas H. Goodwin, and Admiral Guy C. Gaunt. The head of the unit, Lt. Col. Hugh Cabot, and the head matron, Mrs. Katharine M. Hager, were received by the Duke of Connaught, the King's uncle. The work of the Harvard Unit at General Hospital No. 22 received wide acclaim and commendation. The King acknowledged that "their record can never be forgotten, or remembered without lively gratitude." Field Marshall Douglas Haig expressed his appreciation for "the admirable spirit displayed by all." Arthur James Balfour, British Foreign Secretary, proclaimed to President Woodrow Wilson: "The work of General Hospital 22, the largest hospital unit serving with the British Army, has held a record for skillful and untiring treatment of our wounded. The memory of so much service and self-sacrifice can never pass from us."[3]

When Dr. Brigham sailed home with the Harvard Unit, stowed away in the hold of the ship under his charge were seventeen cases or boxes containing models, appliances, x-rays, photographs and records of the patients whom they had treated in France. The voyage home was "wonderfully smooth," the ship reached Halifax on January 28, and Portland, Maine, on the 29th, where the unit disembarked, arriving in Boston by train. There were about twenty-five doctors and eighty-five nurses in the Unit when it reached

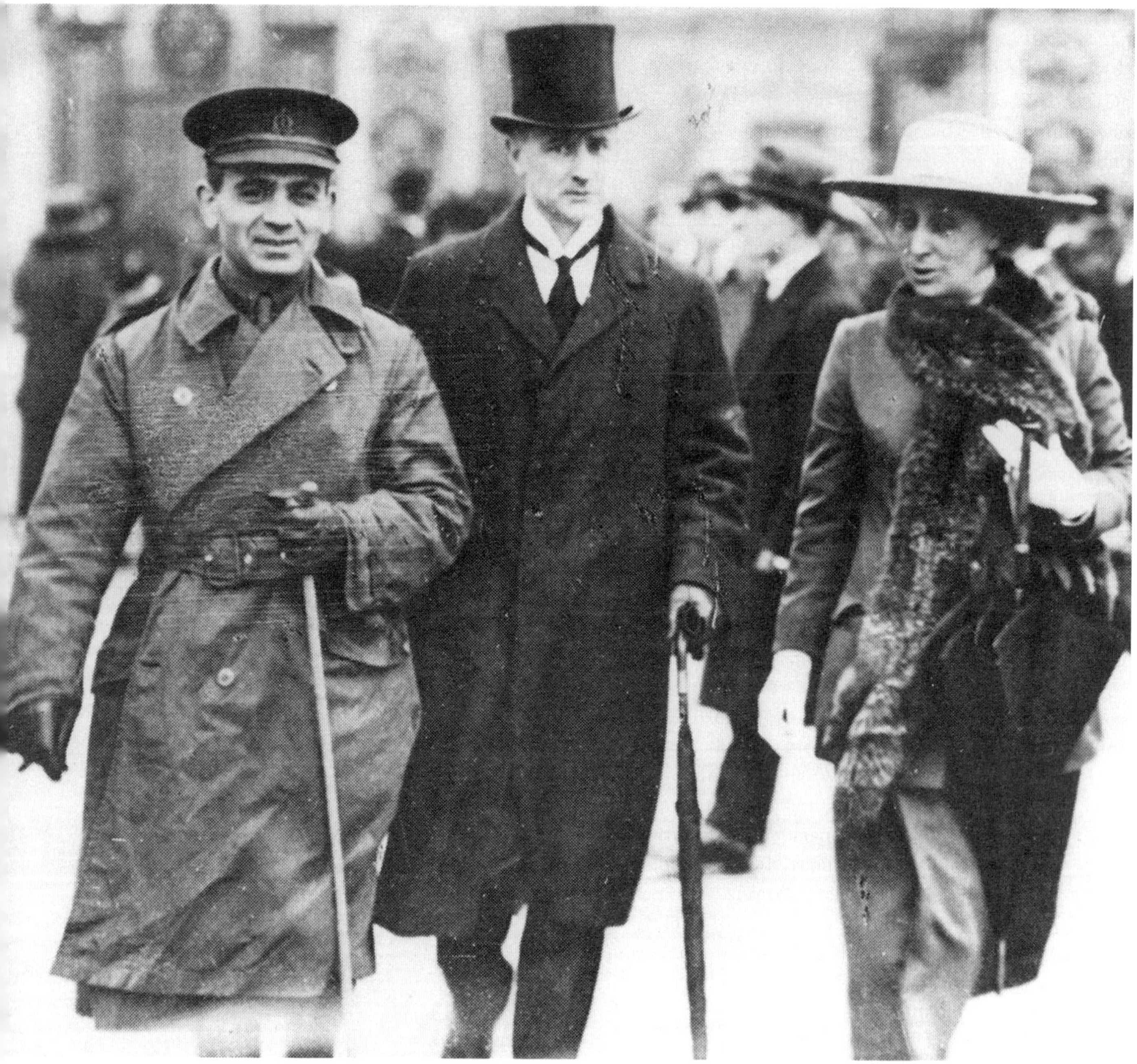

Major Kazanjian accompanied by Dr. and Mrs. W. Warwick James following the ceremony in Buckingham Palace of his investure as a Companion of the Most Distinguished Order of St. Michael and St. George March 15, 1919
The Harvard Medical Library in the Francis A. Countway Library of Medicine

Boston. On February 14, a public reception in honor of the members of the Harvard Unit was held at the Boston Opera House, at which the homecoming address was delivered by Lt. Col. Herbert H. White.[4]

Mailed just before boarding the S.S. *Megantic*, Dr. Brigham's farewell letter to his chief expressed his concern that there be "no obstacles to yourself and Mrs. Kazanjian." He must have known that Sophie Kazanjian was pregnant. Early in February the Kazanjians were in Paris, where she was examined by an American physician, Capt. Francis C. O'Neill, who was serving with the American Red Cross. His letter ominously reported:

> *This is to certify that Mrs. V. H. Kazanjian, wife of Major V. H. Kazanjian, has been a patient under my professional care for the past three weeks. She has so far recovered as to be able to travel to Switzerland, where I have ordered her to proceed during her convalescence, a period of perhaps three weeks. Mrs. Kazanjian is now in the middle of her 4th month of pregnancy and it is absolutely obligatory that she reaches her home in America, before the 6th month.*
>
> *Respectfully,*
> *Capt. F. C. O'Neill, A. R. C.*[5]

The Kazanjians left for Sainte-Croix, Switzerland, which was Sophie's ancestral home. They travelled via Bellegarde, France, near the border between France and Geneva. Mrs. Kazanjian was to remain for a time and rest, but Dr. Kazanjian's presence was "required" by royal command in London for one of the most extraordinary events in his life. Less than a month later, an invitation from the Lord Chamberlain in the form of a post office telegram was delivered to Dr. Kazanjian commanding his attendance "in service dress" at Buckingham Palace on March 15, 1919, at ten thirty in the morning. The honorable and royal occasion was to be his investiture by King

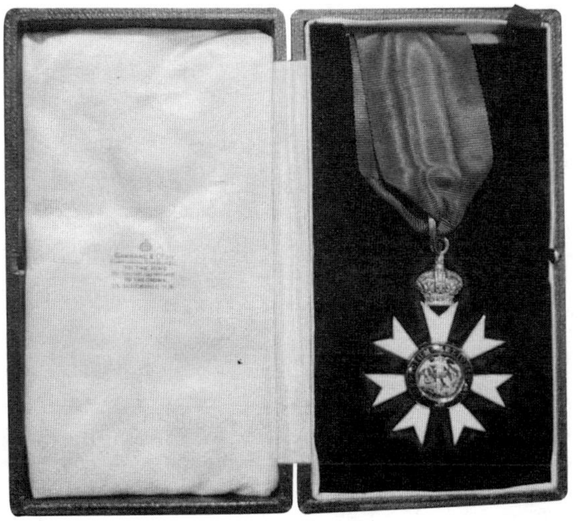

The badge of the Most Distinguished Order of St. Michael and St. George
Loaned by the Kazanjian family H MS c51
Photograph by Dr. Paul Davis

George V as a Companion of the Most Distinguished Order of Saint Michael and Saint George, a lesser knighthood but nonetheless the highest honor that the British Empire could bestow upon a person who was not a British subject.[6]

The motto of the Order was *Auspicium Melioris Aevi*—"an omen of a better age." The badge shows a seven-pointed star with a representation of the Archangel Saint Michael holding a flaming sword and trampling upon Satan, and on its reverse a representation of Saint George on horseback and in armor, with a spear, encountering a dragon. The order, founded in 1818 by the prince regent, who afterwards became King George IV, ranks in the hierarchy of British knighthood between the "most exalted" Order of the Star of India and the "most eminent" Order of the Indian Empire.[7]

The Royal Warrant granting the dignity of Companion of the Order was addressed to "our trusty and well beloved Varaztad H. Kazanjian, Esquire." who was identified as "Temporary Honorary Major of Our Army, Harvard Unit, attached to No. 20 General Hospital, Royal Army

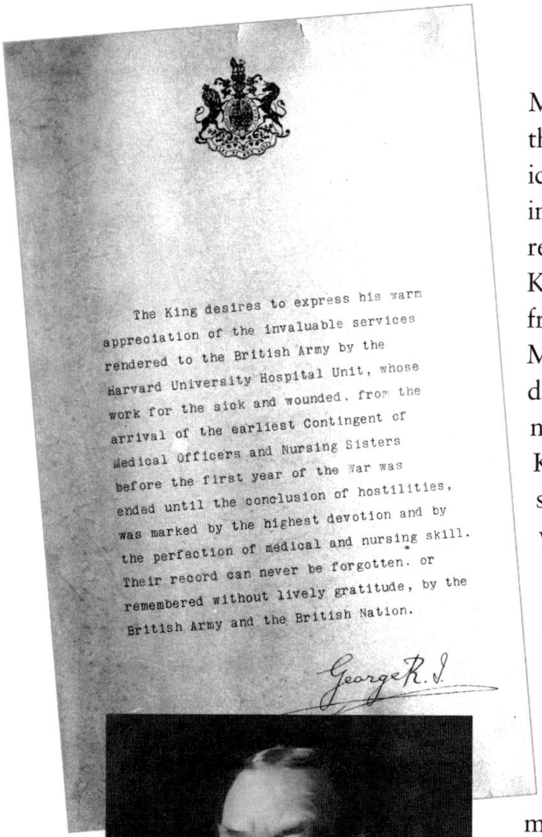

The King desires to express his warm appreciation of the invaluable services rendered to the British Army by the Harvard University Hospital Unit, whose work for the sick and wounded, from the arrival of the earliest Contingent of Medical Officers and Nursing Sisters before the first year of the War was ended until the conclusion of hostilities, was marked by the highest devotion and by the perfection of medical and nursing skill. Their record can never be forgotten, or remembered without lively gratitude, by the British Army and the British Nation.

George R. I.

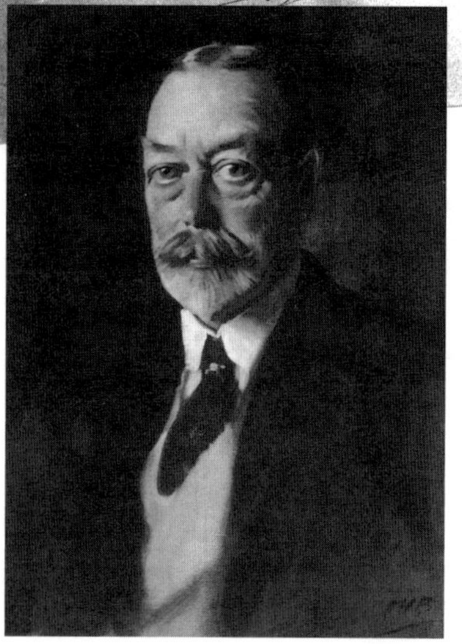

Above: *King George V's proclamation October 10, 1919. "Their record can never be forgotten or remembered without lively gratitude." The Harvard Medical Library in the Francis A. Countway Library of Medicine*

Below: *King George V By Sir Oswald Birley, oil on canvas, ID no. 4013, National Portrait Gallery, London*

Medical Corps." A newspaperman observed that the honorees "who thus met King George, face to face, were impressed by his democratic manner and his cordiality. He gave evidence of a good memory, for in many cases he spoke of some incident connected with the service rendered by the person whom he was decorating." Accompanying Dr. Kazanjian to the ceremony in Buckingham Palace was his British friend and colleague, W. Warwick James, and Mrs. James. Back in Massachusetts, Dr. Kazanjian's sister, Nouvart Roopenian, and her daughter, Flora, were in a South Boston movie theater watching a newsreel. It portrayed a wartime medical officer being honored by King George V. "That's my brother! That's my brother!" Nouvart shouted. "Had Dr. Kazanjian been a British subject," it was said, "he would be known to us today as Sir Varaztad."[8]

"I tried to get decorations for my assistants," Dr. Kazanjian professed. "They did fully as much as I in the work." He felt that Brigham's accomplishments in maxillofacial and jaw surgery were exceptional. "During the entire period," Dr. Kazanjian acknowledged, "he was my right-hand man, and though just out of dental school, showed great skill and resourcefulness . . . and during my absences from the hospital . . . he conducted the department." Dr. Kazanjian also paid tribute to Dr. Brigham's skill "in the development of the mechanical appliances used" and his assistance "in the compilation of the various articles for publication." Dr. Brigham never forgot "the daily life of our Harvard Unit," and he longingly reminisced years later, "Ironically, one might wish to live again in such a community."[9]

"It was the great need at the time that evolved the techniques that made it possible for injured men to speak again, to look something like they had before," Dr. Kazanjian characteristically stated as he diverted attention from himself. "Take the need, add patience and hope, and resourcefulness, and you have the ingredients that bring the surgeon to success in most cases of shattered jaws, paralyzed tongues, or noses shot away." Dr. Kazanjian continued, "As I look back upon those busy days, it is apparent that the principles and methods evolved during World War I for the treatment of maxillofacial injuries had far reaching influence on the surgical treatment of civilian injuries and of acquired and congenital deformities of the face and jaw as well as of other parts of the body." *The New York Times* in 1918 reported, "Science advanced half a century in four years. The war has taught us how to save more lives than the war has cost."[10]

Dr. and Mrs. Kazanjian left Boulogne on April 16, 1919, and after stopping in Paris until the 19th, they travelled via Lyon to

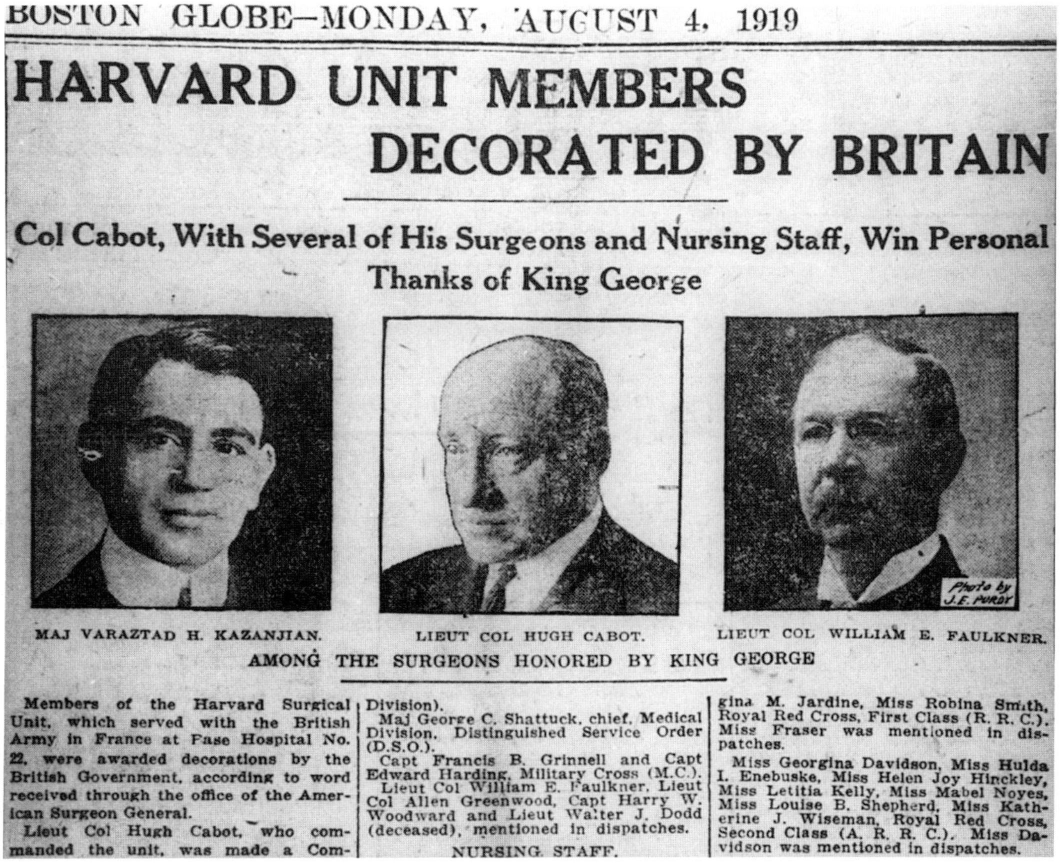

BOSTON GLOBE—MONDAY, AUGUST 4, 1919

HARVARD UNIT MEMBERS DECORATED BY BRITAIN

Col Cabot, With Several of His Surgeons and Nursing Staff, Win Personal Thanks of King George

MAJ VARAZTAD H. KAZANJIAN. LIEUT COL HUGH CABOT. LIEUT COL WILLIAM E. FAULKNER.

AMONG THE SURGEONS HONORED BY KING GEORGE

Members of the Harvard Surgical Unit, which served with the British Army in France at Fase Hospital No. 22, were awarded decorations by the British Government, according to word received through the office of the American Surgeon General.

Lieut Col Hugh Cabot, who commanded the unit, was made a Com- Division).

Maj George C. Shattuck, chief, Medical Division, Distinguished Service Order (D.S.O.).

Capt Francis B. Grinnell and Capt Edward Harding, Military Cross (M.C.).

Lieut Col William E. Faulkner, Lieut Col Allen Greenwood, Capt Harry W. Woodward and Lieut Walter J. Dodd (deceased), mentioned in dispatches.

NURSING STAFF.

gina M. Jardine, Miss Robina Smith, Royal Red Cross, First Class (R. R. C.). Miss Fraser was mentioned in dispatches.

Miss Georgina Davidson, Miss Hulda I. Enebuske, Miss Helen Joy Hinckley, Miss Letitia Kelly, Miss Mabel Noyes, Miss Louise B. Shepherd, Miss Katherine J. Wiseman, Royal Red Cross, Second Class (A. R. R. C.). Miss Davidson was mentioned in dispatches.

Boston Globe, August 4, 1919
The Harvard Medical Library in the Francis A. Countway Library of Medicine

Marseille. On April 24 they boarded the ship *Patria* bound for New York. Still Dean of Harvard Dental School when Dr. Kazanjian returned to Boston, Dr. Eugene Smith was eager to bestow all honors in his power. Through Dean Smith's efforts, on October 1, 1918, the President and Fellows of Harvard College had elected Dr. Kazanjian Professor of Military Oral Surgery while he was still in France, and granted him a leave of absence without salary. This election recognized a remarkable transition, as Dr. Kazanjian's departure from Harvard in 1915 was as head of the Department of Prosthetic Dentistry. He had become a surgeon the long and arduous way. His war experiences had determined "inexorably" the future direction of his career—toward surgery.[11]

In Boston Dr. and Mrs. Kazanjian lived at 25 Hemenway Street, which was also the address of Mrs. Kazanjian's sister, Ida, and her husband, Victor de Bellefroid, the riding master.[12]

While in France Dr. Kazanjian had found a dog "in the war front trenches, homeless and unclaimed." He brought the dog back with him and placed him in the home of another one of Mrs. Kazanjian's sisters, Georgine Malcom, who lived in Belmont, a suburb of Boston. The dog, a mixture of spaniel and Irish setter, made the newspapers when he was reported missing and later

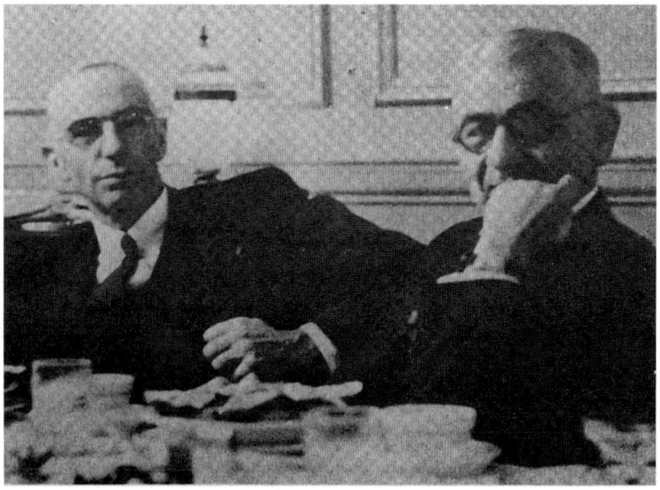

Dr. Robert H. Ivy and Dr. Kazanjian
The Harvard Medical Library in the Francis A. Countway Library of Medicine

found: the dog was described as "bright and intelligent, so much so that he understands both French and English."[13]

In early June, 1919, Dr. Kazanjian delivered a paper, "Prosthetic Appliances in Surgical Treatment of Wounds of the Face and Jaws," before the Section of Stomatology of the American Medical Association at the Association's meeting in Atlantic City, New Jersey. It received an immensely favorable response not only for its content and for its finely executed drawings of his complex appliances, but also by reason of the personality of its author. Gathered together for the first time in the audience were the very surgeons who had treated facial war wounds in the American, Canadian, and British Armies.[14] Among them was Dr. Robert H. Ivy, another outstanding pioneer in plastic surgery, who also delivered a paper and who recalled that occasion thirty-two years later:

> *At that time everyone, like myself, was impressed by the simple modesty of this man who had already achieved so much and who in the years to come was destined to add to his laurels as an outstanding teacher and surgeon. We had been fast friends for thirty-two years and at our rather infrequent meetings I have never failed to obtain something valuable from association with him.*[15]

Dr. Kazanjian was honored as a war hero by the Harvard Dental Alumni Association, as it honored all alumni who served humanity in the war. The occasion was both impressive and elegant. It was held at the Boston City Club on June 18, 1919. The speakers included Harvard President Emeritus Charles W. Eliot, Dean Smith, and Dr. Potter. "We were willing to chance our lives with the millions who were standing fast to prevent the advance of the enemy," Dr. Kazanjian declared. "Throughout the period of our service overseas," the Association "constantly gave moral and material aid, and encouraged us in many dark and trying hours."[16]

At this time Dr. Kazanjian was considering returning to Europe to practice dental surgery in England. During the summer of 1919 he corresponded with the General Council of Medical Education and Registration in London: "I expect to be in England and Europe in the summer of 1920 and would like to make the necessary preparations," he wrote. He anticipated that he would be "admitted to the final examination for license in Dental Surgery without further certificates." The British had always held Dr. Kazanjian in high esteem and they regarded him with deep affection. Dr. John Converse, who had studied under Dr. Kazanjian, relates an incident illustrating the devotion that the British had for his mentor. During World War II Dr. Converse was with a group of surgeons at a reception in London during a deafening air-raid. While "the anti-aircraft guns were blasting away," he recounted. "Sir Harold Gillies was there. No one could hear. I introduced myself: the magic word 'Kazanjian' penetrated through the din."[17]

In October 1919, Boston University School of Medicine admitted Dr. Kazanjian into the third year class that was being enrolled. He had been credited for the first and second years there "without hindrances or condition." Dr. Kazanjian also applied to the Harvard Medical School for admission as a third year student. "My purpose in studying medicine is to prepare myself to practice oral and facial surgery, a specialty in which I am deeply interested," he wrote in his letter to the assistant dean. He made it clear that he planned to continue his private practice while a medical student. It seems obvious, in retrospect, that pursuing a medical education was a necessary step he had to take at that time if he was to continue doing the work he had begun in France under the exigencies of wartime conditions, which could not be carried over to peacetime practice without the credentials of a medical degree. Otherwise, he simply would not be allowed to work outside of the traditional area restricted to the dentist—the mouth—at least in America.[18]

Sophie Kazanjian's time had come for the delivery of their child, and she was admitted to the Massachusetts Homeopathic Hospital on August 4, 1919. The following day a Caesarian section was performed, and a daughter, Hélène, was born. The days that followed were fateful to the extreme. Sophie Kazanjian's condition became increasingly grave; peritonitis had developed, which was further complicated by acute myocarditis. She failed and died five days later, on August 10. The premature and sudden loss of his wife was the utmost tragedy that could befall Dr. Kazanjian. He was deeply in love with Sophie. Not yet thirty-four years old, she was in the prime of her life. Dr. Edward Malcom, who was a child at the time, retained the memory of "the hushed shock of it all" when his aunt Sophie died. She was a person who was "very strong in character."[19] President Lowell, of Harvard University, wrote:

> *"I was very much grieved to hear of your wife's death. I know how closely bound together you were, and how she was everything to you. One would like to bring a little comfort to you in your desolation if it were possible. There are multitudes of men to whom you have made life bearable who would like to do so, and who must be feeling intense sympathy with you, if in their distant homes they knew of your bereavement. I hope the child will grow to be a consolation to you, as you abundantly deserve."*[20]

Dorothy Brierly wrote from England: "Your dear little wife was always so awfully kind to us all, and was a very favorite with everyone," Brierly had worked with Dr. Kazanjian in France as a nurse or aide. "We always thought how devoted you were to each other." Lilla Simpson wrote: "She was always so full of life and happiness. I like to think of her as she was at the chateau, always interested in us and our doings, and always so sympathetic. I was very fond of her—indeed we all were." Simpson asked for a photograph "to have some tangible remembrance." The new-born daughter, Hélène, was initially cared for by Victor and Ida de Bellefroid, who had no children of their own.[21]

Notwithstanding the difficult and painful circumstances of his life at the time, in the fall of 1919, when he was forty years old, Dr. Kazanjian matriculated at medical school for the second time in his life. This time it was at Harvard, where he was admitted as a member of the third year class. "Harvard was wise," Dr. John W. Cooke observed, "but not over-generous in accepting him." It must have seemed so anti-climactic and paradoxical to him. He became simultaneously a medical student, a professor, and a practitioner—an arduous, fatiguing, and demanding undertaking. His innate qualities of perseverance, "steady endeavor," and a "fierce determination to excel—the heritage of the persecuted"—prevailed. "Self pity," he once asserted, "has no place in the aggressive mind."[22]

After he had been in medical school for about six months, Dr. Kazanjian was called to Washington, D.C. on a political mission to help plead the cause of Armenia before the United

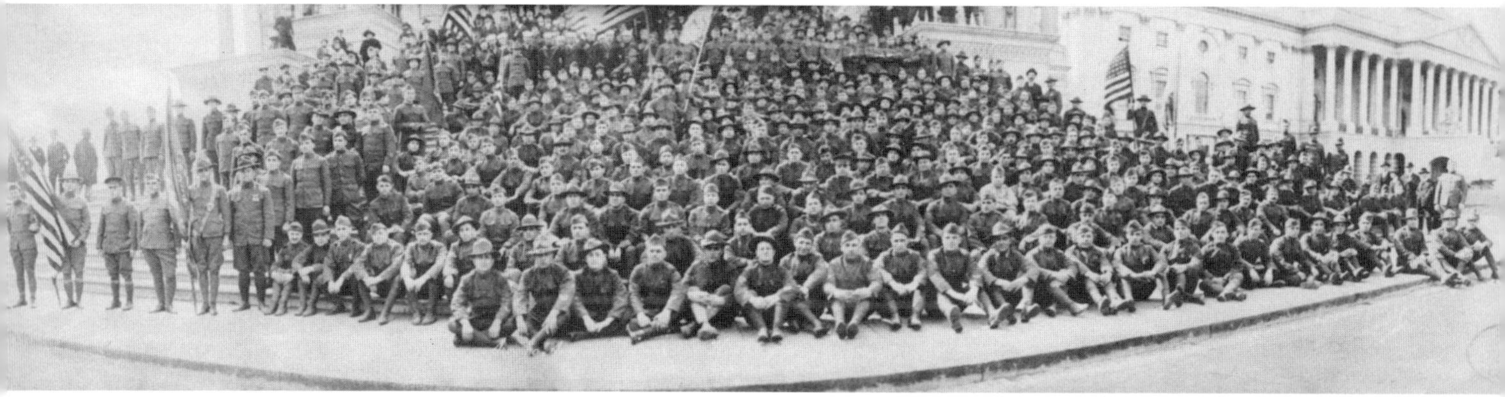

Armeno-American veterans, Washington, D.C., April 14, 1920
Photograph by S. Arakelyan, Cambridge, Mass.
Courtesy Armenian Library and Museum of America., Watertown, Mass.

States government. On April 14, 1920, a delegation of some 500 members of the World War I Union of American Veterans of Armenian Birth assembled on the steps of the Capitol, in uniform. On that day a strongly worded memorial petition was presented to the President of the United States and to Congress calling for the official recognition of the Republic of Armenia, which had gained its independence in 1918. The spokesman for the delegation was Dr. Varaztad H. Kazanjian.[23]

Senator Henry Cabot Lodge, the Chairman of the Committee on Foreign Relations had the entire memorial read to the Senate and reproduced it in the *Congressional Record*. It said in part:

> *We, therefore, respectfully urge our Government to take the necessary measures for the immediate protection of the Armenian people, now in imminent danger, to furnish them with adequate means of self-defense, and to provide them with facilities for the repatriation of the Armenian people, so that they may resume their normal life, and to extend immediate recognition to the republic of Armenia, already in existence.*[24]

On April 23, 1920, the United States formally recognized the Armenian Republic as a de facto government. Dr. Kazanjian's support and prestige had been vital to the success of the undertaking. The Allies had previously granted recognition on January 23, 1920.[25]

Back in medical school, Dr. Kazanjian was understandably quieter than usual and was "saddened and discouraged" by the loss of his wife. To his fellow medical students, he was "just a quiet dentist seeking a medical degree, and nothing more." Characteristically, he never volunteered information about himself and apparently was never asked.[26] His position and stature were dramatically changed with a rather singular and unforeseen incident, which occurred in his second and final year a few months before his graduation. A clinic for medical students was being held at the surgical amphitheater of the Peter Bent Brigham Hospital. It was a most impressive occasion, since the demonstration was being conducted by two distinguished visiting British surgeons.

As the demonstration was proceeding, one surgeon in glancing up at the assembled students paused in disbelief for a fraction of a second and, firmly grasping the arm of his partner, pointed directly at one of the students. These two British surgeons "with greater haste than dignity" rushed up and physically dragged "the quiet, black haired little dentist" down the stairs of the amphitheater. Kazanjian was presented as the one who had taught the British surgeons the very technical skills that they were demonstrating. "I remember vividly the episode," Dr. James H. Townsend, one of his classmates, related. "From then on he was our class hero." The scene was also recounted by William B. Castle, later of "intrinsic-extrinsic factor" fame, who was also in the Class of 1921. Dr. John W. Cooke described this as "just one more in a long list of experiences" that he had never heard Kazanjian mention.[27]

While the identity of the British surgeons cannot be confirmed, as the clinic was an informal affair, two strong possibilities suggest themselves: Dr. George E. Gask, professor of surgery in London University and until recently Colonel R.A.M.C., and Sir Robert Jones of Liverpool. Dr. Gask served as Visiting Surgeon Pro-Tempore at the Peter Bent Brigham Hospital from March 20 to April 3, 1921. He lived in the resident quarters and was "on intimate terms with the house staff . . . . His visit will be long remembered, for it made a bright spot in the year's work," Harvey Cushing wrote in the annual report of the Brigham Hospital for 1921. Gask was stationed at General Hospital No. 7 at St. Omer, near Boulogne, during the war. He and Cushing were friendly. Gask's specialty was the treatment of wounds of the chest and lungs. "Gask was not only an extremely able surgeon and a man of imperturbable character, he was moved by a deep sense of mission to improve the education of younger surgeons." He was created a

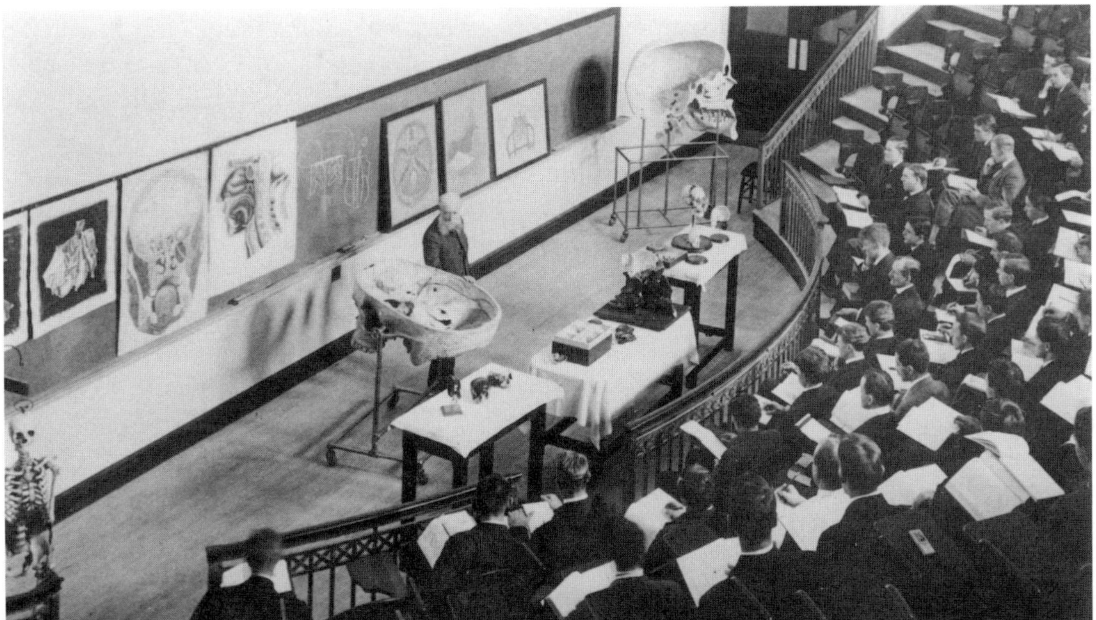

Amphitheater with Dr. Thomas Dwight (1843-1911) lecturing students at Harvard Medical School. This might well have been the amphitheater where the visiting British surgeons recognized Dr. Kazanjian. The Harvard Medical Library in the Francis A. Countway Library of Medicine

Companion of the Order of Saint Michael and Saint George in 1919, the same year in which Dr. Kazanjian was so honored. Sir Robert Jones was in New York in October 1919, where he addressed the Clinical Congress of the American College of Surgeons, and was a frequent visitor to the States. He served as major general in the war as an inspector of military orthopedics.[28] As a result of this incident, the patterns of Dr. Kazanjian's life were repeated. One moment he was quietly unnoticed in the background; the next he was a hero.

While still in medical school, Dr. Kazanjian was appointed lecturer in the Harvard-Forsyth Post-Graduate School of Orthodontia (1919-20). The Trustees of Peter Bent Brigham Hospital appointed him Dental Surgeon in 1920, an office he resigned in 1922, and the Boston City Hospital appointed him Visiting Surgeon for Oral and Plastic Surgery on February 4, 1921. Even as a medical student, Kazanjian maintained his position as Professor of Military Oral Surgery in the faculty of medicine and is so listed in the Announcement of the Medical School of Harvard University for 1919-20. His home address was 25 Hemenway Street in Boston. The Harvard Dental School class of 1921 dedicated their yearbook, *The Mirror*, to him "in acknowledgment of his miraculous work in the world war and the added respect his work brought to the dental profession." During his spare time while in medical school "he is treating special surgical cases at the [dental] school."[29]

Among his teachers in medical school were many faculty members whose lives had touched his, particularly during the war. Professor Lowell was still Harvard President; Dr. Eugene H. Smith was still Dean of the Dental School; Dr. Harvey Cushing was Mosley Professor of Surgery; Dr. William H. Potter was Professor of Operative Dentistry; Dr. Edward H. Nichols was Professor of Clinical Surgery; Dr. David Cheever was Assistant Professor of Surgery; and Dr. Maynard Ladd was Instructor of Pediatrics. Dr. Walter B. Cannon was the George Higginson Professor of Physiology at the Harvard Medical School while Dr. Kazanjian was a student. Professor Cannon had been in France in 1917 where he was "unravelling the mystery of shock." He was in Camiers and at Base Hospital No. 5 for a period of time and had been in contact with Dr. Harvey Cushing. There is no information to indicate that Drs. Cannon and Kazanjian met in France in 1917, although it is possible.[30]

Kazanjian became "the class hero" to his fellow classmates of 1921. "Fifteen years older than the rest of us," his classmates stated, "he was a friendly avuncular figure of true distinction." In the years after graduation, he kept up his cordial relationship with his classmates who observed, "Kay and Marion [Kazanjian's second wife] have added wonderfully to the spirit of our incisive five year reunions, including our climactic 50th by entertaining all of us in a warm and friendly relationship in their lovely home in Belmont."[31]

The 280th commencement of Harvard University was held on June 23, 1921. It was a "particularly humid day." Dr. Kazanjian was among the ninety-eight students awarded the degree of Doctor of Medicine—Medicinae Doctor. Madame Marie Curie was present and welcomed on June 20, but Harvard had not honored her with a degree as had Yale and other institutions. One of the persons upon whom the degree of Doctor of Science was conferred was Sir Robert Jones, "the orthopedic surgeon who patiently and silently showed the way to restore the usefulness and comfort of the cripples of the war."[32]

In 1921, Kazanjian established a private practice in Boston at 400 Marlborough Street in plastic surgery of the face, surgical prosthesis and oral surgery. He had gained proficiency in surgery "in the hard school through the slippery fingers of blood,"[33] but he needed the authority of an M.D. degree. The medical degree that was awarded Dr. Kazanjian was a key that would open many doors in his future.

NOTES

1 *The [London] Times*, February 4. 1919; Richard Locke Hapgood, *History of the Harvard Dental School* (Peterboro, N. H.: Transcript Printing Co., 1930), p. 128. A letter from the Headquarters of R. A. M. C., dated January 14, 1919, attests that Major Kazanjian had satisfactorily completed his service "and ceased duty on the hospital being closed," (V. H. Kazanjian Archive in The Francis A. Countway Library of Medicine, folder PAM-21.) Ferdinand Brigham, "Harvard Goes to War," *Harvard Dental Alumni Bulletin* 24, no. 4 (1964): 103, relates that an estimate of the total number of patients who passed through his hands was 2,500, while Hapgood, *Harvard Dental School*, sets the number at 3,000. See also "Special Awards of the American Society of Plastic and Reconstructive Surgery, and of the Foundation of the Society of Plastic and Reconstructive Surgery," *Plastic and Reconstructive Surgery* 9, no. 4 (April 1952): 290-299.

2 *Massachusetts General Hospital, Memorial and Historical Volume* (Boston 1921), p. 74 (Base Hospital No. 6 was a distinctively Massachusetts General Hospital unit.); Benjamin Castleman, David C. Crockett, and S. B. Sutton, eds. *The Massachusetts General Hospital, 1955-1980* (Boston: Little, Brown, 1983) p. 233; Letter from Lt. Gen. C. H. Burtchaell, General Headquarters, British Armies in France, to V. H. Kazanjian, March 26, 1919, in the Kazanjian Archive, Section IV. General Sir Charles H. Burtchaell succeeded General Sir Arthur Sloggett as Director General of the Medical Services, British Armies in active service (Harvey Cushing, *From A Surgeon's Journal* [Boston: Little Brown, 1936], p. 363); W. G. Macthlerson, *Medical Services General History* (London: His Majesty's Stationery Office, 1923), contains information on the transfer of command of D.G.M.S.

3 *Boston Herald*, January 31, 1919, Extra edition, p. 3, col. 1. Lt. Gen. Sir Thomas H. Goodwin succeeded Lt. Gen. Sir Alfred Keogh as Director General, Royal Army Medical Service, late in the war. Earlier he had been in charge of a neighboring hospital to No. 22. Admiral Sir Guy Gaunt was the representative to the United States of the Director of Naval Intelligence for Great Britain. Also, Hapgood, *Harvard Dental School*, pp. 128-129; Proclamation by King George V, October 10. 1919, in the Kazanjian Archive, PAM-14; Communication dated January 31, 1919 from Field Marshall Haig to the Secretary, London War Office, commending "the valuable services rendered by the Harvard University Hospital," from the Army General Headquarters, Kazanjian Archive, PAM-21; Letter from Arthur J. Balfour to Woodrow Wilson, December 18, 1918, Kazanjian Archive, folder C-464.

4 Letters from Dr. Ferdinand Brigham to "Dear Old K," the first one undated, but probably January 20, 1919, and the second dated February 5, 1919, Kazanjian Archive, folders C-42 and C-43; *Boston Herald*, January 31, 1919.

5 Letter from Dr. F. C. O'Neill, "Médecin-en-Chef du Comité Franco-Américain pour la Protection des Enfants de la Frontière," February 14, 1919, Kazanjian Archive, folder C-501. It is on American Red Cross stationery.

6 Letter from the United States Passport Bureau, Paris, February 11, 1919 (in French), Kazanjian Archive, folder C-840. The Kazanjian Archive (folder PAM-14) contains a copy of the post office telegram, the ticket admitting the bearer to Buckingham Palace, a copy of Dr. Kazanjian's Royal Warrant of the Order, and the Statutes of Most Distinguished Order of Saint Michael and Saint George.

7 *The Encyclopaedia Britannica,* 11th ed, v. 15, p. 861, section on knighthood. A photograph of the badge appears on p. 860.

8 The Royal Warrant was "given at our Court at Saint James . . . this third day of June, one thousand, nine hundred and eighteen," Kazanjian Archive, folder PAM-14. See also newspaper article headed "Harvard Unit Honored," Kazanjian Archive, folder PAM-21 (There is no identification as to the date or name of the newspaper, and portions of the article are missing); John Hughes, "Special Report—The Eyes of Armenia, Missions of Mercy," *The Armenian Reporter Int'l*, January 11, 1997, p. 14. Newsletter for Plastic and Reconstructive Surgery 6:2 (March 1969) p.2, col. 1.

9 Hapgood, *Harvard Dental School*, p. 129; V. H. Kazanjian, unpublished paper read before the Harvard Dental Alumni Association meeting on

June 18, 1919. A letter from V. H. Kazanjian to Herbert H. White, February 28, 1917, urging the promotion of Dr. Brigham to captain ("he deserves recognition") is in the Kazanjian Archive, folder C-446. Dr. Frederick Caldwell, the other associate, headed the section on General Dentistry. He arrived in May 1916, succeeding Dr. Frank H. Cushman, who had completed his term of service in January 1916. Dr. Caldwell remained until August 1919, six months after Dr. Kazanjian left for home. Dr. Ferdinand Brigham returned to practice dentistry in the United States in 1919, but left for France after one year and associated in Paris with Dr. Frank Stahl for twenty years. In 1940 he returned to practice in the Boston area, where he remained a close friend and collaborator of Dr. Kazanjian. He died in 1975. Also, Brigham, "Harvard Goes to War," p. 105; and Robert H. Ivy, "The Mysterious Dr. Valadier," *Plastic and Reconstructive Surgery* 74, no. 4 (1971): 369.

10 John M. Converse, "The Extraordinary Career of Dr. Varaztad Hovhannes Kazanjian," *Plastic and Reconstructive Surgery* 71, no. 1 (January 1982): 140-141; V. H. Kazanjian, "Remembrance of Things Past," *Plastic and Reconstructive Surgery* 35, no. 1 (1965): 12. The Harvard Unit of General Hospital No. 22 Association would meet for reunions until at least 1953. Also, *The New York Times*, Sunday Editorial Section, December 29, 1918, p. 4, cols, 1-6.

11 The Kazanjian Archive, folder WW-1266, contains copies of railroad tickets from Boulogne to Paris, Paris to Marseille, and embarkation slip from the ship *Patria* from Marseille to New York, April 24, 1919. See also folder C-660. In June 1922, Kazanjian was elected Professor of Clinical Oral Surgery. The official change of title was signed by Francis W. Hunnewell, Secretary, Board of Overseers, Harvard University, September 25, 1922. Also, Stephen Plumpton, "Kazanjian," *Dental Magazine and Oral Topics* 84, no. 5 (October 1967): 207.

12 *Boston Directory* 1920, p. 905, 1921, p. 941, and 1922, p. 956. Dr. Kazanjian is listed as a Professor, Harvard Medical School, residing at 25 Hemenway St., Boston. Also, *Fourteenth U. S. Bureau of the United States Census, 1920 City of Boston*, v. 107, ed (enumeration district) 198, sheet 13, line 83 lists him and his five-month-old daughter, Hélène, as a lodger at 25 Hemenway Street, Boston.

13 A newspaper article headed "Dog From Trenches Understands Both French and English," with no further identification except the year 1919, is in the Kazanjian Archive, folder M-24.

14 Official program of the Scientific Assembly of the Seventieth Annual Session of the American Medical Association, Atlantic City, June 10-13, 1919. Section of Stomatology, pp. 87-90. Dr. Kazanjian's paper was delivered on June 13 and published in the *Journal of the American Medical Association* 73, no, 17 (October 25, 1919): 1265-1271, and in the *Dental Summary,* as noted in the previous chapter. The papers delivered in the Section were discussed (pp. 933-934) by Dr. V. P. Blair, who wrote, "The work of Dr. Kazanjian was known to all of the Allies. . . . It is impossible to give an intelligent discussion, in the 400 words allotted, of the vast amount of work he has presented." Dr. C. W. Waldron and Dr. Fred H. Albee were the other discussants. Dr. Kazanjian was back in Atlantic City a month later, where he delivered his paper, "Observations on War Surgery of the Facc and Jaws," before the New Jersey State Dental Society which met July 16-18. The paper was published in *Dental Cosmos* (March 1920): 3-15. Also, Robert H. Ivy, *A Link with the Past* (Baltimore: Williams & Wilkins, 1962), p. 49. Information on the Section on Stomatology of the American Medical Association can be found in the taped interviews with Dr. Robert Ivy conducted by Dr. Robin Anderson in 1970, and by Dr. Leo Bernstein on May 24, 1971, National Archive of Plastic Surgery in The Francis A. Countway Library of Medicine. Dr. Ivy chaired the Section of Stomatology in 1923-24. It ceased to function in 1926.

15 "Special Awards of the American Society of Plastic and Reconstructive Surgery, and of the Foundation of the Society of Plastic and Reconstructive Surgery," p. 299. It was at the Atlantic City meeting in 1919, Dr. Ivy wrote in *A Link with the Past* (p. 49), that he first met V. H. Kazanjian, and others who became lifelong friends.

16 A copy of the Program of the Harvard Dental Alumni Association's forty- eighth banquet, June 18, 1919, is in the Kazanjian Archive, folder C-662. See also, V. H. Kazanjian, Unpublished paper read before the Harvard Dental Alumni Association, June 18, 1919.

17 V. H. Kazanjian, letters to Registrar General of the General Council of Medical Education and Registration of the United Kingdom, 30 May 1919 and 3 July 1919, and to Frederick G. Hallett, Director of Examinations, Royal College of Surgeons, July 3, 1919, in the Kazanjian Archive, folders C-649 and C-767. "Some people frankly say that they never expected to see you back," letter from Dr. Ferdinand Brigham to "Dear Old K," dated Feb. 5. 1919. John Marquis Converse, *Kazanjian & Converse's Surgical Treatment of Facial Injuries*, (Baltimore: Williams & Wilkins, 1974) 3rd ed., v. 1, p. ix.

18 Letters to V. H. Kazanjian from Registrar, Boston University School of Medicine, 6 September 1912—24 July 1919, and letter from V. H. Kazanjian to Worth Hale, M.D., Assistant Dean, Harvard Medical School, dated July 10, 1919. in the Kazanjian Archive, folders C-607 and C-667.

19 Standard Certificate of Death, Commonwealth of Massachusetts Register No. 7823, filed August 14, 1919, E. W. M. Glenen, Registrar. Funeral services for Sophie Kazanjian were held at Appleton Chapel, Harvard University, Cambridge, Massachusetts, on August 13, 1919, with interment at Mount Auburn Cemetery. *Boston Globe*, August 12, 1919, p. 5, col 2; M. Verazin, "Professor Varaztad H. Kazanjian: His Surgery During the Great War," *Hairenik Monthly* 8, no. 2/95 (Sept. 1930): 162-163 (in Armenian); Interview of author with Dr. Edward Malcom, August 5, 1995, Boothbay Harbor, Maine, in the author's possession.

20 Letter from A. Lawrence Lowell to V. H. Kazanjian dated August 16, 1919, Kazanjian Archive, folder C-264.

21 Letters from Dorothy S. Brierly to "My dear Major Kazanjian," dated February 1, 1920, from Yorkshire, England, and from Lilla Simpson to Major V. H. Kazanjian, December 31, 1919, Kazanjian Archive, folders C-41 and C-389; letter from Dr. Edward Malcom to the author, Boothbay, Maine, November 28, 1994.

22 John W. Cooke, "Kazanjian and Harvard," *Harvard Dental Alumni Bulletin* 3, no. 2 (January 1943): 26. The announcement of the Medical School of Harvard University for 1919-20, p. 13, lists Kazanjian as Professor of Military Oral Surgery residing at 25 Hemenway Street, Boston; Plumpton "Kazanjian," p. 207; Ivan Sandrof, "World's Most Famous Plastic Surgeon," *Worcester Sunday Telegram*, January 12, 1958, Feature Parade section, p. 3; Avedis Derounian, "Noted Surgeon Prescribes Industry," *Armenian Spectator*, February 7, 1935.

23 *New York Times*, April 15, 1920, p. 10, col. 7.

24 *Congressional Record*, April 12, 1920, Senate no. 5644 and 5645, contain the entire memorial petition.

25 *New York Times*, April 24, 1920, p. 1, col. 2; Gregory Aftandilian, *Armenia: Vision of a Republic, The Independence Lobby in America* (Boston: Charles River Press, 1981), p. 43.

26 Cooke, "Kazanjian and Harvard," p. 26.

27 In "Kazanjian and Harvard," John Cooke writes that Dr. Harvey Cushing was present, "accompanied by two high-ranking officers from the Royal Army Medical Corps." John M. Converse, "The Extraordinary Career of Varaztad H. Kazanjian," *Plastic and Reconstructive Surgery* 71, no. 1, (January 1982): ix, states that "Dr. Cushing's guests were Sir William Osler and Sir Robert Jones." However, Sir William had died in late 1919, although Jones, who died in 1933, is a likely candidate. Also, Walter C. Guralnick, et al., "V. H. Kazanjian, A Pioneer in Dentistry and Plastic Surgery," *Harvard University Gazette*, May 2, 1975, p. 9. This was "the official faculty minute." Guralnick, in "Varaztad H. Kazanjian, M. D.," *New England Journal of Medicine* 292, no. 15 (April 10, 1975): 807, quotes William B. Castle as saying: A distinguished visiting British surgeon was discussing a case of severe facial injury. He remarked that he wished that he could have the benefit of Kazanjian's opinion. Whereupon, urged by adjacent classmates, to our excited delight "Kay" stepped down from the ranks of the audience to the floor of the amphitheater and fulfilled the visitor's express wish.

28 Peter Bent Brigham Hospital *Eighth Annual Report for the Year 1921* (Cambridge, Mass.: University Press, 1922), pp. 62, 162; Cushing, *From a Surgeon's Journal*, pp. 329, 331, 332; John F. Fulton, *Harvey Cushing, a Biography*, (Springfield, Ill.: Thomas, 1941), p. 477. For a biographical sketch of George Ernest Gask (1875-1951), see *Plarr's Lives of the Fellows of the Royal College of Surgeons of England,* Supplement 1930-1951, by Sir D'Arcy Power and W. R. Le Fanu, pp. 314-315. Also, Robert Jones, "Joint,

Nerve and Other Injuries in War Surgery," *Surgery, Gynecology and Obstetrics* 30, no. 1 (January 1920): 1-2; and "A Few Surgical Lessons of the War," *British Medical Journal* 2, no. 12 (November 8, 1919): 587-590, addressed to the American College of Surgeons. For biographical information on Jones, see "Great Teachers of Surgery in the Past," *British Journal of Surgery* 54, no. 2 (February 1967): 85-90.

29 Letters from Alfred P. Rogers, Dean of the Harvard-Forsyth Post Graduate School of Orthodontia, to V. H. Kazanjian, undated, Kazanjian Archive, PAM-4; from J. B. Howland, Superintendent, Peter Bent Brigham Hospital to V. H. Kazanjian, February 14, 1920, folder PAM-4; V. H. Kazanjian to J. B. Howland, September 30, 1922, folder C-756; and from Thomas A. Forsyth, Secretary, Boston City Hospital to V. H. Kazanjian, February 4, 1921, folder C-601.

30 Cushing, *From a Surgeon's Journal*, p. 112; also, Saul Benison, A. Clifford Barger and Elin L. Wolfe, "Walter B. Cannon and the Mystery of Shock: A Study of Anglo-American Co-Operation in World War I," *Medical History* 35 (1919): 217-249.

31 *Harvard Medical School Class of 1921. Fifty Years in Retrospect, A Biographical History 1921-1971*, p. 28; Kazanjian Archive, folder C-666 and C-668. At the 40th reunion of the class, a silver tray inscribed as follows was presented to:

Dr. and Mrs. Varaztad Kazanjian
with love and appreciation
from your friends in the
Class of 1921
Harvard Medical School
May, 1961

32 *Harvard Alumni Bulletin* 23, no. 38 (June 30, 1921): 904-905; Harvard University Medical School, *Commencement Program*, 1921, Harvard Medical Archives in The Francis A. Countway Library of Medicine, XXI and XXII, Archives AB13:2. For biographical sketches of the members of the Class, see *Harvard Medical School Alumni* 1921. Kazanjian Archive, folder C-668. Also Harvard Medical School Class of 1921, *1921-1961 Fortieth Reunion Report* and Harvard Medical School Class of 1921, *Fifty Years in Retrospect, A Biographical History,* 1921-1971, copies of which can be found in both the Harvard Medical Archives and the Kazanjian Archive, folder C-668; *Harvard University Gazette* 16, no.39 (June 18, 1921): 187.

33 Kazanjian Archive, folder M-1. V. H. Kazanjian, "Problems of Prosthetic Restoration Following Injuries to the Face and Jaws," *Military Dental Journal* 2 (June 1922): 18, lists his address as 400 Marlborough Street, Boston. Also, Sandrof, "World"s Most Famous," p. 4.

CHAPTER NINE

The Gentle Genius of Plastic Surgery[1] V. H. Kazanjian: 1921 through World War II

The clinical materials from Dannes-Camiers—records, models, photographs, etc.—were preserved for succeeding generations by Dr. Brigham. He had carefully helped transport the material in boxes to Boston where they were soon safely "resting under lock and key in the basement of the dental school." Some of them did not remain in storage for long. Dr. Kazanjian exhibited his plaster masks, casts, and photographs of war injuries to the face and jaw in Boston at the seventy-second Annual Meeting of the American Medical Association, at which he was awarded a Certificate of Honor. He also delivered a paper before its Section on Stomatology on July 10, 1921, titled "Notes on Plastic Surgery of the Lips," which focused on gunshot injuries to the face. This was all the more remarkable as it was written while he was still a medical student.[2]

Following his graduation from medical school, Dr. Kazanjian commenced a private practice of plastic surgery in Boston, concentrating on surgery of the face, surgical prosthetics and oral surgery. As was noted in the prior chapter, in 1921 and for a few years after the war, his first office was located at 400 Marlborough Street in Boston's Back Bay. During this time he took the U.S. Civil Service Commission Physician Grade A examination and passed it successfully. By 1924, he had moved his office to 224 Commonwealth Avenue in Boston; and in 1925, and continuing for the remainder of his professional career, his office was situated at 475 Commonwealth Avenue, on tree-lined Kenmore Square in Boston's Back Bay, in a building devoted primarily to medical offices. Dr. John Converse, who began an association with Dr. Kazanjian in 1935, described it as "a modest office."[3]

As for Kazanjian's affiliation with Harvard, in 1922 his academic appointment in the dental school was changed from Professor of Military Oral Surgery to Professor of Clinical Oral Surgery,[4] and this remained his title until 1941, when he was named Harvard's first Professor of Plastic Surgery.[5] Dr. Kazanjian's first hospital appointment came in November 1921, when he was designated Graduate Assistant in the Laryngological Clinic of the Out-Patient Department of the Massachusetts General Hospital; in 1922, he was appointed Dental Surgeon at the Peter Bent Brigham Hospital; and in 1923, he was made Assistant in the Laryngological Department of the M.G.H. and appointed also to the staff of the Laryngological Department of the Massachusetts Eye and Ear Infirmary, where the resident physician was Dr. Frederick A. Washburn, whom he had previously encountered in France. In the years following, he was appointed Visiting Physician for Oral and Plastic Surgery at the Boston City Hospital (1923), Consulting Surgeon of the Cambridge City Hospital (1925), and subsequently to similar posts at several other Boston-area hospitals.

Dr. Kazanjian's long affiliation with the M.G.H. and Massachusetts Eye and Ear

Infirmary has been commented on by a later colleague, Dr. Bradford Cannon:

> *In 1922 [i.e., 1923] he joined the staff of the Eye and Ear Infirmary as a Clinical Assistant in the Department of Laryngology, and in the following years an ever-increasing number of plastic cases were treated at the Infirmary.*

The hospital's records consistently cite Dr. Kazanjian's "startling" results in treatment of face, neck, and scalp. In his annual report of 1930, Dr. Harris P. Mosher, then Chief of Laryngology at the Infirmary, reported: "Dr. Kazanjian's . . . work continues to increase in complexity and brilliance."

During this period the Plastic Clinic was established at the Massachusetts General Hospital under Dr. Kazanjian. The clinic eventually merged with the service in plastic surgery offered at the Infirmary and from that time has been a joint project of the two hospitals. Patients came to the clinic from considerable distances, for it was a pioneer of its kind in the New England area. In 1931, Dr. Kazanjian was named Surgeon for Plastic Operations at the Eye and Ear Infirmary and was Special Consultant in Plastic Surgery at the General.[6]

Dr. Kazanjian undoubtedly established very early the routine that Dr. Converse described at the time he became associated with Kazanjian in the mid-thirties, when, as he related, Dr. Kazanjian operated virtually every day of the week, including Saturdays, beginning at 8 a.m. and continuing until 1 p.m. Dr. Converse confessed that he would become "quite exhausted" on those days when he assisted, and he depicted Dr. Kazanjian's surgical ability as "astounding." Dr. Kazanjian operated "without any wasted movements," "very decisively and fast." On Saturday and Monday mornings, Dr. Kazanjian operated at the Massachusetts Eye and Ear Infirmary, when he treated "most of the clinic patients who required facial plastic surgery."

Dr. Converse once asked Dr. Kazanjian how he performed a very difficult and delicate opera-

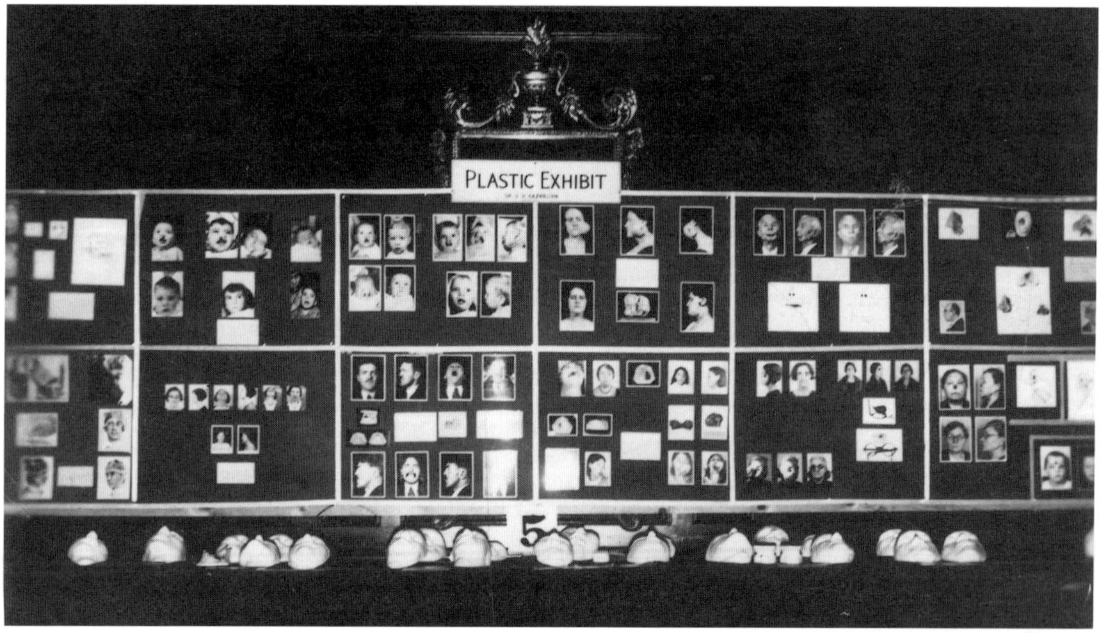

Dr. Kazanjian's exhibit at the 1921 American Medical Association annual session in Boston
The Harvard Medical Library in the Francis A. Countway Library of Medicine

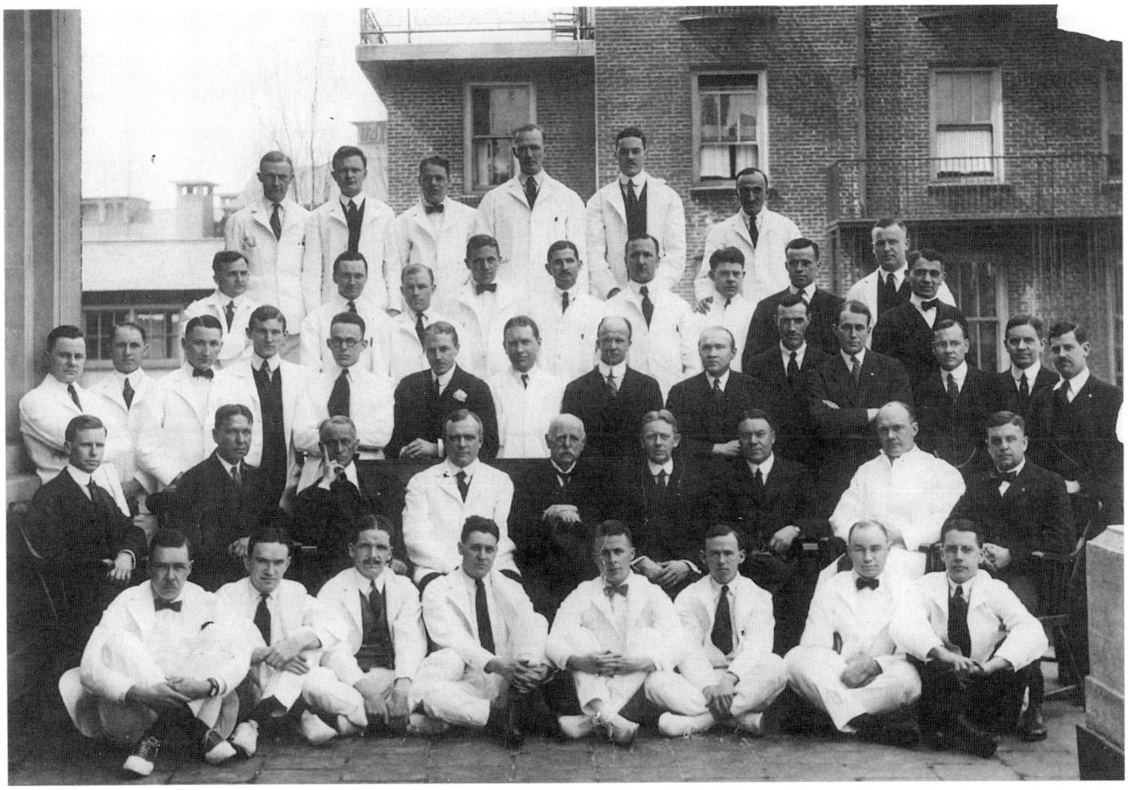

Surgical staff of the Peter Bent Brigham Hospital 1921-22.
Dr. Kazanjian is the first man on the right (with bow tie) in the second row from the top.
The Harvard Medical Library in the Francis A. Countway Library of Medicine

tion of removing a large facial birthmark, leaving "a relatively inconspicuous fine scar." Dr. Kazanjian's reply was, "You must do it just right."[7] He had not received the traditional formal surgical residency training. As a consequence, his original techniques were acquired through "observation and empiricism" and were "necessarily innovative" but "sound." He was "imaginative" and "resourceful" yet unconventional, and he continuously sought to "improvise new methods." "From a practical point of view," a later student, Dr. Richard C. Webster reported, "the Massachusetts Eye and Ear Infirmary accorded much more value to Dr. Kazanjian and his teachings, and it was in the fields of ophthalmology . . . and in otolaryngology . . . that Dr. Kazanjian was more appreciated." Otolaryngologists considered him "responsible for establishing facial surgery at the Massachusetts Eye and Ear Infirmary" and acknowledged that he is "considered by many to be the father of modern facial plastic surgery."[8]

Dr. Kazanjian's work was considered to have had a mysterious quality, an idea which he deflated. "It always amuses me that young surgeons think there is something mysterious about plastic surgery," Kazanjian asserted. "There is nothing mysterious about it. First you must know general surgery." Richard Webster felt that Dr. Kazanjian was "totally in command of the three dimensions involved in maxillofacial and prosthetic work" and that he "knew more than most men at his time about local flaps and tissue shifts." Converse recalled during his training "a group of general surgeons . . . gathering around V. H. Kazanjian to watch him cut a large split-thickness graft freehand." "That little Armenian," a number of surgeons remarked to Dr. Converse, "is really very clever." Converse attributed this patronizing mindset to "the parochial attitude by New Englanders at the time toward foreigners." It was also Dr. Kazanjian's humble nature, Converse believed, that "made it difficult for him to believe that he had risen so high in his chosen profession." The phrase Dr. Kazanjian often used, deferential in tone, to describe his feeling about the care of his patients, was "I had the privilege of treating."[9]

Dr. Kazanjian was "an outsider," Dr. Robert Goldwyn has written. "Being an outsider is not a total disadvantage," he opined, "for him . . . it is an advantage." Dr. Goldwyn points out that "the history of plastic surgery has been made by poachers and hybrids . . . those of impure pedigree." He also depicts Dr. Kazanjian's life as an allegory, a symbolic representation, of a man who not only crossed frontiers as an important immigrant but who discovered "new territory" in his specialty as well. Dr. Kazanjian "was by no means a person preoccupied with power. . . . He was all substance and no image . . . puffery was not part of his person," Dr. Goldwyn has further observed. His humility was such that "Hospital personnel who worked around him were unaware of his eminence."[10]

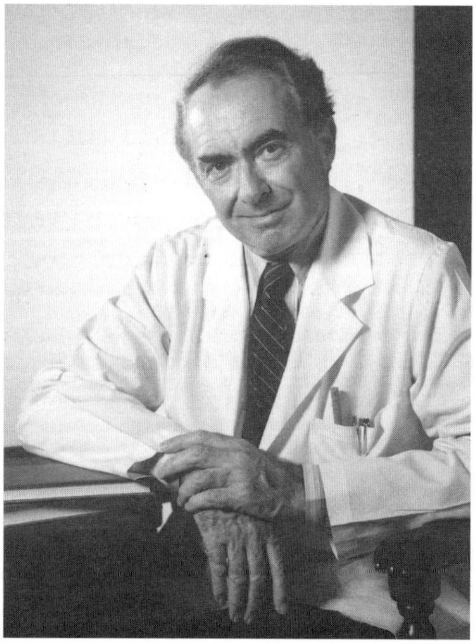

Dr. Robert M. Goldwyn
Photograph by Karsh, Ottawa, 1985

Although he possessed an excellent command of the English language, Kazanjian's speech was marked by a pronounced Armenian accent that he retained long after he lost proficiency in his native tongue.[11] This made it difficult for him to explain what he was doing during operations. Some of his colleagues tended to consider him "just a dentist," and referred to him as "Katzie" or "Kay." Dr. Converse reported that a general surgeon at M.G.H. replied to the mother of a physician who was considering specialty training in plastic surgery, "Oh yes, we used to have some sort of a dentist around here who did that type of work." This betrayed a profound "lack of appreciation by the other surgeons of what Doctor Kazanjian had accomplished." It was an expression of latent jealousy.[12]

Certain surgeons acknowledged and appreciated the advances that plastic surgery had made possible during World War I "but they had an incomprehension and a prejudiced opinion about the need for plastic surgery during peacetime." It had a "lowly reputation, a marginal status," and plastic surgeons felt that they "have had to fight hard for the modest rung of the ladder that we occupy." Even Dr. Joseph E. Murray, "after winning the Nobel Prize," was thought of primarily "as a general surgeon who had an interest in plastic surgery." Vilray Blair was once asked by his friend, Dr. Borden S. Veeder, "just what is a plastic surgeon?" Blair replied, "Just a damn fool who takes on things that no one else will."[13]

Nonetheless, when all else failed for the general surgeons, there was always "Kay," one of his colleagues reflected. Still another added, he was "all doctor, all medicine," and would even sneak into his office on weekends to work. But in spite of this, Richard Webster declared, "Actually, Dr. Kazanjian in reality was never accepted by the general surgical world here in Boston" and, "his creativity and brilliance could not be denied nor could his record and so he was granted honors but never a real service at the General." At the end of World War II, Webster related, he had approached Dr. Kazanjian with the desire "to form a plastic surgical service of worth." Dr. Kazanjian responded that "the climate here in Boston was totally unsatisfactory for such a venture."[14]

In his 1967 survey of plastic surgery in the early decades of the twentieth century, John Converse refers to some of the problems encountered by would-be plastic and reconstructive surgeons in the period between World War I and World War II, and even for a long time afterwards. After alluding to the dramatic advances that had been made in the first world war, Converse related that "Gillies told me that following the closure of Queen's Hospital in Sidcup, Kilner and he wondered how they were going to be able to continue to specialize in the field of plastic surgery." And he added, "When one thinks of a tremendous development of plastic surgery during the past twenty-five years it is difficult to realize that there was so little demand for the services of the plastic surgeon in the early 1920s." But things began to change, gradually. Converse points out that after the war national and international congresses began to include in their scientific programs papers concerned with the methods of treatment of the victims of the war, so that in retrospect one might consider World War I as the beginning of a new era in plastic surgery. In addition, a number of new publications appeared —he cites the important books of John S. Davis (1919) and Harold Gillies (1920)—as well as a growing number of articles on plastic and reparative surgery in the periodical literature. Furthermore, with the advent of peace and a period of relative prosperity, a new branch of plastic surgery appeared that was designated "esthetic" and "cosmetic." He mentions Jacques Joseph, an orthopedic surgeon in Berlin, who from early in the century pioneered a new method of corrective rhinoplasty, which in the early 1920s was brought to the United States by two of his pupils, Gustav Aufricht and J. Safian. In 1921, the American Association of Oral Surgeons was founded, an organization that initially was open only to men like Kazanjian who held both dental and medical degrees and who did most of the work in plastic surgery at that time. (Dr. Kazanjian was elected to membership in 1924.) However, it did not take

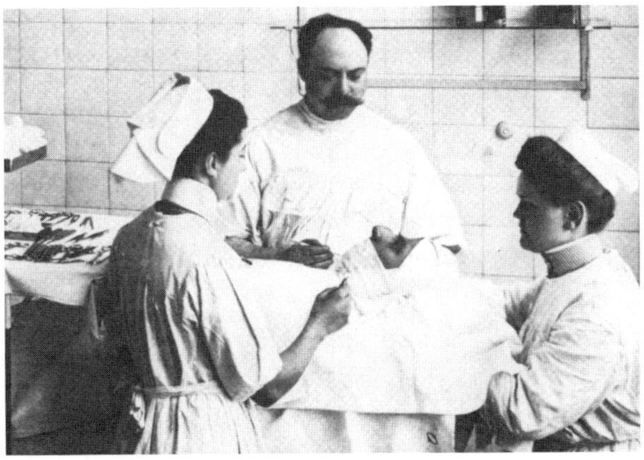

Dr. Jacques Joseph of Berlin, Germany (1865-1934) is remembered as the " father of the art of modern rhinoplasty." His most famous book Nasenplastik und Sonstige Gesichtsplastik Nebst Mammaplastik (Rhinoplasty and Other Facial Plasties, with a supplement on Breast-Plasty), *appeared in 1931.*

During World War I in 1916, Dr. Joseph established a unit devoted to plastic surgery at the Charité Hospital in Berlin. Widely recognized, he was awarded the Iron Cross, second class in 1919. The contributions of Germans to jaw surgery was noteworthy and advanced. Photograph from Paul Natvig, Jacques Joseph Surgical Sculptor, *(Philadelpia: W. B. Saunders Company, 1982)*

long for the dental requirement to be dropped and in time the word *Oral* was also omitted from the Association's title and the American Association of Plastic Surgeons came into being.

But in spite of the hard-won gains, Converse acknowledged, it was "difficult for a young plastic surgeon to realize the flimsy status of plastic surgery 30 years ago" (i.e., in the late 1930s). As Jerome Webster also observed, "At that time the public generally considered plastic surgeons as 'face lifters' and 'nose whittlers.' There were also those who were close to the border of being ethical, if not unethical, in their practice, and some were definitely below that level." Furthermore, Converse related, opportunities for learning plastic surgery were few in the 1930s, preceptorships were not very numerous, and there were few well organized plastic surgery services in hospitals. "The only method of learning was observation and there were well trodden paths to St. Louis, Baltimore, New York, Boston and London."[15] It can be presumed that most of the adverse conditions described by Drs. Converse and Webster persisted through much, if not all, of Dr. Kazanjian's professional career, although he was a loner who was little interested in or affected by organizational meetings and politics, preceptorships, competition, and the like. When he commenced practice as a plastic and oral surgeon in the early 1920s he undoubtedly soon had all the work he needed or could handle, due to his special dental and surgical skills, the reputation he had earned as a miracle man during the first world war, and his ability to take on and successfully complete difficult cases and problems that others were not competent or willing to assume.

Before the conclusion of this description of Dr. Kazanjian's initial career in the 1920s, a curious incident should be mentioned that was connected to his World War I treatment of British soldiers. Dr. Kazanjian was with a group of doctors at dinner in Niagara Falls, in upstate New York in 1923. As the food did not please him, he left the group and found another restaurant. There, as often happened, the waitress asked him his name, and when he told her, the astonished woman said, "There is a man in the kitchen who knows you and is looking for you." Peering through the kitchen window was D, one of the British soldiers whom Kazanjian had treated in France during the war. His wounds had not healed as well as he wished, so he had travelled to America with only the magical name Kazanjian to go on. He ended up in Buffalo, where his sister lived, to begin his search. In this small restaurant his search quickly and fortuitously ended. Dr. Kazanjian arranged for D to be admitted to a Veterans Hospital in Boston, where he successfully completed his former patient's treatment.[16]

However, the year 1923 was far more memorable for another event that occurred in Dr. Kazanjian's life, his second marriage. On August 23, at age forty-four, he was married in New York City to Marion Victorine Hanford, born twenty-nine years earlier in London, the daughter of Malangthon Hanford and Alice V. Gouriet. At the time of their wedding, she resided in Lowell, Massachusetts, and had completed a business executive training course, "the results of which are very much in evidence." She was secretary to the Dean of the Harvard Medical School.[17]

Dr. and Mrs. Kazanjian had two children, Dr. Joan H., a physician born in 1926, and Victor H., an attorney, born in 1927, and five grandchildren. Of the Kazanjian children, at this writing, only Hélène K. Sargeant survives. Their grandson, The Reverend Victor H. Kazanjian, Jr., an Episcopal priest, became Dean of Religion and Spiritual Life at Wellesley College. He lived with his grandparents in Belmont, Massachusetts, as a young adolescent and shared his "visceral" memories with the author. He was very close to his grandmother, Marion, and remembered her as being "formidable" and "very good in business." She "ran the show" and she managed the family, which freed her husband from many of the day-to-day responsibilities.

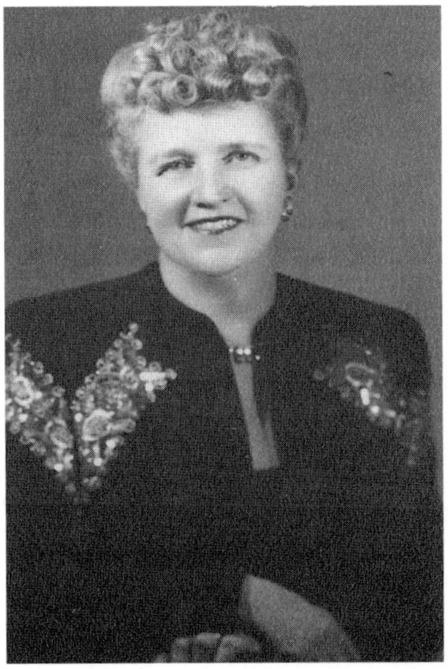

Marion Kazanjian
Abraham Pollen Archives and Roll Book Library, Massachusetts Eye and Ear Infirmary

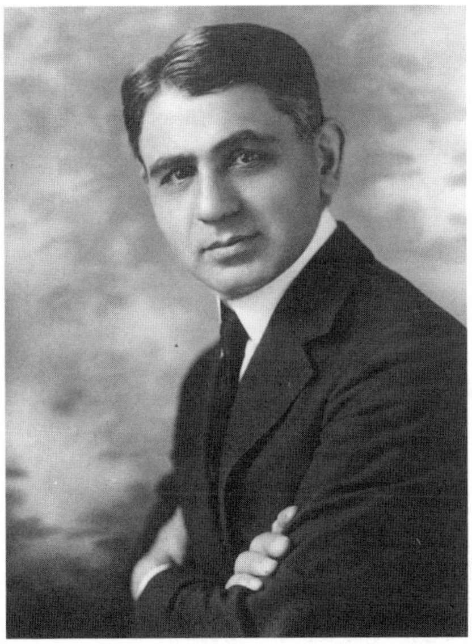

Dr. V. H. Kazanjian 1922
The Harvard Medical Library in the Francis A. Countway Library of Medicine

She would have been one of the great women of her time, her grandson prophesied, "had she lived in another era." He particularly remembers hearty breakfasts prepared by Dora, the live-in maid and cook, a virtual member of the family. Once his grandmother asked if he planned to marry an Armenian. He even learned to prepare Armenian food. Marion Kazanjian may have taken on the formal air of a doctor's wife in the outside world, but that all fell away at home where there was a lot of play, and hugging, Victor recalled. She was a passionate Red Sox fan and even wore the team's cap on her eightieth birthday. At home Dr. Kazanjian was "Papa" to his grandchildren and was very gentle and warm, playful and funny. The medical life was the outer trapping. It was the family life that was all important. The non-negotiable and clear lesson that was imparted to the children and grandchildren was to take responsibility and help others.

"Be gentle and be wise," the Reverend Kazanjian remembered his grandfather advising him. "They are the two things that really matter," but these are "not the qualities which the world rewards." Life cannot "be free of suffering, to be fully human is to suffer and yet to be fully human is also to experience unimaginable joy." The grandson never forgot these moral lessons. In one paper, "Beyond Tolerance," Mr. Kazanjian recognizes "the atrocities committed against the people whose body is mine," and his dreams are haunted by them. It was the image of his grandfather's "face shining with hope, love, compassion and life" that was the saving grace. "Here was a man who had experienced the depth of human cruelty and emerged with a belief in the possibility of the healing of mankind." He lived life above the limitations of his ethnic heritage.[18]

Marion Kazanjian volunteered her time, talents, and commitment to several charitable causes, particularly as a volunteer at the Massachusetts Eye and Ear Infirmary. During World War II, she served as treasurer of the Boston Uptown Branch of the British War Relief Society. She was vice-president of the Mount Auburn Hospital Auxiliary and chair of the Ladies Visiting Committee of the Massachusetts Eye and Ear Infirmary for many years as well as chair of community service to camps and hospitals of the Metropolitan Chapter of the American Red Cross. She was honored by the Ladies' Visiting Committee of the Massachusetts Eye and Ear Infirmary for thirty years of service. During her term as chair, she opened a gift shop at the hospital. She also served on the board of trustees of the Belmont Hill School and was treasurer of the summer residents' committee of the New London, New Hampshire Hospital.[19]

The Kazanjians lived in a brick house, which they built in the late 1920s or early 1930s at 191 Clifton Street in Belmont. The furniture was hand-carved by Charles Najarian, a master craftsman in wood with outstanding talents. "Each authentically designed, carefully constructed and beautifully carved piece has been a continuing source of pleasure for us," Dr. Kazanjian wrote. "Charlie, you and I have an equal talent—we are both carvers," he commented. "Our hands are equally skilled to do our special work and we have much in common." Najarian was an Armenian immigrant born in 1888 in the town of Hussenig in the Kharpert province of Turkey, where, for 300 years, Najarians were master woodworkers. He had arrived in Boston in 1912.[20]

Dr. Kazanjian continued to be a familiar figure at the Harvard Dental School and never lost his interest in oral surgery and maxillofacial prosthetics. He was one of twelve alumni presented with the School's Centennial Award in 1967. To one Harvard dental student, Wallace J. Gardner (DMD '39), Dr. Kazanjian was a "gift of God" and never forgotten even sixty years later.

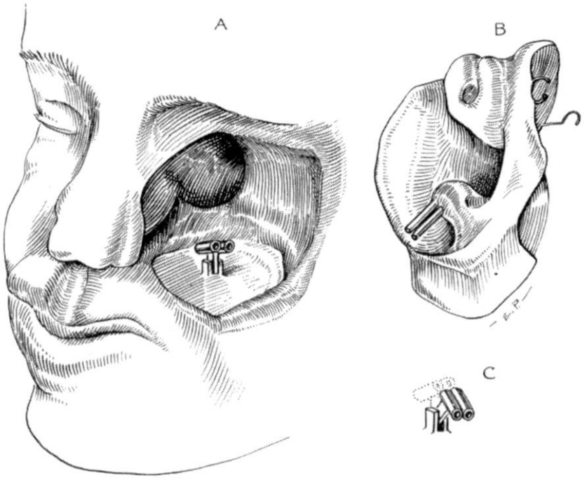

Diagram of large maxillofacial prothesis. On inner surface of facial prothesis were two parallel wires which fitted into tubes on maxillary prothesis. The two sections in position supported each other firmly. V. H. Kazanjian, Prothestic Restoration of Congenital and Aquired Deformities of Hard and Soft Palate, Journal of Oral Surgery, *v. 5 (July 1947) 200*

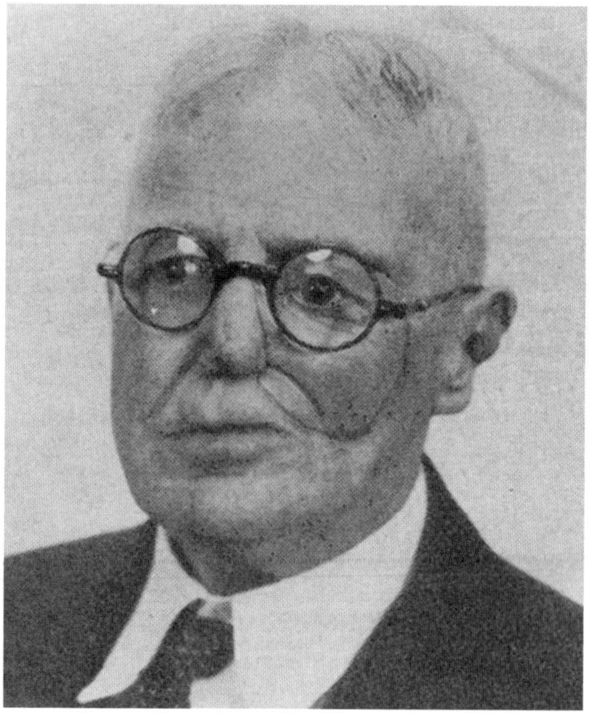

Gardner worked with him for four months in surgery class in his fourth year. "Words just cannot portray my utter amazement at the scope of his ability," Gardner related. Gardner approached one of Dr. Kazanjian's patients whose "face looked quite normal" until he was asked to remove his upper full denture, and out came "an eye — his left cheek — half his nose — and part of his ear." "This was a whole new world for me," Gardner confessed, but Dr. Kazanjian "acted as if he had done nothing out of the ordinary. . . . his actions were so precise, assertive and 'God given' but administered with grace, great calm and humility." Dr. Gardner served in the United States Navy during World War II and was assigned to the United States Marines: "All of these things pale into insignificance when compared with my incredible good fortune to have had the opportunity to work with Dr. Kazanjian."[21]

Dr. Henry Kaplan, who entered Harvard Dental School in 1944, remembered that during his first year, his class in anatomy was assigned to the Massachusetts General Hospital surgical area on Saturday mornings to observe Dr. Kazanjian operate. The students did not consider their instructor to be "a hale fellow well met," but respected him as a "legendary figure" who exerted a major influence on the class. The dean of the dental school, Dr. Leroy M. S. Miner, admired him greatly. To Kaplan, Dr. Kazanjian was "almost saintly," with a "very kind and sweet face" and a "very humble" manner. His lectures to the fourth-year class on fractures were not most of the students' "cup of tea." Dr. Carnig Thomason recalled, "You had to know your stuff. He was tough in the clinic." He would often ask his students, "What do I do now, Doctor?"[22]

Alexander Pope, in "An Essay on Criticism,"

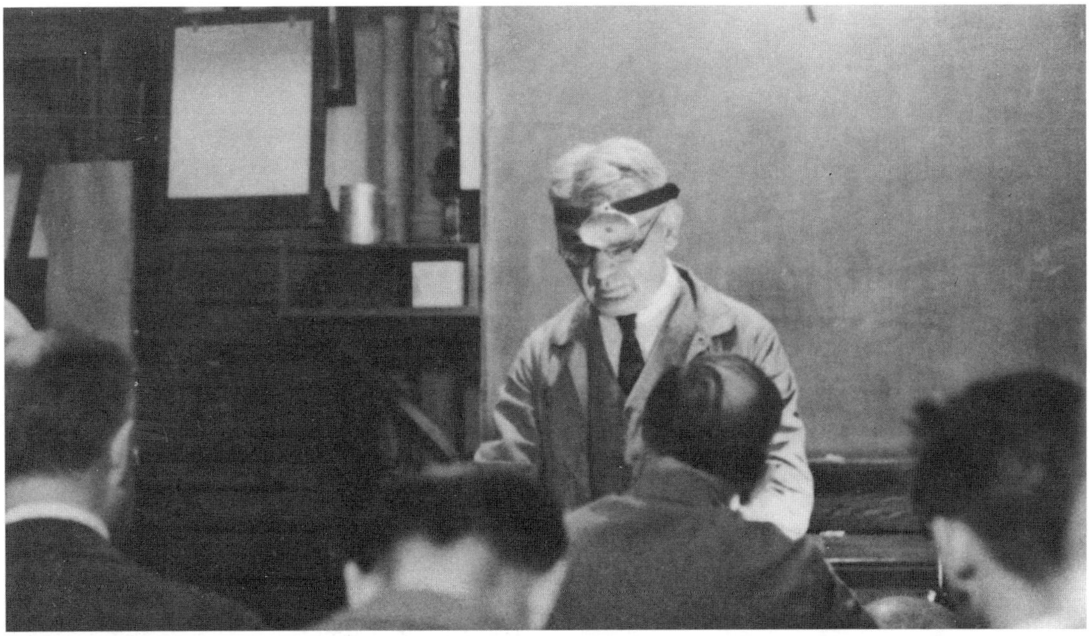

Dr. Kazanjian in the classroom
The Harvard Medical Library in the Francis A. Countway Library of Medicine

admonished, "Let such teach others who themselves excel." Kazanjian's teaching ability was not oratorical eloquence. Rather his success was due to the originality and soundness of the techniques that he demonstrated and to his innate sincerity and humble nature. His students valued what he taught more than the way that he taught it. "He gave freely of his time and talent, saying that he was complimented when anyone wanted to learn from him." Dr. Ralph L. Carney wrote to Dr. Kazanjian after taking a course given by him in 1928, "You unquestionably have something with which you should set the nose and throat world on fire. I wish you had a little more conceit and did more to cram it down our throats." Many oral surgeons "owe him a great debt not only for his inspiring guidance but also for the friendship and support given to them by a man of deep understanding and generosity." Plumpton from Glasgow called his contribution "incalculable."[23]

Dental students were taught by Dr. Kazanjian the importance of the medical aspect of dental practice while his medical students learned "that dentistry can contribute a great deal, especially in the surgical treatment of face and jaw deformities." Dr. Richard C. Webster, who graduated from Harvard Medical School in 1943 and served his residency in the Burns and Plastic Surgery Unit at the Massachusetts General Hospital and at the Massachusetts Eye and Ear Infirmary, was asked to "scrub in" with Dr. Kazanjian beginning in 1944. Dr. Webster (1918-1994) later formed his own clinic in Brookline and served on the staff of many hospitals and is remembered as a leader in cosmetic surgery. Dr. Webster "found him a generous and great teacher." At the end of a day, he would send his office staff home "so that he could finish some thought or teaching concept with me."[24]

Over the years, Dr. Kazanjian willingly gave freely of his knowledge and experience to others. Nonetheless, only a handful of students and others remained close to him. The first, John Marquis Converse, who, it was noted before, became associated with him in 1935, was born in San Francisco in 1909 and traced his American ancestry to the year 1634. His father, George Marquis Converse, was a physician who served in France during World War I and was in charge of preventive medicine in the Public Health Service of the American Expeditionary Force. After the war, the senior Converse remained in Paris and became head of the American Ambulance Hospital in Neuilly. His son was educated in France. By 1935, he had received a dental degree from the Paris School of Stomatology and an M.D. from the Faculty of Medicine in Paris.[25]

Converse wrote from Paris on February 4, 1935, a "rather brash letter to Kazanjian: 'I'm young and healthy and full of beans and really ready to go!'" The letter was written on the recommendation of Dr. Ferdinand Brigham, then practicing dentistry in Paris, and Dr. Samuel Jackson of Philadelphia, who had served in France in the United States Army during World War I and knew Kazanjian. It was Dr. Kazanjian's work during World War I that prompted Dr. Converse to write to him. "I intend to make oral maxillofacial and plastic surgery my life work, and as you are considered the master on that part of surgery, I am hoping to have the privilege of becoming one of your pupils," Converse confessed in his letter. In response, Dr. Kazanjian arranged with Dr. Mosher, Surgeon-in-Chief of the Massachusetts Eye and Ear Infirmary, for Dr. Converse to be admitted as a resident in surgery from 1935 to 1938 on Dr. Mosher's service. Dr. Kazanjian also arranged for him to serve as assistant in surgery at the Massachusetts General Hospital from the end of 1935 through 1936. Dr. Converse returned to Paris following his residency and in the period that followed visited the most important plastic surgeons in Europe and eventually settled in New York. From these beginnings under the tutelage of Dr. Kazanjian, Dr. Converse advanced to become the Lawrence D. Bell Professor of Plastic Surgery at the New York University College of Medicine, Director of the Institute of Reconstructive Plastic Surgery at New York University Medical Center, Chairman of the Department of Plastic Surgery at Manhattan Eye, Ear and Throat Hospital, and Director of Plastic Surgery at Bellevue Hospital until his death in 1981. At the completion of his residency in 1938, Dr. Converse wrote to Dr. Kazanjian, "I realize how very fortunate I was to work with a man like yourself . . . I am indebted to you . . . . All these things I shall never forget."[26]

When Dr. Converse first began working with Dr. Kazanjian in 1935, his mentor was fifty-six years old. "His white hair . . . belied his tremendous activity," Converse recalled many years later. The writer, Avedis Derounian, recorded his impressions of Dr. Kazanjian that same year. "He was a short man, trimly dressed . . . his full head of hair, neatly parted, had turned mellow grey. His brows were prominent. He wore brown rimmed glasses over soft brown eyes. His face — square and straight-jawed — was smooth textured and of habitual studious and content expression." Dr. Converse related an incident that had occurred while he was in New York before going on to Boston that did not bode well for the direction he was about to take in medicine. His father had corresponded with a physician friend who invited him to dinner. "Now, young man, what are you going to do?" his host asked. When told that his guest intended to be trained as a plastic surgeon, the physician fell silent. "How disappointing it must be for my old friend, George, to have a son who wants to become a plastic surgeon," he finally remarked.[27]

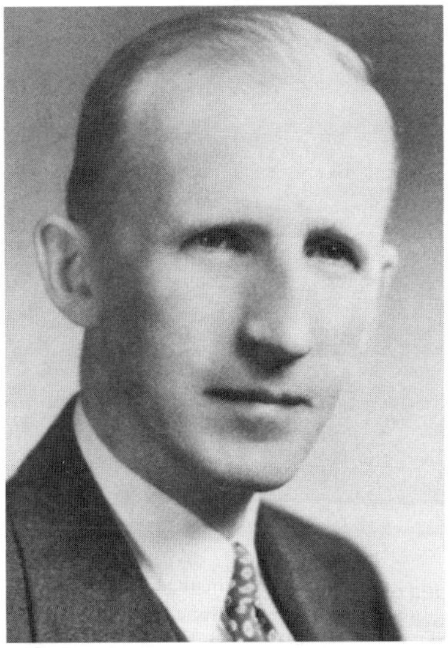

Dr. Edgar M. Holmes, Jr. (1902-1997)
Photograph from Mark L. Cheney, Facial Surgery: Plastic and Reconstructive *(Baltimore: Williams & Wilkins, 1997) p. 7*

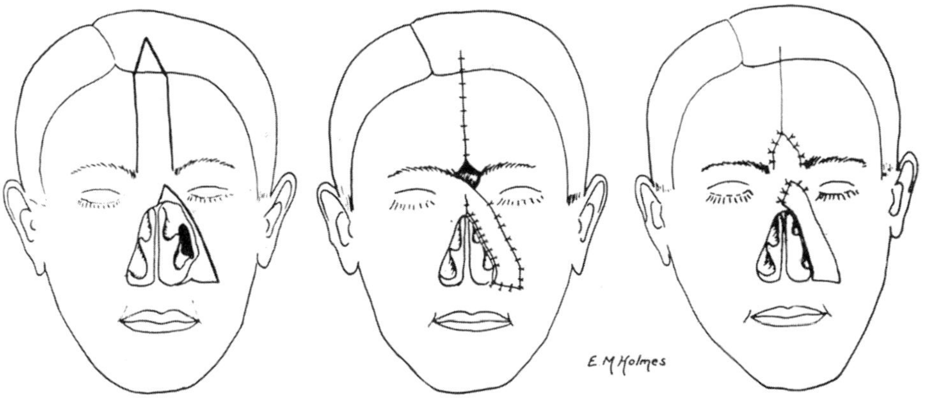

Diagram showing a median forehead flap which was used to partially close the left side of the nasal opening. Drawn by Dr. E. M. Holmes
Varaztad H. Kazanjian, "Restoration of the Nose, Lip, and Maxilla by Surgery and Prothesis," Plastic and Reconstructive Surgery, 2:6 (November, 1947): 534

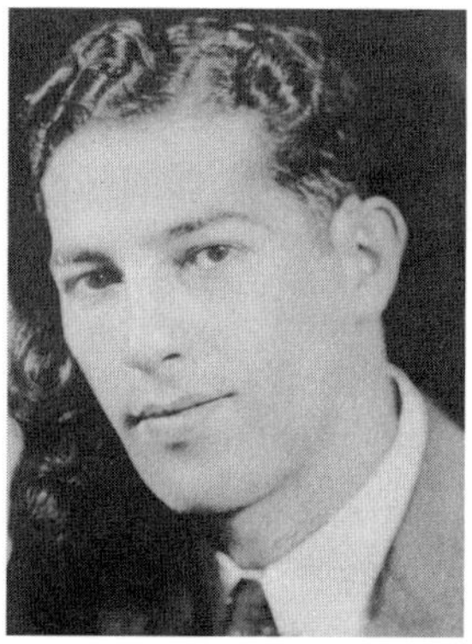

Dr. Kenneth Kazanjian, (1906-1977)
Courtesy Andrea Pogarian

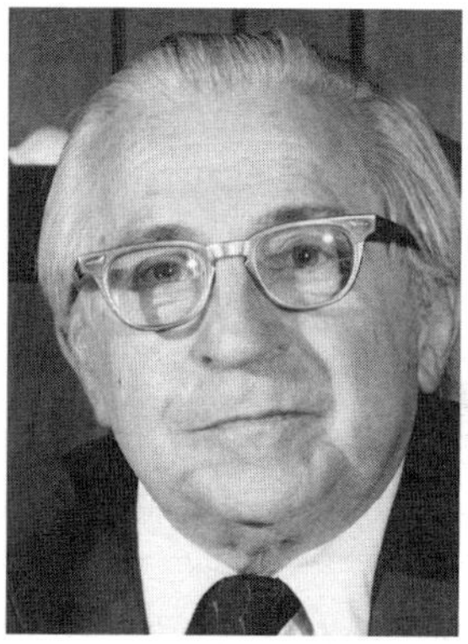

Dr. Richard C. Webster (1918-1994)
Courtesy Mrs. Richard Webster and Dr. Raffi Der Sarkissian

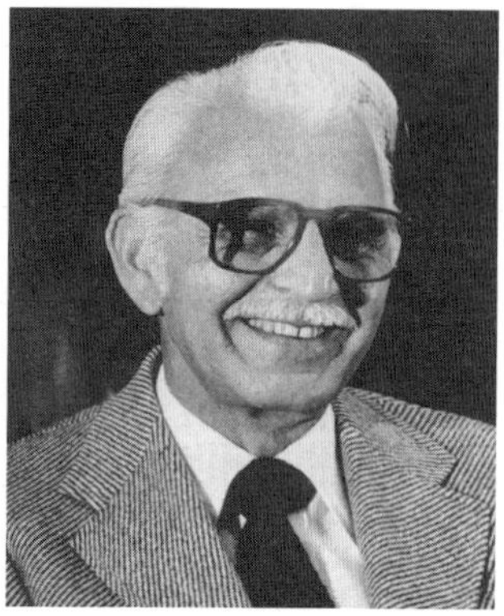

Dr. Aram Roopenian (1914-1990)
Photograph from Abraham Pollen Archives and Roll Book Library, Massachusetts Eye and Eye Infirmary. Reproduced in Cheney, *p. 9*

Dr. Edgar M. Holmes, Jr. (1902-1997) was another facial plastic surgeon in Dr. Kazanjian's intimate professional circle. After World War II, Dr. Kazanjian was asked "to train two younger staff surgeons [at the Massachusetts Eye and Ear Infirmary] who had an interest in plastic surgery, Drs. Edgar Holmes and Aram Roopenian were chosen." Drs. Kazanjian and Holmes collaborated in the writing and publication of at least five articles in the facial surgical literature. The illustrations accompanying these papers were expertly and finely drawn by Dr. Holmes. Dr. Holmes succeeded Dr. Kazanjian as chief of the Facial Plastic Surgery Services at the Massachusetts Eye and Ear Infirmary and is remembered as "a skilled surgeon and excellent teacher."[28]

It had always been Aram Roopenian's desire to "follow in the footsteps" of his uncle and for many years he had worked closely with him, "scrubbing in" with all surgical cases. Dr. Roopenian graduated from Tufts University Medical School in 1942, served as an intern in general surgery at the Boston City Hospital until 1943, and completed his residency in otolaryngology at the Massachusetts Eye and Ear Infirmary in 1944. He afterwards served as a captain in the U.S. Army Medical Corps in the Pacific theater of operations, where he performed surgery on facial wounds in a field unit. Upon his discharge from the service in 1946, he joined his uncle's practice. Dr. Roopenian, whose skill in performing the rhinoplasty procedures was unrivaled, later succeeded his uncle as Chief of Plastic Surgery at the Massachusetts Eye and Ear Infirmary. From his uncle, Dr. Roopenian learned to make plaster molds of the upper part of the face which proved very useful in planning his rhinoplasty surgery. Following his uncle's retirement, Dr. Roopenian joined forces with Dr. William G. Lavelle and Dr. Theodore Jacobs in the private practice of otolaryngology in Boston. His career ended in 1980 when he was involved in an automobile accident that left him unable to continue his practice. He died in 1990 and is remembered as "a handsome, quiet and unassuming person who loved teaching," and was an "unusually wonderful person."[29]

Prior to Dr. Kazanjian's association with Drs. Webster and Roopenian, he had as his associate his nephew, Kenneth A. Kazanjian, whose father, Alexander, was Varaztad Kazanjian's half brother. Kenneth, along with Alexander's family, moved to South Boston in 1911 and to Watertown in 1930. Following his graduation from the Harvard Medical School in 1931, he was on the staff of the Massachusetts General Hospital, the Massachu-

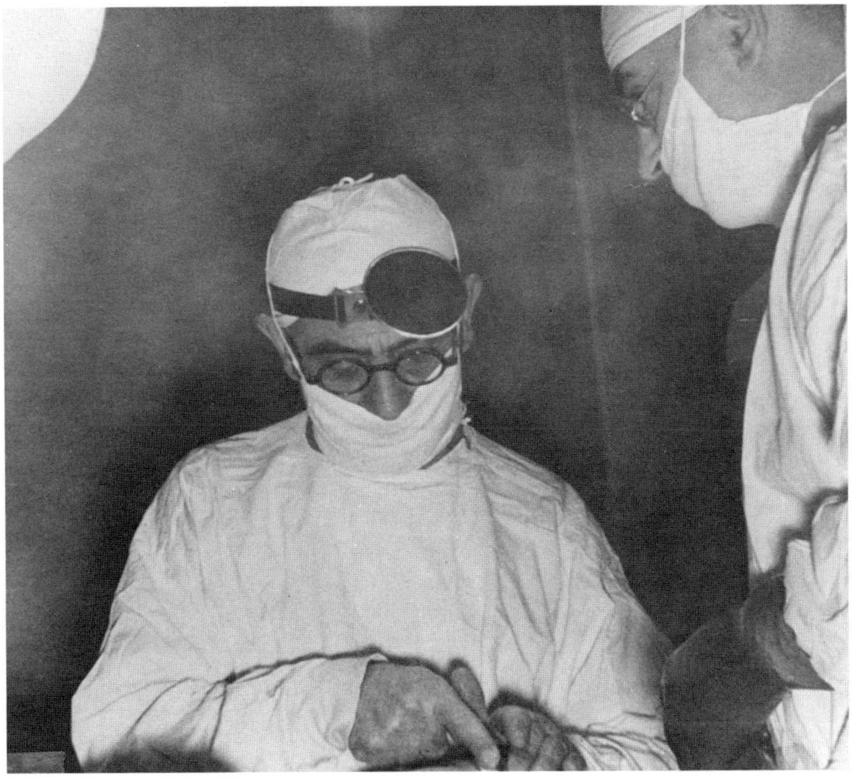

Dr. Kazanjian in the operating room
The Harvard Medical Library in the Francis A. Countway Library of Medicine

setts Eye and Ear Infirmary, and several other local hospitals. He served as a major in the Army Medical Corps during World War II. His obituary described him as a "noted dermatologist and plastic surgeon." He left his uncle's practice in 1945 and opened his own office in an adjacent suite at 475 Commonwealth Avenue. Their practices were dissimilar. Dr. Varaztad did not emphasize face-lifts, believing that patients should grow old gracefully.[30]

The professional associates of Dr. Kazanjian's office were supported by a staff, some of whom had served for decades. Evelyn Bateman, R.N., performed the duties of secretary from 1920 to 1963. She was succeeded by Priscilla Greene. Louise Linehan Roopenian, who had married Deron Roopenian, the son of Dr. Kazanjian's sister Nouvart, worked from 1930 on. Among her duties was the taking of the patient's photographs and making models. Basil Brownell, chauffeur for about fifty years, drove the large Buick that ferried Dr. Kazanjian around Boston to hospitals and appointments. Jessie Robertson, R.N., was Dr. Kazanjian's operating room nurse. She retired in 1962 and was succeeded by Marilyn Betts. Virginia Ring was medical secretary from 1944 to 1948.[31]

Bradford Cannon was another who, while not directly trained in plastic surgery by Dr. Kazanjian, was inspired by him to become a plastic surgeon, associated in many ways with him after qualifying as one, and who during his long career experienced final acceptance of plastic surgery both nationally as well as in Boston and at the Massachusetts General Hospital. Dr. Cannon related in a recent retrospective glance that "My first exposure to plastic surgery was as a medical student [at the Harvard Medical School] when I watched Varaztad H. Kazanjian, DMD, MD, reconstruct a nose with a forehead flap — the ancient Indian method. I was greatly intrigued. A decade later, I became his fast friend, . . . and professional colleague, and, in 1941, I succeeded him as chief of the Plastic Clinic at the Massachusetts General Hospital (MGH), Boston." The son of Harvard's famous physiologist, Walter Bradford Cannon, who had investigated the problem of shock in France in the last year of the Great War while Kazanjian was repairing soldiers' faces, Cannon in 1935 chose the Barnes Hospital in St. Louis for his internship training, rotating through general surgery and afterwards undertaking a residency training program. During his first assignment as an intern at the St. Louis Shriner's Hospital, where he first observed the devastating contractures following untreated deep burns, he met Barrett Brown, who became his first clinical teacher.

Cannon points out in his memoir that during the 1930s there were no formal residencies in plastic surgery. "Most of us, exposed to a handful of plastic surgeons in the United States, chose the specialty after completing a general surgical residency. Our specialized training consisted of assisting in an informal plastic surgical preceptorship." In 1938, he went on, "an opportunity arose, which I seized at once, to join the renowned 'three *B*'s' of plastic surgery: Vilray Blair, MD, Barrett Brown, MD, and Louis Byars, MD, all in St. Louis." His next year and a half was full of extraordinary exposure to almost every conceivable type of plastic and reconstructive surgical problem, from congenital anomalies to head and neck cancer and a variety of traumas. "Blair and Brown had demonstrated how large sheets of 'split skin grafts' could be cut. Learning this technique put me in a unique position when I demonstrated it on my return to Boston, where 'pinch grafts' prevailed."

On Cannon's return to Boston in 1940, he was appointed assistant surgeon by Edward D. Churchill, Chief of Surgery at the MGH, and assigned to the Plastic Clinic. "Kazanjian headed the clinic and proved to be a most delightful and generous leader. He had difficulty explaining to the unprepared observer what he was doing and why, but, to the prepared observer his moves were logical and quite original. He and I worked closely at the MGH and at the Harvard Dental School, where he was an honored senior faculty member." When, a few months later, he and Kazanjian were asked to deal with the enormous backlog of patients under the state's Crippled Children's Program, they chose to establish a new, autonomous clinic at the Mount Auburn Hospital in Cambridge, and the program they set up lasted for thirty-four years. "To have done cosmetic procedures at the MGH in the 1940s would have been frowned on," Cannon reported, remarking that it was quite a contrast to the 1980s, when the MGH welcomed these paying patients.

Returning to Boston in 1946 after nearly four years of army service, Dr. Cannon "still found the MGH reluctant to accept a plastic surgical program." As a result, the clinic at Mount Auburn Hospital was reactivated. In 1960, Cannon related, there were signs that the MGH was beginning to recognize the need for plastic surgery experience in a general surgical residency program, and two surgical residents were assigned to work with him. "Final recognition of plastic surgery as a specialty came in 1970, when a formal residency was established." His and Dr. Kazanjian's specialty had at last taken its place among the respected surgical sub-specialties at the hospital.[32]

Dr. Kazanjian published approximately eighty articles, along with occasional book reviews, in the twenty-four year period extending from 1922 through 1945, or an average of three or four per year. While these concentrated on maxillofacial problems, they related more specifically to plastic surgery of the face and jaws: to gunshot injuries, injuries to the face resulting from automobile accidents, to prostheses, to

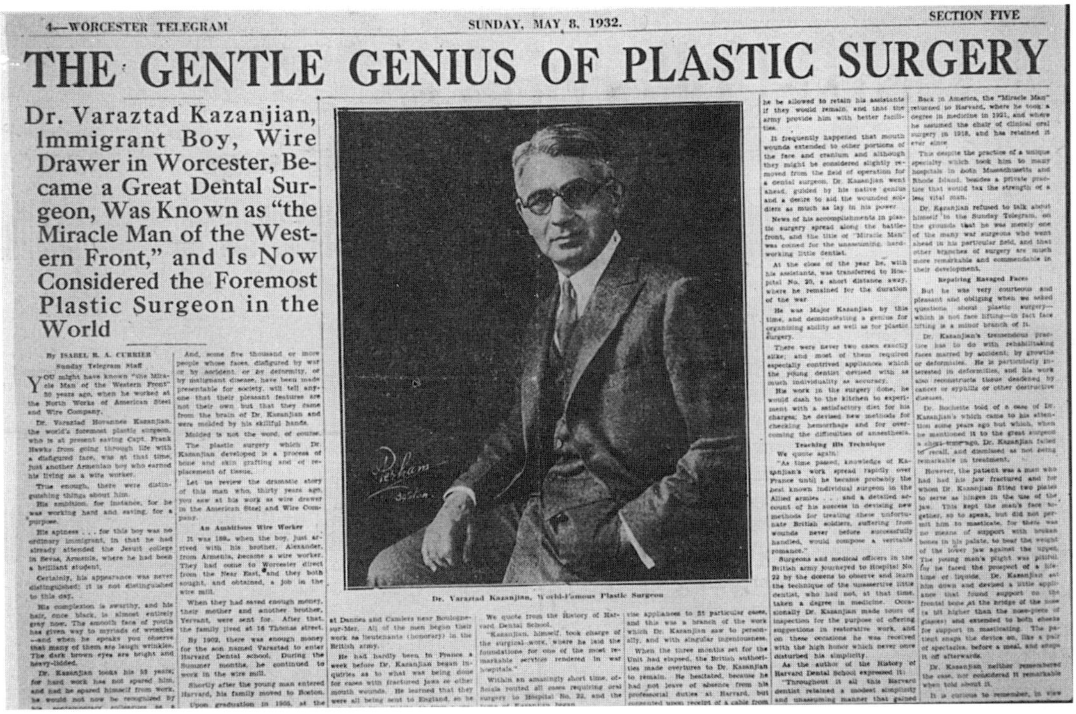

4—WORCESTER TELEGRAM SUNDAY, MAY 8, 1932. SECTION FIVE

THE GENTLE GENIUS OF PLASTIC SURGERY

Dr. Varaztad Kazanjian, Immigrant Boy, Wire Drawer in Worcester, Became a Great Dental Surgeon, Was Known as "the Miracle Man of the Western Front," and Is Now Considered the Foremost Plastic Surgeon in the World

By ISABEL R. A. CURRIER
Sunday Telegram Staff

YOU might have known "the Miracle Man of the Western Front" 30 years ago, when he worked at the North Works of American Steel and Wire Company.

Dr. Varaztad Hovannes Kazanjian, the world's foremost plastic surgeon, who is at present saving Capt. Frank Hawks from going through life with a disfigured face, was at that time, just another Armenian boy who earned his living as a wire worker.

True enough, there were distinguishing things about him.

His ambition, for instance, for he was working hard and saving, for a purpose.

His aptness . . . for this boy was no ordinary immigrant, in that he had already attended the Jesuit college in Sevas, Armenia, where he had been a brilliant student.

Certainly, his appearance was never distinguished; it is not distinguished to this day.

And, some five thousand or more people whose faces, disfigured by war or by accident, or by deformity, or by malignant disease, have been made presentable for society, will tell anyone that their pleasant features are not their own but that they came from the brain of Dr. Kazanjian and were molded by his skillful hands.

Molded is not the word, of course.

The plastic surgery which Dr. Kazanjian developed is a process of bone and skin grafting and of replacement of tissue.

Let us review the dramatic story of this man who, thirty years ago, you saw at his work as wire drawer in the American Steel and Wire Company.

An Ambitious Wire Worker

It was 189., when the boy, just arrived with his brother, Alexander, from Armenia, became a wire worker. They had come to Worcester direct from the Near East, and they both sought, and obtained, a job in the wire mill.

Dr. Varaztad Kazanjian, World-Famous Plastic Surgeon

Worcester Sunday Telegram, *May 3, 1932, Section Two, p. 4*
Reprinted with permission from the Worcester Telegram & Gazette

problems concerning cancer of the mouth, to cleft palates and the resulting speech problems, and to facial bone fractures. The majority were written by Dr. Kazanjian alone, especially in his early years of practice, but later on a number were published in collaboration with others. In 1932, for example, he published an article on prostheses of the mouth and face in collaboration with A. T. Rowe and H. A. Young; and in 1938, he cooperated with his fellow dental school teacher Kurt H. Thoma in contributing a chapter on fractures to the facial bones to the eleventh edition of Charles L. Scudder's *The Treatment of Fractures*, a standard text in its day. From 1940 on, a few of his articles appeared with John Converse as secondary author as well as articles written in collaboration with Somers H. Sturgis, Carl W. Waldron, Douglas B. Parker, Moses S. Strock, and Edgar M. Holmes. Many of these articles, written in the 1920s and 1930s, would be cited as references in a book by him and John Converse, *The Surgical Treatment of Facial Injuries*, which first appeared in 1949. Thus, while Dr. Kazanjian was busy in these years, treating patients and teaching students, he found time to write about interesting cases and procedures that he had developed to improve the treatment given to his patients. His innovative surgery, his development of new and original methods and appliances for repair and treatment, and his teaching and writing set him apart from most plastic surgeons and dentists of his era, whose sole or chief concern was caring for their patients.

From late in the nineteenth century, science had begun to afford significant aid to medicine in understanding and controlling a number of serious diseases, so that by the late 1930s there arose a feeling of optimism that medical science was on the threshold of achieving additional significant gains. The founding of the science of bacteriology in the 1870s and 1880s and the subsequent development of vaccines and antitoxins had resulted in the prevention or control of several devastating infectious diseases, and the implementation of public health measures had brought about other remarkable advances as well. From early in the twentieth century the emerging science of biochemistry had begun to provide a better understanding of the role of nutrition in health and disease, especially through the perception of a previously unrecognized group of constituents in most foods in their natural states, called vitamins. In 1922, Frederick Banting and his group at the University of Toronto suddenly and dramatically isolated the hormone insulin from animal pancreases, making it possible for the first time to maintain patients suffering from diabetes who previously had no hope of survival. Then, just a few years later, George Richards Minot and his colleagues at Harvard developed a cure for the devastating disease, pernicious anemia, and continued to make inroads on other forms of the anemias. These and other dramatic gains, achieved in a period of only fifty or sixty years, made it seem that, truly, there was no end in sight so long as medicine continued along this scientific path — and a few began to think of extending these advances to the field of dentistry also.

In the mid 1930s, a number of officials at Harvard University, including its president, James Bryant Conant, himself a brilliant chemist and scientist, Leroy M. S. Miner, dean of its dental school, and C. Sidney Burwell, its medical dean, believed that science might prove useful also in advancing dentistry. They questioned the advisability of continuing to train students to repair the damage caused by tooth decay when the progress recently made in a number of fields of medicine indicated that a far better approach to the ravages of tooth decay would be to attack the underlying problem through research programs aimed at understanding the root cause of caries in the first place and finding the means to prevent or retard it. In addition, they thought it advisable to equip the dentists of the future with more rigorous training in medicine and science. Based on the experience of the past sixty years, this would enable them to cope with the problems and methods of research that were thought to be necessary in this quest. With this in mind, these officials formulated a plan to reorganize the Harvard Dental School for the mission at hand. It was a drastic plan in its formulation and implementation and one that would have a serious impact on the dental school, its faculty, and its alumni that, in the eyes of some, still has not completely run its course.

On May 10, 1939, a committee known as the Burwell Committee announced its plan to reorganize the Harvard Dental School into the Harvard School of Dental Medicine. The program was to begin in 1940, and graduates were to receive both the M.D. and D.M.D. degree. The basic four-year course was preserved, but an additional year was required to acquire the technical skills needed in dentistry. "The fat was in the fire," Dr. and later Dean James Morse Dunning wrote in his 1981 history of the Harvard School of Dental Medicine,[33] the source of much of this information. (Dr. Dunning was later to play an integral role both nationally and in Massachusetts in leading the long and ofttimes bitter campaign for the fluoridation of drinking water to prevent or inhibit tooth decay.) During the five years required, the students would receive three and a half years of dentistry.

In the deliberations leading up to this ultimate decision, Dean Miner was in favor of a slow, cautious approach. His view was to introduce a few of the "new style" students into the program each year and build it up gradually. Conant, on the other hand, saw no reason for delay and opted for a fast and complete break with the past. On

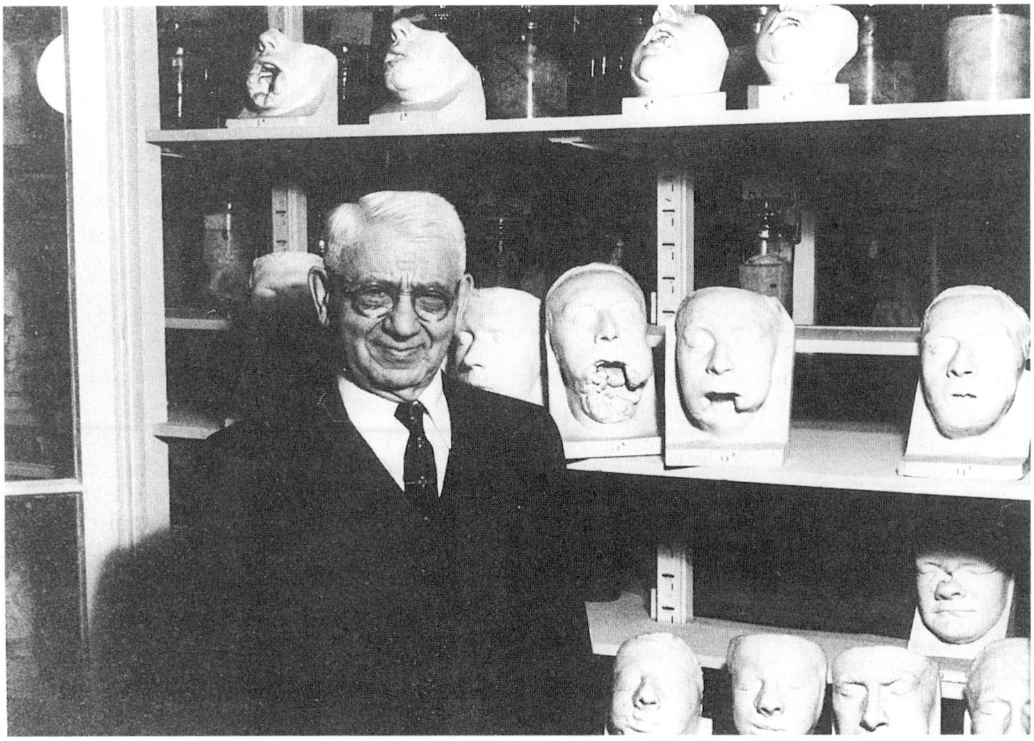

Dr. Kazanjian and plaster models of patients
The Harvard Medical Library in the Francis A. Countway Library of Medicine

February 27, 1940, President Conant announced, in the process of reorganization, that the entire staff of the dental school was to be "separated from the University" with a new staff to be later announced. (It was reported, based on information provided by one who was on hand at the meeting, that Dr. Conant started out by praising the faculty as one of the best in the country, but then added, "as of five o'clock this afternoon you're all fired," or words to that effect.)[34] Many observers referred to that day as "Black Monday." Quite naturally, the move did not go over well with the alumni of the school, who were quite proud of the outstanding reputation that their institution had attained, or with its distinguished faculty as well. Harvard was called "a bargain basement of degrees" and concern was expressed that dentistry would be submerged and that the graduates would be "illegitimate off-springs not acceptable to either dentistry or medicine."

In the reorganized Oral and Plastic Surgery Department, Dr. Kazanjian became Professor of Plastic Surgery, Dr. Bradford Cannon, Instructor in Plastic Surgery, Dr. Kurt H. Thoma, Professor of Oral Surgery, Dr. Harold A. Kent, Assistant of Oral Surgery, and Charles A. Brackett, Professor of Oral Pathology. The staff was divided into two groups: one concerned with maxillofacial-plastic surgery with Drs. Kazanjian and Cannon. The other was concerned with oral surgery with Drs. Thoma and Kent. Dr. Thoma was appointed to serve as chair of the combined department. The program was in some ways poorly thought out. Few students receiving both the M.D. and D.M.D. degree would choose other than to practice medicine, which indeed proved to be the case in the early years. Then, with the outbreak of total war in late 1941, the plan and the school would languish for much of the 1940s decade. Eventually, Dr. Dunning wrote, Harvard "decided to alter the procedure" and to "place the attainment of the dental degree ahead of the medical degree." This put the ball back in dentistry's court. Dr. Kazanjian expressed his concern that the finest dental school in the country was in danger of being closed; and while this did not happen, its student body (and future alumni) became very small — perhaps a fourth or a fifth of its size in prior times — in the half century following. The reorganization of the school and the problems that followed put a pall on its past alumni who were quite vocal in their opposition to the move. The protests and criticisms still have not died down, over sixty years later.

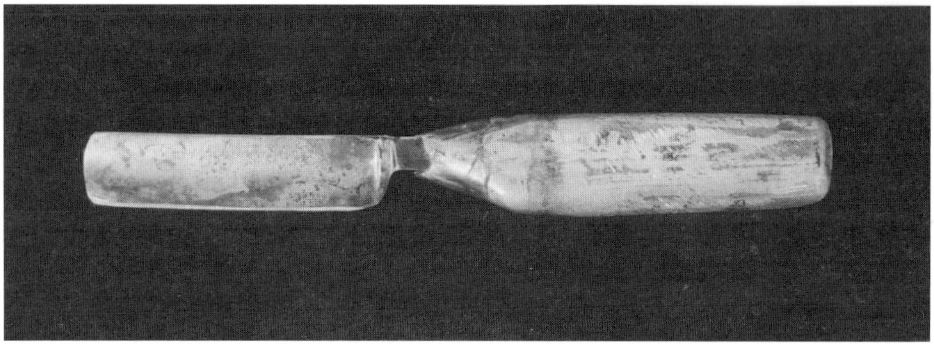

Skin grafting instrument improved by Dr. Kazanjian On loan by the Kazanjian family to The Harvard Medical Library in the Francis A. Countway Library of Medicine Photograph by Dr. Paul Davis

The 1939-1940 reorganization caused other modifications in the Harvard Dental School. By 1925 one of the most comprehensive museums of its kind had been established at the Harvard Dental School with Dr. Adelbert Fernald as curator. A large and important section of the museum was devoted to Dr. Kazanjian's collection of life-sized casts of his World War I patients. Following the implementation of the reorganization of the Dental School, and in the "chaos" that ensued, staff and others became concerned with the future of the museum. A major portion of its contents, including George Washington's gold denture teeth, were "carried off." Dr. Kazanjian rescued his models and other materials that he had deposited earlier.[35]

By the late 1930s, Varaztad Kazanjian was beginning to garner honors. In 1937, he was elected President of the American Academy of Dental Science, and in 1940, he was chosen President of the American Association of Plastic Surgeons. "For the most part," Dr. Richard C. Webster has written, "he did not join with those who really ruled plastic surgery and who, to a large extent, dictated its course in an organized way. He was a quiet man who stayed largely out of the politics of the field; he had little to say about others and no special aptitude for policy making. He let his result, his writings, and his teaching speak for him. Because of this, I learned little about the nonmedical side of plastic surgery until later." What Dr. Webster learned when he went into private practice in 1947 and began going to plastic surgery meetings "was that there was a power structure and that its leadership came largely from St. Louis."[36]

Another honor bestowed on Varaztad Kazanjian in this period was the decision of the World's Fair Commission to have his name inscribed on the Wall of Honor at the New York World's Fair held in 1939-1940. This was the way chosen by the Commission to recognize the foremost foreign-born representatives of the various nations in the United States. The dedication of the wall took place on September 20, 1940. The speaker, Dr. Edward C. Laudemann, Professor of Philosophy at the New School for Social Research, related: "Our past record as a people is irrevocably associated with the fact that we are heterogeneous. Our future destiny will likewise be determined by this fact: either we demonstrate that strength may come from heterogeneity, or we succumb to the deadly rule of uniformity. The testing time has arrived. In actuality we are at this moment making a declaration to the world. We are saying . . . 'We prize the contributions which our foreign-born citizens have made to our culture. . . and we believe that in their hearts they carry a deep and unswerving devotion to American ideals.'"[37] Another speaker was Avedis Derounian, whose topic was "Contributions of the Armenians in America."[38] Dr. Kazanjian was living proof that the American dream was not a myth.

Dr. Kazanjian neither denied his ethnic background nor Anglicized his name. "Why should I change my name?" he responded to a reporter's question. "I was asked to do so when I first entered medicine. By changing my name do I change my color, myself? I have been respected more for retaining my basic Armenian loyalties. And I am happy that I have." He added, "Of course, one can expect rebuffs. But that's all in store for a minority people . . . Self-pity has no place in the aggressive mind. Self-pity is little less than mental suicide. Armenians ought to study hard, work hard and concentrate on the achievement of an ideal. All this should be done without being constantly conscious that they are Armenians in America."

Kazanjian felt that William Saroyan adapted himself well. "I approve of his attitude. He is honest. He is not a hyphenated Armenian . . . Saroyan is teaching Armenians to face the facts as they are — and not to entertain themselves with sentimentally nationalistic notions. Saroyan had adapted himself to America, yet he has fully retained his Armenian identity."[39] When one Armenian, Carnig Thomason (Harvard School of Dental Medicine, '43), was about to begin dental practice, he asked Kazanjian for advice. Thomason confided that he was planning to practice in Watertown, where there was a heavy concentration of Armenians. Kazanjian quickly retorted, "Mistake." He advised Thomason to begin practice first in a location away from Armenians and establish a reputation, and then later return to Watertown, where he was more likely to be respected by his fellow Armenians.[40]

At the time of the attack on Pearl Harbor on December 7, 1941, Varaztad Kazanjian was sixty-three years old, too old, by far, for active service in the conflict that followed. Besides, he had done his part several decades earlier, in the War to End All Wars, and outstandingly. His service to his country at this second trying time of need would be to stay at home and care for a civilian population that was largely deprived of its medical profession by the necessities of war. However, he may have contributed marginally to the war effort in helping train physicians for war surgery through his appointment in 1945 to the Graduate School of Medicine at the University of Pennsylvania, where he served until 1959, first as Guest Lecturer in Oral Surgery and later as Visiting Lecturer of Maxillofacial Surgery.[41]

NOTES

1 The designation of Dr. Kazanjian as "the Gentle Genius of Plastic Surgery" was first used in an article written by Isabel Currier in the *Sunday Worcester Telegram*, May 3, 1932, p. 4, cols. 1-6. The term "plastic surgery" is derived from the ancient Greek word "plastikos," which means "molded or given form."

2 This clinical material is now part of the Varaztad H. Kazanjian Archive in The Francis A. Countway Library of Medicine, folder C-43. The American Medical Association's Certificate of Honor for Dr. Kazanjian's exhibit at the 1921 meeting is preserved in the Kazanjian Archive, folder PAM-21, See also the *Program of the Scientific Assembly of the Seventy-second Annual Session of the American Medical Association*, Boston, June 7-10, 1921 (Chicago: Press of the A.M.A., 1921), p. 100. Courtesy A.M.A. Archives, Chicago.

3 *Boston Directory*, 1926, p. 1374; John M. Converse, "The Extraordinary Career of Varaztad Hovhannes Kazanjian," *Plastic and Reconstructive Surgery* 71, no. 1 (January 1982): 138.

4 Letter from Frances W. Hunnewell, Secretary, Harvard University Board of Overseers, to Varaztad H. Kazanjian, September 25, 1922, Kazanjian Archive, folder C-667 (this appointment carried over to the medical school as well); also, folder C-660, which contains the record of his appointment as Professor of Military Oral Surgery on Sept. 30, 1918.

5 He was appointed Professor of Plastic Surgery, Emeritus, in 1947.

6 Massachusetts General Hospital, *The News*, no. 108, January 1952, p. 2. A chronological listing of Dr. Kazanjian's professional appointments is included as an addendum to this book.

7 Converse, "Extraordinary Career," pp. 141-142. Also interviews by the author of Dr. Bradford Cannon, June 3, 1996, Boston, and November 11, 2002, in Lincoln, Mass., in the author's possession.

8 Robert M. Goldwyn, "Dr. Varaztad H. Kazanjian: Relevant or Irrelevant to Our Times?" paper delivered to the American Society of Maxillofacial Surgeons, Seattle, Wash., September 24, 1991. p. 10, in the author's possession; John Marquis Converse, *Kazanjian & Converse's Surgical Treatment of Facial Injuries*, 3rd. ed., vol. 1, p. ix; Letter from Dr. Richard C. Webster to Dr. Robert M. Goldwyn, June 4, 1975, in the author's possession; Mack L. Cheney, *Facial Surgery: Plastic and Reconstructive* (Baltimore: Williams & Wilkins, 1997), pp. 3, 6 (Section by William W. Montgomery and Mack L. Cheney).

9 Pam Hait, "History of the American Society of Plastic and Reconstructive Surgery, Inc. 1931-1994," *Journal of Plastic and Reconstructive Surgery* 94, no. 4: 13A; Letter from Richard C. Webster to Robert M. Goldwyn, June 4, 1975; John M. Converse, "Plastic Surgery: The Twentieth Century, The Period of Growth, 1914-1939," *Surgical Clinics of North America* 47, no. 2 (April 1967): 268. See Varaztad H. Kazanjian and John M. Converse, *The Surgical Treatment of Facial Injuries,* 2d ed., p. 435, for the technique of free-hand split thickness grafts and "Extraordinary Career," p. 142; Goldwyn, "Relevant or Irrelevant," p. 12.

10 Goldwyn, "Relevant or Irrelevant," pp. 10, 13-14, 21.

11 Letter from Hélène K. Sargeant to Dr. Robert M. Goldwyn, November 7, 1991, a copy of which is in the author's possession.

12 Converse, "Extraordinary Career," p. 142. Joseph E. Murray, *Surgery of the Soul* (Canton, Mass.: Science History Publications, 2001), p. 60. observed: "Dr. Kazanjian was not particularly welcome there [MGH] either because he was considered by many to be 'just a dentist'." Also, Walter C. Guralnick, Obituary: "Varaztad H. Kazanjian," *Harvard Dental Alumni Bulletin* 35, no. 1 (February 1975): 20-21; Interview with Dr. William W. Montgomery, John W. Merriam Professor of Otology and Laryngology at Harvard Medical School, on April 20, 1999, in Boston, in the author's possession. Dr. Montgomery related that he was considered a hero among the staff of Massachusetts Eye and Ear Infirmary because Dr. Kazanjian allowed him the freedom to observe his operations any time. This was permitted because Dr. Montgomery had

successfully treated a post-operative complication on one of Dr. Kazanjian's patients. Dr. Kazanjian, when operating, would normally cover the operative field if he felt that an untrained person was observing. Dr. Montgomery had extensive personal knowledge of Dr. Kazanjian's presence at the Massachusetts Eye and Ear Infirmary dating back to the 1940s and 1950s. The author's interview with him was arranged by Dr. Cliff A. Mergerian, formerly of the Department of Otolaryngology of the University of Massachusetts Medical School.

13 Interview with Dr. Montgomery; Goldwyn, "Relevant or Irrelevant," p. 11; R. H. Ivy, "Personal Recollections of the Organization and Founders of the American Association of Plastic Surgeons," *Plastic and Reconstructive Surgery* 47 no. 5 (May 1971): 444.

14 Interview by the author of Dr. Richard C. Webster, Brookline, Mass., date unrecorded, in the author's possession; Interview with Dr. Montgomery; Letter from Richard C. Webster to Robert M. Goldwyn. Dr. Kazanjian vacationed at his New Hampshire farm near Lake Sunapee. He was a robust swimmer and a devoted fisherman, and labelled himself "a clumsy gardener" who tramps the woods for wild flowers, *Harvard Medical Alumni Bulletin* 36, no. 3 (Winter 1962): 9.

15 John M. Converse, "Plastic Surgery: The Twentieth Century, 1914-1939," pp. 264-265, 270-271.

16 Ferdinand Brigham, Unpublished manuscript on the Dental Unit of the First Harvard Unit during World War I.

17 Certificate of marriage no. 26332, August 25, 1923, the City of New York, Borough of Manhattan, Municipal Archives; Natalie Gordon, *Boston Traveler*, September 17, 1947, p. 29, col. 4. Mrs. Kazanjian ran "a tight ship at home and office. Dr. Kazanjian did not think much about money." Taped interview by Dr. Robert M. Goldwyn and Madeline W. Mullin of Louise Roopenian, November 22, 1991.

18 Interview by the author of the Reverend Victor H. Kazanjian, Jr., Wellesley, Mass., February 4, 2002, in the author's possession. Also address by the Rev. Kazanjian, delivered at Harvard Memorial Church, "Be Gentle, Be Wise," on December 10, 1995; and a paper, "Beyond Tolerance: the Role of Religion and Spirituality in the Search for Community," given at the Peace Studies Association Eighth Annual Meeting at Earlham College and School of Religion, Richmond, Indiana, April 20, 1996.

19 *Boston Traveler*, September 17, 1947, p. 29, col. 4; Personal communication to the author by the Archivist, Massachusetts Eye and Ear Infirmary; *Belmont Citizen*, October 21, 1960, p. 10, col, 1.

20 *Boston Directory,* 1924, p. 700; 1926, p. 1374; 1930, p. 1396. The 1931 issue, p. 1442, lists his home as "Belmont, Mass." (4 Gorham Road). The 1932 *Boston Directory,* p. 1104, locates his home as 191 Clifton Street, Belmont, Mass. See letter from Varaztad H. Kazanjian to Charles Najarian, October 24, 1968, in the Kazanjian Archive, copy in the author's possession; *Belmont Herald*, Dec. 7, 1972, p. 12, cols. 4-8; Marderos Deranian, *Hussenig* (Belmont, Mass.: Armenian Heritage Press, 1994), p. 180.

21 Letter from Dr. Wallace J. Gardner to the author, October 29, 2001, in the author's possession.

22 Interviews by the author of Dr. Henry Kaplan, May 25, 1998, Rockport, Mass.; of Dr. Walter C. Guralnick, Boston, June 24, 1996; of Dr. Carnig Thomason, July 19, 1995, West Harwich, Mass. (Thomason had been a student at Harvard Dental School from 1939 to 1943); and of Dr. Bradford Cannon, June 3, 1996, in Boston, and November 11, 2002, in Lincoln, Mass. (All interviews in the author's possession.)

23 Alexander Pope, "An Essay on Criticism," line 15, "Let such teach others who themselves excel, and censure freely who have written well," as reprinted in Louis Kronenberger, ed., *Alexander Pope: Selected Works* (New York: Random House, 1951), p. 32. Also, Hait, "History of the American Society," p. 13A; Letter from Ralph L. Carney to Varaztad H. Kazanjian, October 12, 1928, in the Kazanjian Archive, folder C-60; Stephen Plumpton, "Kazanjian," *Dental Magazine and Oral Topics* 84 (no. 5): 207.

24 *Harvard Medical Alumni Bulletin* 36, no. 3 (Winter 1962): 9; Obituary, "Dr. Richard C. Webster," *Boston Globe*, September 28, 1994, p. 5, cols. 5-6; E. Antonio Mangubat, Steve B. Hopping and Richard Smith, "Leaders in Cosmetic Surgery: Richard Curtis Webster," *International Journal of Esthetic Surgery* 5, no. 1 (November 1, 1997): 5-12; Interview by author of

Virginia (Ring) Lane, February 15, 1999, Shrewsbury, Mass., in the author's possession. Mrs. Lane was medical secretary in Dr. Kazanjian's office from 1944 to 1948; Letter from Richard C. Webster to the author, August 9, 1948, from his office at 1101 Beacon Street, Brookline, in the author's possession; Letter from Richard C. Webster to Robert M. Goldwyn.

25 His middle name, Marquis, had been perpetuated in the family from the time of his great, great grandfather, who had fought in the Revolutionary War and had expressed an admiration for the Marquis de Lafayette. Blair O. Rogers, "John Marquis Converse (1909-1981), Obituary," *Annal of Plastic Surgery* 8, no. 4 (April 1982): 144-146.

26 Letter from John Marquis Converse to Varaztad H. Kazanjian, February 4, 1935. Kazanjian Archive, folder C-82 (written on the letterhead of "The American Hospital in Paris"); Rogers, "John Marquis Converse"; p. 343. Letter from John M. Converse to Varaztad H. Kazanjian, October 18, 1938, Kazanjian Archives, folder C-82. "Dr. Kazanjian, because of his personality and his inclination, never had a residency program, and in fact the only person whom he truly trained was Dr. Converse." Robert M. Goldwyn, "The Kazanjian Lecture: What Remains," *Aestheic Plastic Surgery* 18, (1994): 233-241.

27 Converse, "Extraordinary Career," p. 270; Avedis Derounian, "The Noted Surgeon Prescribes Industry," *The Armenian Spectator*, February 7, 1935, original preserved in the offices of *The Armenian Mirror-Spectator*, 755 Mount Auburn Street, Watertown, Mass.

28 Cheney, *Facial Surgery*, pp. 6-7; Interview by the author of Dr. Holmes's widow, Martha, February 4, 2002, Weston, Mass., in the author's possession.

29 Interview by the author of Dr. William G. Lavelle, July 8, 1999, Wellesley Hills, Mass., in the author's possession. Dr. Lavelle is Professor of the Department of Otolaryngology and Head and Neck Surgery at the University of Massachusetts Medical Center, Worcester. It is his view that Dr. Kazanjian and Sir Harold Gillies were the fathers of modern plastic surgery. The author acknowledges the assistance of Dr. Cliff A. Megerian, formerly of Dr. Lavelle's service, in arranging the interview. Also, videotaped interview of Dr. Aram Roopenian conducted by Dr. William G. Lavelle, January 28, 1989, courtesy of the Massachusetts Eye and Ear Infirmary Archives; Obituary, "Aram Roopenian," *The Boston Globe*, January 1, 1991, p. 33, col. 3; letter from Richard C. Webster to Robert M. Goldwyn; Interview by the author of Virginia (Ring) Lane, February 15, 1999, Shrewsbury, Mass., and interview by the author of Dr. Howard Ecker, Boston, Mass. and Dr. Joshua Charles Brooker, January 13, 2003, Brookline, Mass., in the author's possession.

30 Letter of Andrea Pogarian to the author from Brookline, Mass., August 5, 1999, in the author's possession (Mrs. Pogarian is Dr. Kenneth Kazanjian's daughter); Obituary: "Dr. Kenneth A. Kazanjian," *Boston Globe*, September 26, 1977, p. 33, cols. 7-8.

31 Interview by the author of Virginia (Ring) Lane, February 15, 1999, Shrewsbury, Mass.

32 Bradford Cannon, "The Flowering of Plastic Surgery," *Journal of the American Medical Association* 263, no. 6 (February 9, 1990): 862-864.

33 James M. Dunning, *The Harvard School of Dental Medicine: Phase Two in the Development of a University Dental School* (Cambridge, Mass.: The Harvard School of Dental Medicine, 1981).

34 Letter from Richard J. Wolfe to the author, October 13, 2002. In his capacity as curator of Rare Books and Manuscripts at Harvard's Countway Library of Medicine between 1962 and 1997, and as curator of the Harvard Medical Archives, Wolfe reported that he had many conversations with dental school faculty and alumni over the years, including Leroy Miner's widow, about the events that went on in the re-structuring of the Harvard Dental School. The quotation is from an unidentified faculty member whom he remembered having provided this piece of information.

35 Personal communication of Richard J. Wolfe to the author, October 13, 2002.

36 Richard C. Webster, "Cosmetic Surgery: Its Past, Present and Future," *The American Journal of Cosmetic Surgery* 1 (1984): 3-14.

37 Edward C. Lindeman, "Dedication of The Wall of Fame." This and other material on the New York World's Fair, 1940, can be found in the Kazanjian Archive, folder C-746.

38 Derounian, "Noted Surgeon." Kazanjian was not the first Armenian physician to serve in America's wars. Three Armenian physicians, Drs. Garabed Calousdian, Bornig Matteosian and Garabed J. Vartan, treated casualties in hospitals during the Civil War. M. Vartan Malcom, *The Armenians in America* (Boston: Pilgrim, 1919), p. 58. Dr. Mihran Krikor Kassabian (1870-1910) enlisted in the Hospital Corps of the U.S. Army in 1899 during the Spanish-American War, while in medical school. Like Dr. Kazanjian, he was born in Turkish Armenia. He emigrated to Philadelphia and obtained his M.D. degree from the Medico-Chirurgical College of Philadelphia in 1899. He became one of the foremost Roentgen Ray investigators in the world and wrote one of the most comprehensive texts on this new science. Unaware of the danger of radiation, which was little understood at that time, he gave his life to the destructive effects of X-rays and is commemorated in Percy Brown's *American Martyrs to Science Through the Roentgen Rays* (Springfield, Ill.: Charles Thomas, 1936), pp. 86-99.

39 Derounian, "Noted Surgeon." Some Armenians resented Dr. Kazanjian's failure to become actively involved with Armenian causes and organizations. Kazanjian did on occasion accept speaking engagements from Armenian-American groups. In March 1935, for example, he gave a lecture on plastic surgery to a group of young Armenian college graduates who met at regular intervals to discuss scientific problems. The lecture in Cambridge, Massachusetts, was accompanied by "lantern-slide illustrations." It was described in the April 1935 issue of *The Armenian Student.*

40 Interview by the author of Carnig Thomason, July 15, 1995, West Harwich, Mass., in the author's possession.

41 "Special Awards of the Society, and the Foundation of the Society of Plastic and Reconstructive Surgery," *Plastic and Reconstructive Surgery,* 9 no. 4 (April, 1952): 299. Also, letter to the author from Pat Heller, Librarian, University of Pennsylvania School of Dental Medicine, March 6, 1998.

THE WEATHER
Cloudy
Details on Page 2

WORCESTER TELEGRAM

COUNTY EDITION

VOL. XLVI. NO. 277. WORCESTER, MASS., THURSDAY MORNING, APRIL 7, 1932. 22 PAGES TWO CENTS

CURTIS BRINGS NEWS LINDY JR. ALIVE, WELL

SMITH FOES TWIST WORDS, ELY REPLY

Governor Opens Bay State Campaign for 1928 Nominee With Blast at Curley and 'Rooseveltian Misrepresentations'—Stresses Smith's 'If You Want Me, I'll Run'—Answers Wall Street and Power Trust Charges, Says Massachusetts Not So Fickle as Maine, New Hampshire

By JAMES H. GUILFOYLE

METHODISTS IN HONOR TO HEAD OF CONFERENCE

Bishop Anderson, Soon to Retire, Given Purse At Leominster

OFFICERS ELECTED

Today Brings Business Sessions, Veterans of Cross Banquet

LETTER INVITES HOOVER TO GIVE ECONOMY PLAN

House Committee Sends Message to President Pledging Help

WARNS OF POLITICS

$12,000,000 Cut From Interior Department Appropriation

POLICE OF WEBSTER GRANTED PAY CUT

Department Commended By Seletcmen; Janitor Wages Slashed

FITCHBURG MUSIC SUPERVISOR DIES

Miss Emma F. Southwick In Teachers' College Post 10 Years

Capt. Hawks Comes to Worcester

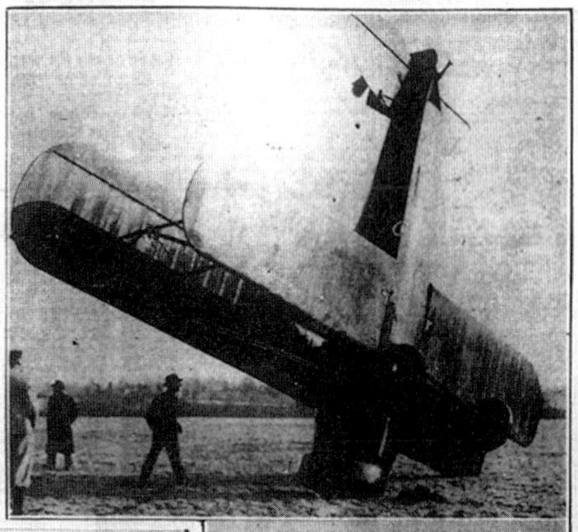

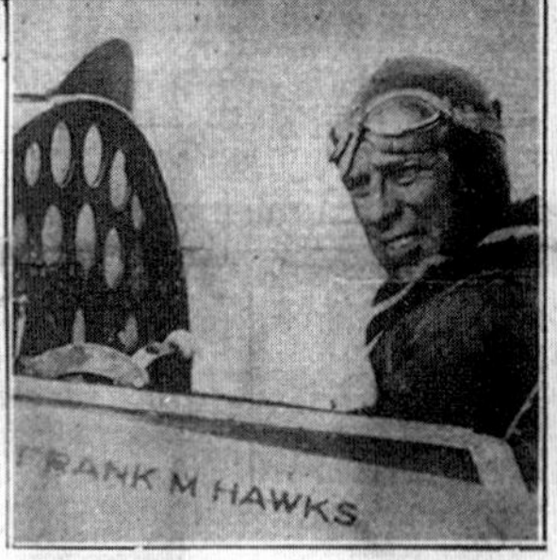

The unorthodox position of the plane in the above photo came about when John Whitin Lasell landed his biplane in a muddy spot at the Worcester airport at North Grafton. The plane nosed over, but without injury to the pilot. Mr. Lasell was flying as escort to Capt. Frank M. Hawks (shown below).

DEPUTIES CAN'T USE BOND FUND

Sheriff Rocheleau Bans Practice; Must File With Agencies

$10,000 REQUIRED

Matter of Protection, Is Stand Which County Official Takes

FRAMINGHAM FIRE LEVELS ICEHOUSES

$20,000 Blaze at Lake Waushakum Is Seen For Miles

Hawks Here From Detroit in 4 Hours, Fresh and Smiling

Need of Faster and Fool-Proof Planes Cited By Speed King—Escort Ship in Slight Mishap at Grafton Airport

Capt. Frank M. Hawks, famous speed king, scorched the ether over Grafton airport yesterday afternoon as he flashed above the hangars at more than 200 miles an hour. His rocket-like ship had cleaved a passage from Detroit in three hours and 55 minutes.

Banking high above the heads of spectators, after circling the field for inspection, he nosed down for a landing. The field was heavy. His wheels, striking the turf at 70 miles an hour, bogged far down the runway, bringing his plane to a sudden stop.

John Whitin Lasell, Whitinsville aviator, driving an escort plane, landed ahead of Captain Hawks to one side of the central runway, leaving a clear field for the visiting flier.

Continued on Page Twenty-Two

VIRGINIAN MAKES KIDNAP CONTACT

Admits Meeting Colonel Lindbergh While Away—Bay State Waters Searched—Hopes Increasing

DARROW SEEKS ANGLO-SAXONS IN JURY QUEST

Defense in Fortescue Case Fights Against Race Prejudice

MANY OBSTACLES

Mrs. Massie May Take Stand in Honolulu Honor Slaying

POLICE TO FIGHT LEOMINSTER CUT

Association Also Votes Against Volunteering Two Weeks' Pay

Today's Features

Worcester Telegram, April 7, 1932, page 1, col. 4, 5, and 6
Reprinted with permission from the Worcester Telegram & Gazette

CHAPTER TEN

Two Notable Patients of the 1930s: Frank M. Hawks and Sigmund Freud

Varaztad H. Kazanjian carried on what is known in medical circles as a "blue stocking" practice. The reputation he had earned through his advanced oral surgical techniques—especially in the making of prostheses—prior to World War I, followed by his accomplishments during that conflict, assured him a continual inflow of patients, not only locally but from all over America and even from abroad. If, for example, the daughter of a Boston Brahmin had been kicked in the face by a horse, it was a good bet that she would wind up under his care for the plastic surgery necessary to restore her flawlessly to her former appearance and beauty. And the same would apply to the son of a wealthy businessman or scion of industry who had been disfigured in an automobile accident or in a sporting contest or to the businessmen or industrialists themselves. For serious injuries to the face or mouth, or in the case of a face ravaged by cancer or another disease or disfigured by a birthmark or birth defect, Dr. Kazanjian was the one who was frequently recommended by the family physician as the *ne plus ultra* for the necessary reparative work that would be required. While he did ordinary day-to-day work and charity work as well and treated people from all walks of life, for those who could afford it—although his fees were no higher than those of other leading plastic surgeons—his services were considered the best that money could buy.

In the treatment of many thousands of cases over his nearly fifty-year career following graduation from medical school, Dr. Kazanjian understandably had many notable patients; however, two stand out, because of the international renown attached to them, as fitting examples: the aviator, Frank M. Hawks, and the neurologist and founder of psychoanalysis, Sigmund Freud.

Frank M. Hawks

From the earliest years of the twentieth century the eyes of the world were drawn skyward: in 1903, two brothers from central Ohio had achieved powered flight, and the public soon became enraptured with the novelty and daring of the airplane.[1] While many predicted that this fad would not last, in 1908, after the Wrights took a two-seater biplane to France and powered it off the ground, flew it for two circuits, and landed it again before a crowd of invited witnesses, everyone agreed that aviation was here to stay. The antics of pioneering pilots in the years following endowed this newfangled toy with the atmosphere of a circus, so that flying assumed the aura of public entertainment. World War I, with its engagements of aviators in mortal combat in the sky, like medieval knights in armor jousting in tournaments, added color and romance and dash and a unique excitement to the mystique of flying. Then, in the aftermath of the war, barnstorming and stunt flying by many ex-service pilots in cheap surplus Curtiss Jennies and their daredevil tricks like wingwalking enthralled the public even more, making aviation seem, like a Spanish bullfight, an exciting contest between man and death. But more rational minds foresaw the commercial and military potential of the airplane and began a relentless search for safer and more efficient machines; in their quest, the setting of new speed and distance records across nations and oceans in ever-improving airplanes became a frequent, seemingly everyday occurrence that played on the heartstrings of a fascinated public. In America, the publicity-seeking press made the names of Jimmy Doolittle, Glenn Curtiss, Charles Lindbergh, Colonel Roscoe Turner, Admiral Richard Byrd, Wiley Post, and others, household words. But for a few years in the late 1920s and early 1930s no name was more synonymous with speed in the air than that of Frank M. Hawks — characterized in popular magazine accounts as "Slide Rule Hawks Speed Demon" and the "World's Greatest Salesman of Speed."[2]

Born in Iowa in 1897, Francis Monroe Hawks always had a flair for the dramatic.[3] While attending grammar school in Minneapolis he played juvenile roles with a stock company in St. Paul; and at the end of his freshman year in high school he went on the road with a touring company that played the Northwest. Following Frank's graduation from high school, the Hawks family moved to Long Beach, California, where Frank qualified as a pilot in 1916. In 1917 he joined the aviation section of the U.S. Army Signal Corps, and was stationed at various flying fields in California and Texas as an instructor until his resignation in 1919. After working for a season on a ranch in Montana and as an athletic director and instructor at a Chicago junior high school, he found the lure of aviation too attractive to resist and obtained employment with a fishing tackle manufacturer in Michigan, delivering its products by air to dealers in the Midwest and barnstorming in each town he visited to reduce the cost of delivery. In 1920, he returned to California and took jobs as a mechanic and later as chief pilot for airplane manufacturers in Los Angeles. During this time, he did local passenger flying and made charter trips and barnstorming tours, besides participating in flying meets (and he also gave Amelia Earhart her first ride in an airplane.) He and a fellow flyer subsequently engaged in stunt flying, one of their stunts being the first successful refueling of an airplane by another in flight.

In 1928, after engaging in a variety of flying jobs, one as a pilot in the oil fields of Mexico, Hawks set out to better the transcontinental speed records. On February 4-5, 1929, he flew non-stop from Los Angeles to Roosevelt Field on Long Island in 18 hours, 21 minutes and 59 seconds. Then, on June 27-29, he flew from Roosevelt Field to Los Angeles in the record time of 19 hours and 2 minutes and the next day set a new West-to-East record of 17 hours and 43 minutes, making the round trip in 36 hours and 45 minutes flying time. On August 6, 1930, he followed these achievements by flying from Curtiss Field at Valley Stream, Long Island, to Los Angeles in the elapsed time of 14 hours, 30 minutes and 43 seconds, with five intermediate stops for fuel. He made the return trip, August 13th, from Los Angeles to Curtiss Field in 12 hours, 25 minutes and 3 seconds, with three stops for fuel. The total flying time was 11 hours, 40 minutes and 30 seconds. In addition to his transcontinental records, Hawks set 214 point-to-point records in the United States, Europe, and Latin America and also made some notable achievements as a glider pilot. In 1930, he was awarded the Harmon Trophy as the outstanding aviator in the United States for that year and also received decorations from the French and Swiss aero clubs. In 1931, he published a book entitled *Speed*. In 1932 he was made a lieutenant commander in the U.S. Naval Reserve air force.

On April 6, 1932, Hawkes was the main attraction at a speaking engagement at Mechanics Hall in Worcester, Massachusetts, under the auspices of the Worcester Council of the Boy Scouts of America.

The next day, after breakfasting with M. Whitin Whitehall, a member of the Scout executive committee who was mainly responsible for inviting him to speak, Hawks was driven to the airport by his host. Upon examination of the field, Hawks and Whitehall found that it had become boggy and very soft in many areas. While landing there the previous day in his private red-and-white "Mystery Plane," after a three-hour flight from Detroit, Hawks's plane had become mired in the soft ground and he narrowly escaped overturning it. He attempted an initial take-off by using a dirt road that cut across the field as a runway but was unable to negotiate its short, 450-foot length. Nonetheless he decided to attempt a take-off from the field itself in order to hop to Boston, refuel and fly on to New York, where he intended to complete preparations for a solo flight to Puerto Rico the following week. After the plane was rolled from the hangar and inspected, Hawks donned his flying clothes and climbed into the cockpit for a farewell picture. Although the owners of the airport expressed serious concern over the prospects of a successful take-off from a runway of less than 700 feet, Hawks taxied his plane into position and began his take-off but could not get airborne in time to lift over the stone wall. The plane ripped through a hedge at an estimated speed of fifty miles per hour, struck a large stone wall and rocks at the east side of the field and overturned. Hawks was pulled unconscious from the wreckage of his plane with blood pouring from his face and rushed in a private automobile to City Hospital in Worcester. Upon preliminary examination, he was found to have suffered serious fractures of the jaw and a possible skull fracture, as well as multiple deep cuts to the face. The incident became the subject of reports appearing on the front page of an Extra edition of the *Worcester Telegram* that day and on page one of *The New York Times* on the following day.[4]

A column published on page one of the *Telegram* the next day[5] reported that while state and federal aviation inspectors were concluding their investigation of the accident, Dr. Ernest L. Hunt, chief of the City Hospital's surgical staff, issued a statement that the aviator would recover, but would have to remain in the hospital for five or six weeks. A complete diagnosis of Commander Hawks's injuries, based on x-rays, had revealed that his lower jaw was fractured in two places, that his nose was fractured, and practically all of his teeth in the lower jaw had been knocked out or badly damaged. In

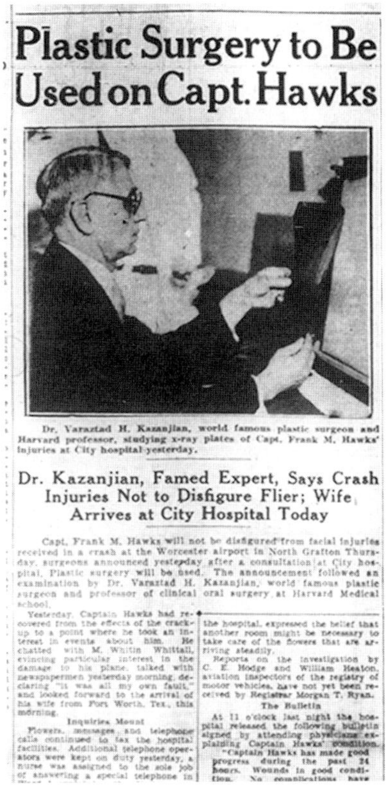

Plastic Surgery to Be Used on Capt. Hawks

Dr. Varaztad H. Kazanjian, world famous plastic surgeon and Harvard professor, studying x-ray plates of Capt. Frank M. Hawks' injuries at City hospital yesterday.

Dr. Kazanjian, Famed Expert, Says Crash Injuries Not to Disfigure Flier; Wife Arrives at City Hospital Today

Capt. Frank M. Hawks will not be disfigured from facial injuries received in a crash at the Worcester airport in North Grafton Thursday, surgeons announced yesterday after a consultation at City hospital. Plastic surgery will be used. The announcement followed an examination by Dr. Varaztad H. Kazanjian, world famous plastic surgeon and professor of clinical oral surgery at Harvard Medical school.

Yesterday, Captain Hawks had recovered from the effects of the crack-up to a point where he took an interest in events about him. He chatted with M. Whitin Whittall, evincing particular interest in the damage to his plane, talked with newspapermen yesterday morning, declaring "it was all my own fault," and looked forward to the arrival of his wife from Fort Worth, Tex., this morning.

Inquiries Mount

Flowers, messages and telephone calls continued to tax the hospital facilities. Additional telephone operators were kept on duty yesterday, a nurse was assigned to the sole job of answering a special telephone in

the hospital, expressed the belief that another room might be necessary to take care of the flowers that are arriving steadily.

Reports on the investigation by C. E. Hodge and William Heaton, aviation inspectors of the registry of motor vehicles, have not yet been received by Registrar Morgan T. Ryan.

The Bulletin

At 11 o'clock last night the hospital released the following bulletin signed by attending physicians explaining Captain Hawks' condition.

"Captain Hawks has made good progress during the past 24 hours. Wounds in good condition. No complications have

Worcester Telegram, April 9, 1932, page 1, col. 4 and 5
Reprinted with permission from the Worcester Telegram & Gazette

addition, he had suffered raw gasoline burns on one arm and shoulder. Mrs. Hawks, notified of her husband's injuries by the Associated Press on the day of the crash, had started out for Worcester by train from Fort Worth, Texas, at 4 p.m. that same day and was expected to arrive in Worcester on Saturday morning, but might switch to an airplane if she encountered delays. (The *Times* report of the 8th related that at first she had considered going by plane, but after she had talked with Commander Hawks's physician and with a friend in Worcester, she said that her husband's condition was not regarded as alarming.)

The *Telegram* also reported that messages had been pouring into City Hospital from all over the country since the previous afternoon. Members of the Morrow family — that is, the Lindbergh family, the accident occurring a little over a month following the kidnapping of the Lindbergh baby son, who was still missing — had called from New Jersey, and Will Rogers had telegraphed from San Francisco, while piles of unopened messages had accumulated. By late afternoon on the day of the crash, Hawks's room was crowded with flowers. Semi-conscious, unable to talk, and not permitted to see visitors, he feebly acknowledged telephone calls when they were repeated to him. An accompanying column by Walter M. Merkel, a *Telegram* staff reporter,[6] related that the speedster's jaw was so fractured that he had to write out his wants. And it reprinted a telegram in which Will Rogers had sent the following message:

> *Sure glad that nothing broke but your jaw, that will keep you still awhile. If I broke my jaw I could still write gags. What's the matter with you anyhow, are you getting old and brittle? I have turned over a couple of times and nothing hurt but all of the iron work of the plane. You are a sissy, that's what you are.*
>
> —Will Rogers

A long article appeared on page one of the Saturday morning, April 9, *Worcester Telegram*, which included a picture of Dr. Kazanjian studying x-ray plates at City Hospital the day after Commander Hawks's injuries. It was reported that on Friday the surgeons had announced at a press conference that it had been determined after an examination and consultation by Dr. Kazanjian, "world famous plastic surgeon and professor of clinical oral surgery at Harvard Medical School," that Hawks would not be disfigured from the facial injuries he received in Thursday's crash and that plastic surgery would be employed to avoid that result.[7] It also reported that Hawks had recovered from the effects of the crack-up so as to be able to follow the events about him. He had talked with Mr. Whitehall and related that he was looking forward to the arrival of his wife. A bulletin had been released at 11 p.m. the previous night, reporting that Hawks had made good progress during the previous twenty-four hours; that his wounds were in good condition; that no complications had arisen; that his pulse and temperature were within normal limits; and that he was comparatively comfortable and in good spirits. It then reported that "Dr. Kazanjian, with Dr. Ernest L. Hunt, attending surgeon, Dr. Max Ginns, dental surgeon, and Dr. Edward J. Crane, house surgeon, examined Captain Hawks' injuries. Dr. MacIver explained to newspapermen that Dr. Kazanjian is recognized as the foremost oral surgeon in the world, having made a name for himself during the World War in reconstructing the shattered faces of wounded soldiers."

At the conclusion of his examination, the article went on, Dr. Kazanjian answered all questions gracefully, declaring that "Captain Hawks' injuries are largely superficial, though severe. It will be necessary to use plastic surgery to restore his face to normal, but this can be done so that there will be scarcely a scar. His speech will not be affected by his injuries. I think his rapid recovery is a reasonable expectation." Asked if the right side of Commander Hawks's face, so cruelly lac-

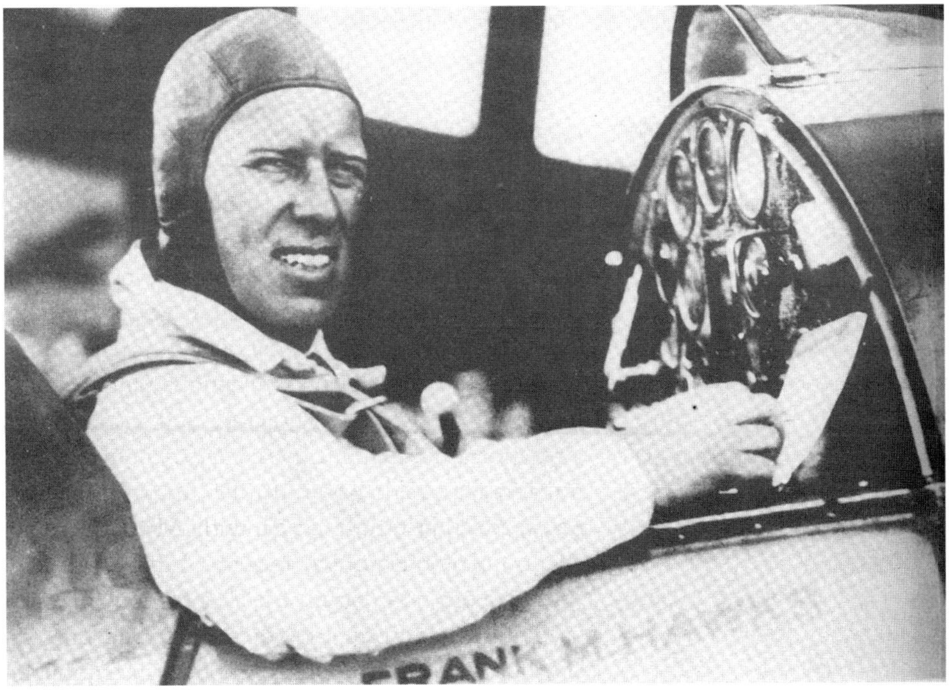

Frank M. Hawks "Now I am a fairly good-looking chap;" Hawks said after his treatment by Dr. Kazanjian, "Never was before, you know." Photograph from Chelsea Fraser, Famous American Flyers, *(New York: Thomas Y. Crowell, 1941) p. 222, Brown Brothers photo*

erated, would be paralyzed, Dr. Kazanjian shrugged his shoulders and replied: "It is too soon to tell the extent of the injury to the muscles and nerves." In the final part of this lengthy article appeared Hawks's version of the crash, and his feelings of responsibility for it:

> *It was my own fault for attempting to make a takeoff without a run of sufficient length over the soft ground. I knew the point where the field ended on the east side, but I thought that I could get off before I got there. I had gotten the plane off the ground, but my propeller struck a bush which slowed down the speed sufficiently so that the plane dropped onto the ground again, when I lost all my flying speed. It all happened in a jiffy. I don't remember that I cut off the ignition switch, but I don't think that I had time to do so.*

He then admitted that he knew all the time he was taking a very close chance. "If it hadn't been that I had to be in New York so to complete plans for the Puerto Rico trip I was going to make next week, I wouldn't have tried to get away. I'd have left the damn plane there until the field hardened up."

> *It was my first crack-up which resulted in injuries that I've ever had in my 15 years of flying. The first thing I knew when the plane went over was when I came to in the car just before we got to the hospital.*
>
> *When I found that the runway on the road was too short, it seemed best to me to take the east and west runway, heading east. I thought that I had distance enough to get off but that bush which got in my propeller threw me down again. I always said that if it was my fault when I cracked up, I'd say so and not try to pass the buck. This was all my own fault and the management was not to blame at all.*
>
> *Just as soon as the doctors say that I'm healed up, I'm going back to flying again. Why not?*

On April 19 the *Boston Herald* also published a special dispatch it had received the prior evening that reported many of the same facts, but with a few additions.[8] It reported that the operation to restore the airman's face would not take place for several days, indicating that Dr. Kazanjian wished to wait a day or two for any possible change in his condition. "Although speaking with difficulty because of his broken jaw and bandages, Captain Hawks readily entered the conversation this afternoon on the hospital bed. He was cheerful and optimistic that he would be out within a short time." The article concluded with a brief notice that Kazanjian had served during the war with the British Expeditionary Force as a specialist for the jaw and face and that he was a visiting surgeon for oral and plastic surgery at the City Hospital in Boston and on the staff of several other Greater Boston hospitals.

The next news item on Hawks's case appeared on April 17, when *The New York Times*[9] and other newspapers reported that Hawks had been taken to Phillips House of the Massachusetts General Hospital the previous day in order to undergo plastic surgery. He was accompanied on the ambulance trip from Worcester City Hospital by Mrs. Hawks and Speed, his Aberdeen terrier. In the two weeks that followed he underwent two operations at the hands of Dr. Kazanjian. Then, on May 4, the *Times* published another brief report on the case.[10]

> BOSTON, May 3. —*Captain Frank Hawks, speed king of the air, who nearly lost his life in a plane crash in North Grafton several weeks ago, will undergo next week a third operation on his jaw, which was shattered, and his face, which was badly torn. The operation in Massachusetts General Hospital is to remove fragments of bone still remaining and to relieve the pull of flesh on one of his eyes caused by one of the wounds "healing tight." Dr. A. V. [sic] Kazanjian, plastic surgeon, at Harvard Medical School, will perform the operation.*

On June 6, *The New York Times* reported on the successful outcome of the operation, stating that Commander Hawks "came out of hospital, played a round of golf and began plans to resume his career in the clouds."[11] On June 15, the same paper reported that "yesterday Hawks made his first long flight since his accident. He left Floyd Bennett Field for Boston for consultation with his physician, flying a Lockheed Sirius."[12] Finally, in a special report it received from Chicago on December 27, the *Times* related that Hawks had passed through Chicago that day on United Airlines flight en route from Fort Worth to New York. He was on his way to the Phillips House in Boston, where he would undergo another operation, this one to remove scars from his face and reset his jaw. He planned to return to San Antonio, Texas, in two weeks to test a new plane, a low wing Northrup, in which he planned to circle the globe.[13]

As to Hawks's later career, in 1935 he reportedly went to China on a six months' leave of absence from the Texas Pipe Line Company to demonstrate the Curtiss bomber to the Chinese government. On his return, he resigned from the company to devote his full time to the construction of the monoplane, Time Flies, designed by him and Peter Miller. In the winter of that year he became vice-president of the Gwinn Aircar Company of Buffalo, New York, and thereafter devoted his time to the development of the Aircar. He suffered fatal injuries in an airplane crash at East Aurora, New York, and died in Buffalo on August 23, 1938. It seems likely that had his fatal accident not occurred or had he survived it, he would have gone on to more significant accomplishments and would have made an even greater name for himself in the war that America entered three years later.

Sigmund Freud

"Man has, as it were, become a kind of prosthetic God," Sigmund Freud wrote in his book, *Civilization and its Discontents*, the second edition of which appeared in 1931. "When he puts on all his auxiliary organs he is truly magnificent; those organs have not grown on him and they still give him much trouble at times."[14] This was a pointed reference to the extreme difficulties Freud was experiencing with the maxillofacial prosthetic appliance he had been wearing since 1923. In that year he had undergone a radical cancer operation of the jaws for the removal of a tumor. A portion of his upper and lower jaw as well as a section of his soft palate had been removed.[15] In a letter Freud had written to Ernest Jones on April 23, 1923, he related:

> *I have detected two months ago a leucoplastic growth on my jaw and palate right side, which I had removed on the 20th. I am still out of work and cannot swallow. I was assured of the benignity of the matter but as you know, nobody can guarantee its behaviour when it be permitted to grow further. My own diagnosis has been epithelioma but was not accepted. Smoking is accused as the etiology of this tissue-rebellion.*[16]

Freud's predisposition toward smoking spanned most of his adult life. As early as 1893, he was writing to his physician, "I am not obeying your smoking prohibitions. Do you really consider it such a great boon to live a great many years in misery?"[17] His attitude in this regard is best illustrated in the following letter written by him on February 12, 1929:

> *I began smoking at the age of 24, first cigarettes but soon exclusively cigars, and am still smoking now (at 79 1/2), and very reluctant to restrict myself in the pleasure. Between the ages of 30 and 40 I had to give up smoking for a year and a half because of heart trouble which may have been [due to] the effect of nicotine, but was probably a sequel to influenza. Since then I have been faithful to my habit or vice, and believe that I owe to the cigar a great intensification of my capacity to work and a facilitation of my self-control. My model in this was my father who was a heavy smoker and remained one till his 81st year.*[18]

Freud's cancer was treated from 1923 to 1938 principally, but not exclusively, by Dr. Hans Pichler, a compassionate oral surgeon in Vienna, who was described as "the best head surgeon in Europe."[19] He was involved in Freud's treatment both as surgeon and prosthodontist. Pichler "kept regular notes of the case, every visit being recorded and the details entered with an admirable exactitude."[20]

During the summer of 1931, H. G. Wells, the English novelist and historian, visited Freud and remarked "that Freud's name was as important in the history of thought as the name of Charles Darwin's."[21] That year marked the seventy-fifth anniversary of Freud's birth. He had been awarded the Goethe Prize the previous year, which had "altered the public attitude toward him into 'reluctant recognition'." Freud's attitude toward the prize was one of open apathy, and he claimed that he would much have preferred a "bearable prosthesis which did not try to turn into the end and chief aim of existence."[22] Referring to his prosthetic appliances, Freud perceived, "It is like the pursuit of happiness," adding that "you think you already have it in your grasp and it is always gone again."[23] Dr. Max Schur, Freud's physician from 1928 to 1938, called the prosthesis "the monster."[24] On one occasion, Freud was asked to speak French, but refused, saying pathetically, "My prosthesis doesn't speak French."[25]

"I detest my mechanical jaw," he declared on his seventieth birthday, "because the struggle with the mechanism consumes so much precious strength. I prefer a mechanical jaw to no jaw at all. I still prefer existence to extinction." Freud devel-

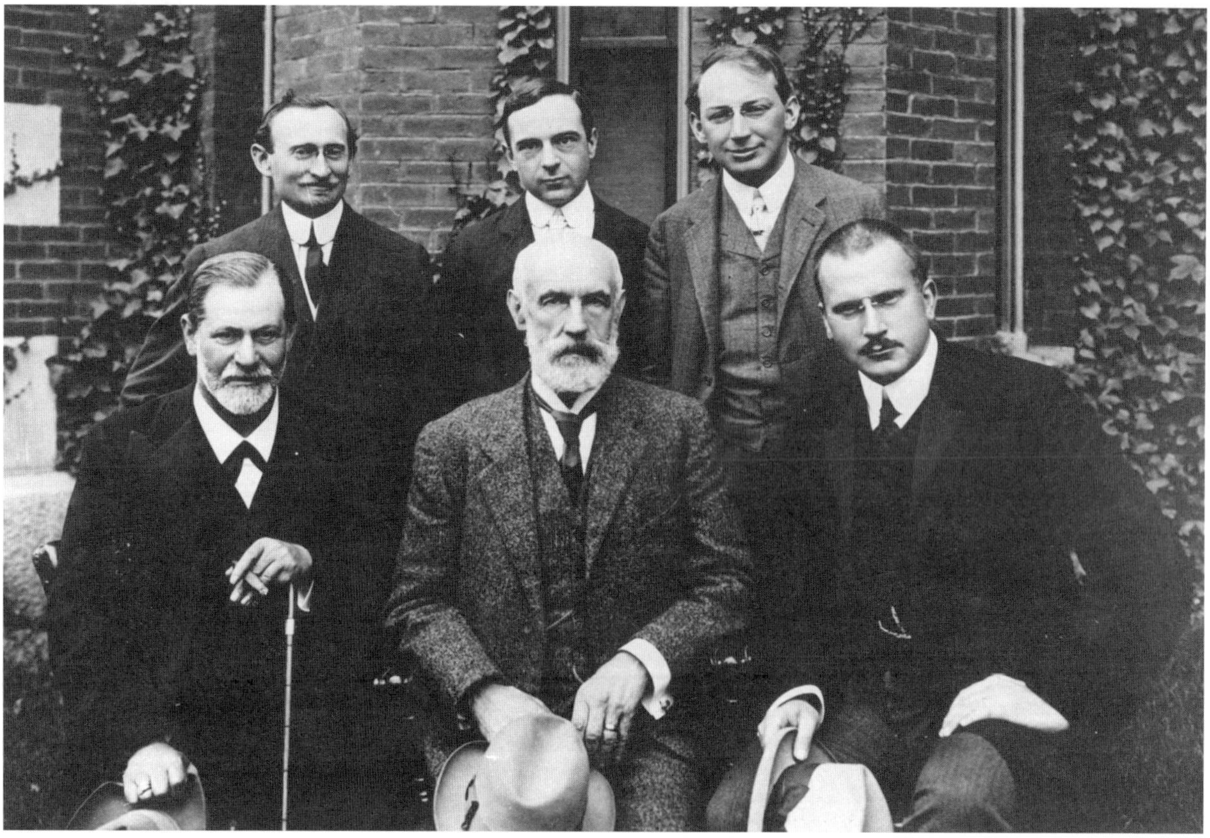

Freud at Clark University, Worcester, Mass., Sept. 1909, where he delivered the "Five Lectures Upon Psychoanalysis." This was the only trip which he made to the United States.
Upper row: A. A. Brill, Ernest Jones, Sandor Ferenczi
Lower row: Sigmund Freud (with cigar), G. Stanley Hall, Carl Jung
Courtesy Clark University Archives

oped the "habit of keeping his prosthesis in its place with his thumb, this . . . produced rather the impression of philosophical concentration."[26] Freud's speech "sounded like a cleft palate patient left untreated. . . . In addition, his hearing suffered."[27] "I disclose," Freud wrote to Lou Andres-Salome shortly before July 10, 1931, "that I have meanwhile experienced all kinds of disagreeable things with my prostheses, which, as usual, has suspended my higher interests."[28]

In 1928, Pichler inserted the fifth prosthesis which he had made and which Freud found as "being too thick and cumbersome." Freud wrote to Jones on July 1, 1928, "Pichler's efforts to provide me with a better prosthesis have caused me a great deal of suffering during the past year and the outcome is quite unsatisfactory. So I have at last yielded to pressure from many sides to turn to someone else."[29]

The new dentist who fabricated another prosthesis was Dr. Hermann Schroeder, Director of the Dental Institute of the University of Berlin. The frequent and extended trips which Freud was forced to make to Berlin were exhausting. As a result, a dentist in Vienna, Dr. Joseph Weinmann, who had spent time with Schroeder, cared for Freud locally. "Later in 1930 he (Freud) went back to Berlin," his physician Max Schur reported, "and underwent three months of torture in an attempt to get more lasting relief from a new prosthesis built by Schroeder."[30] But relief was not in sight.

During this desperate time in 1931, two of Freud's close associates, Dr. Ruth Mack Brunswick and Princess Marie, conceived the plan to bring relief to their mentor. Princess Marie (1881-1962) was a student and personal friend of Sigmund Freud and of his daughter, Anna. She was an eminent psychoanalyst in her own right. In 1938, it was she who "at considerable risk and sacrifice, not only insured his [Freud's] personal security but was responsible for the fact that the Nazis permitted him to leave Austria." She was the great granddaughter of Lucien Bonaparte, Emperor Napoleon's eldest brother. In 1907 she had married Prince George of Greece, and was known as "the greatest heiress in France." Dr. Ruth Mack Brunswick (1899-1946), a native of Chicago, graduated from Radcliffe College and from Tufts Medical School in 1922. Immediately after graduation, she went to Vienna, where she attended the Vienna Psychoanalytic Institute. She became a member of Freud's intimate circle and practiced psychoanalysis in Vienna while teaching at the Institute. Beginning in 1938, she practiced in New York, where she died at the age of forty-seven. Her father was Julian Mack, a judge of the United States Circuit Court of Appeals.[31]

The events that followed have been recorded by Ernest Jones:[32]

Dr. Brunswick had heard that Professor Kazanjian of Harvard, a man reputed to possess magical talents, was attending a dental congress in Berlin (it was, in fact, Paris, not Berlin),[33] and everyday she telephoned him begging him to come to see Freud. He was persistent in refusing but then Ruth Brunswick and Marie Bonaparte, who was also in Vienna, put their heads together. The former got her father, Judge Mack, who was on the Board of the Overseers of Harvard University, to use his influence by cable, and the latter took the train for Paris, caught the unwilling magician on his way home, and brought him back with her, "so to speak on a lead," accompanied by Dr. Weinmann,[34] who had attended the Congress.

Dr. Kazanjian recalled these events in an interview which was recorded twenty-seven years later, in 1958:

> *In 1931, I was invited to two international dental meetings, one in London and one in Paris. I left with my family, consisting of my wife and daughter, and arrived in London on July 19, 1931. I had not been in the hotel for an hour when I was paged. A telegram had arrived from Judge Mack in which he asked me whether I would not go to Vienna to see Prof. Freud for a consultation. I should communicate with Mrs. Brunswick for details [Judge Mack's daughter]. I had gone to Europe for only one month with my wife and a small child and I was not allowed to spend more time and had to return to the United States. Dr. Brunswick, who was trained in Boston, told me of Prof. Freud's whole condition and his difficulties. Nevertheless, I had to refuse and told her that I could not go to Vienna since I had the responsibility of attending the Congresses and had to go home with my family. When she heard that we were going to Switzerland and would stay at Ste. Croix, she asked me to get in touch with Princess Marie of Greece. This I did and telephoned her as soon as I arrived in Ste. Croix. She gave all the details of Freud's sickness and it was clear that he had a cancer of the upper jaw and that his physicians were trying to make a prosthetic appliance to cover the missing parts of the palate so he could talk, swallow, and smoke. She invited me to go as her guest to Vienna and I could not refuse this offer. I went to Vienna and as soon as I arrived Freud and his family were ready for my examination.*

I examined Prof. Freud and saw that the appliance used wasn't suitable.[35]

Before attending the Dental Congress in Paris, Dr. Kazanjian treated Freud in Vienna on July 31 and August 1, 1931. He altered the existing prosthesis and inserted two provisional ones. He returned to Vienna after the Congress and continued his treatment of Freud.

The following entries are from the *Diary of Sigmund Freud*, 1929-1939:

Armenian dentist from Boston Fri 31 July 1931

With the appearance of this "Armenian dentist," Ruth Mack Brunswick resolved that Freud's prosthesis should be improved. She persuaded him, with great difficulty, to come to Vienna briefly before the congress. Kazanjian agreed to look at Freud's prosthesis, but did not make any promises about returning after the congress.

Freud's prosthesis was the bane of his life. He had grown skeptical about the possibility of improvement, but had not entirely given up hope and consented to the consultation. Afterwards he wrote to Eitingon that Kazanjian ". . . inspires great confidence and is a shy man with a smile like Charlie Chaplin." (Freud- Eitingon 3.8 1931)[36]

New prosthesis Kazanjian Sat 1 August 1931

Freud's first response to Kazanjian's preliminary work was amazement: "And now the unbelievable has happened! In 1 1/2 days—Friday and Saturday—today is Monday, the magician has completed a provisional prosthesis, which is only half as big and heavy as the previous one, with which I can chew, speak and smoke at least as well as before." (Freud-Eitingon 3.8. 1931)[37]

"Prof. Kasanjian [sic] reduced and narrowed existing prostheses considerably and finally made 3 prostheses," Pichler recorded. "One of hard rubber, two with back part of soft rubber. These have doubtless the great advantage that they cannot lever the front teeth. Patient speaks much better with soft-rubber prostheses but cannot smoke with it at all and bites his tongue."[38]

At the Eighth International Congress of Dentists held in Paris on August 2-8, Kazanjian presented a paper, "Surgical and Prosthetic Treatment of the Mandible." Dr. Robert H. Ivy, who also delivered a paper at the Congress, reported, "One day we missed Kazanjian and he later told me he had been taken by Pichler to Vienna to make a new prosthesis for Sigmund Freud." Elsewhere it is recorded that "After the Paris congress, Kazanjian did not want to return to Vienna, partly because of his family. However, Ruth Brunswick and Marie Bonaparte inveigled him into coming despite his—and Freud's—resistance: Ruth offered him his equivalent normal income of $5,000 a month and the Princess exhorted him to come 'with wife and daughter also in tow' from Paris to Vienna and paid for their stay at the luxurious Cottage Sanatorium."[39]

Kazanjian was planning to work on Freud only until the last week of August. He notes, in the entry for Monday, 10 August, 1931, "After the continual extensions of his treatment with Schroeder in Berlin, Freud must have welcomed this strict timetable. He submitted passively to the treatment undeterred by the long years of torture and giving in to other people's insistence."[40]

One of the prostheses which Kazanjian fabricated after his return to Vienna is preserved in the Freud Museum in London. Dr. John C. Davenport has carefully identified and described the Kazanjian appliance. It is creatively designed and superbly crafted, weighing only 54 grams, much lighter than some of the previous appliances.[41] It has a gold base. The saddle areas supporting the porcelain teeth were made of a combination of red, pink and black rubber vulcanite.[42] It was held in place with metal clasp arms with female attachments that engaged their male extra-coronal counterparts that were in the mouth. The posterior portion obturator section extended into the soft palate. It was fabricated of rubber vulcanite in two sections, which were joined by a means of two gold prongs, similar to an electrical plug as it engages a wall socket, allowing the prosthesis to be inserted in two sections and permitting a joint-like mobility.[43]

"In fact, he [Kazanjian] 'read' his new patient" well, concluded Professor Dr. Branislav Dimitrijevic maxillofacial surgeon and prosthodontist of Belgrade. He "couldn't do anything against the political pressure" that had been brought to bear, forcing him to change his mind and to go to Vienna to treat Freud. "He did his best" but he well knew that the chance for success was slim.[44] "A classmate of mine, Dr. Blumgart, a professor of Medicine at Harvard, asked me in 1929 or 1930," Dr. Kazanjian revealed, "whether I could go to Europe to make a special prosthetic appliance for a prominent person. I had to refuse this request since it was a very time-comsuming affair to make such a device."[45]

Dr. Kazanjian left Vienna on August 29, 1931. The entry in Freud's diary of that day reads:

> *Kazanjian had reduced an existing prosthesis and produced three new rubber ones. Pichler generously lent him his laboratory, but Kazanjian had had to do all the construction work on the plate himself: there were no trained assistants and many unavailable materials had to be sent by Marie Bonaparte from Paris.*

The day after Kazanjian's departure Freud wrote:

> *The magician left me yesterday. I am not feeling so wonderful, but anyway speech is better. I should anticipate further progress on growing accustomed to the new thing. It does not seem possible to do anything more for me."* (Freud-Eitingon 30.8.1931)[46]

The extensive surgery performed on Freud made the construction of a functional and comfortable prosthesis impossible.[47]

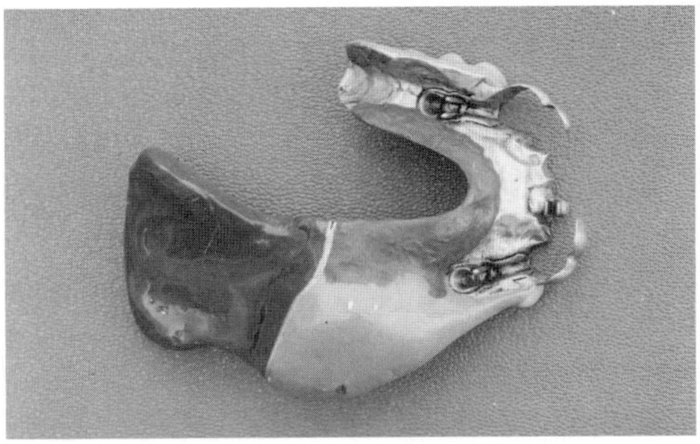

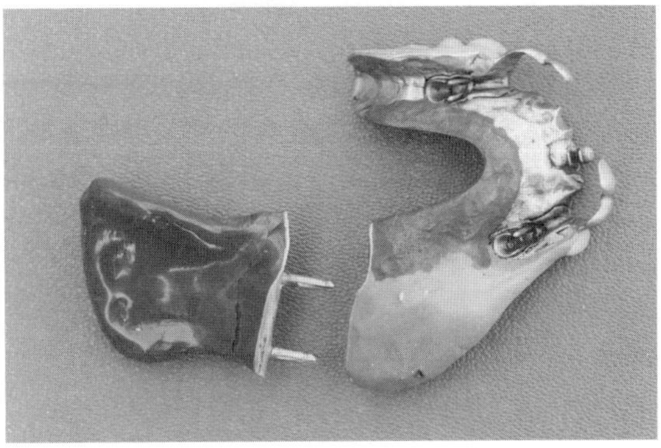

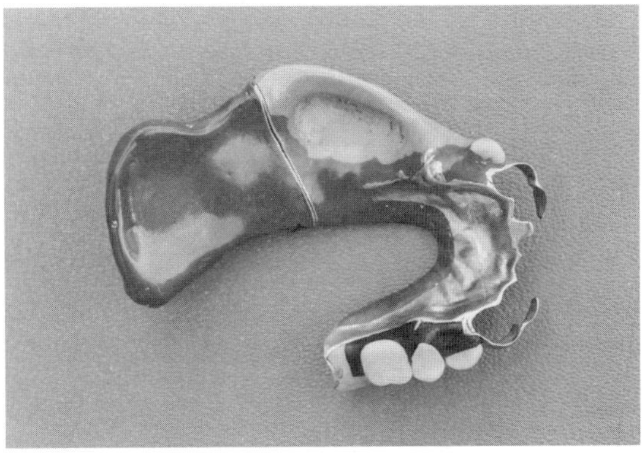

Views of Freud's prosthesis provided by Kazanjian in 1931

Top: *Tissue surface with the two sections joined*
Middle: *Tissue surface showing the sectional design and double pin attachment. The two sections are unjoined*
Bottom: *External surface with the two sections joined*

Courtesy Freud Museum, London, Michael Molnar, Research Director

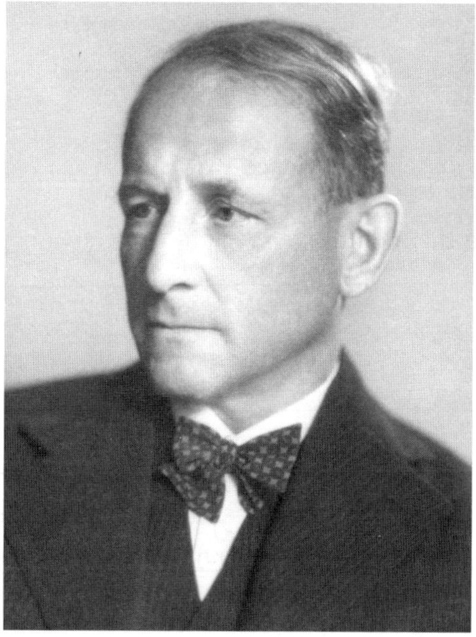

Dr. Hans Pichler (1887-1949)
Osterreichische Nationalbibliothek, Vienna

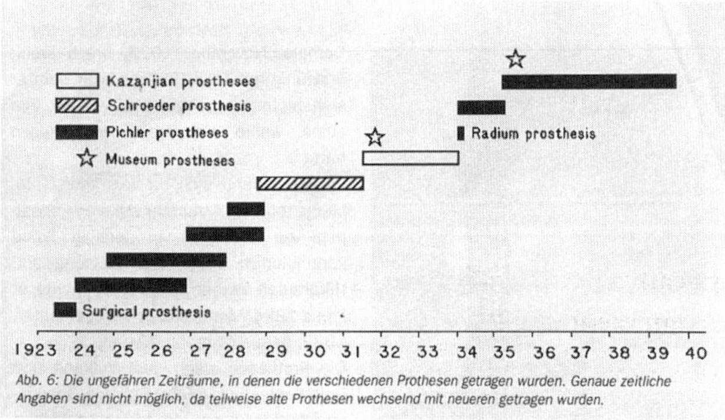

Chart illustrating the various Freud prostheses, their duration of use and by whom fabricated. Kazanjian's prostheses were in use from 1931-34.
J. C. Davenport, British Dental Journal *172:5, March 1992*
Permission from Dr. Davenport and the publishers of the British Dental Journal

"I was asked how much my stay in Vienna would cost and I said that my income in the United States was $5,000 per month," Dr. Kazanjian disclosed. "Dr. Brunswick willingly approved and there was no special difficulty encountered with the financing. She generously paid the bill without my asking for it." Dr. Kazanjian never had the opportunity to see Vienna during his stay of twenty days. He worked on Freud's prostheses "from morning to midnight. Sometimes I worked with Freud for 3-4 hours. I saw Freud every day and in some days two or three times. I worked on an adjustable appliance which could be modified in accordance with the changes the surrounding tissue would under-go."[48]

Kazanjian's appliance served Freud for three years, about as long as Schroeder's had previously. A premalignant lesion appeared in 1934 and radium therapy was required. Because the Kazanjian prostheses contained metal, they could not be used in the presence of radium for fear of secondary radiation. A new all-vulcanite prosthesis was constructed by Pichler to carry radium to the site of the lesion.[49]

Pichler treated Freud sixteen times in 1923, seventy-four times in 1924, and ninety-four times in 1932.[50] Even with this succession of visits, Freud expressed a wish to be treated more frequently, stating that "he felt neglected" by Pichler.[51]

Both Kazanjian and Pichler had entered surgical practice by way of dentistry. Pichler studied at the Northwestern University School of Dentistry in Chicago under Dr. Greene Vardiman Black, "the Father of Modern Dentistry," and translated Black's textbook, *Operative Dentistry*, into German.[52] By contrast, it was Kazanjian's early experience and facility in prosthetics that marked the difference in training and orientation of the two men, although both were influenced by the theories and writings of Claude Martin of Lyon, France (see Chapter 3). The relationship between Kazanjian and Pichler remained cordial. "I guess you will remember our patient, Sigmund Freud," Pichler wrote to Dr. Kazanjian in 1948.

"I have thought of you often," Dr. Kazanjian responded, "and I remember how generous you were in giving me the use of your office when I was in Vienna."[53]

It was in 1934, a year "surprisingly free from surgical intervention," Romm observed, "that Freud outlined his last major work, *Moses and Monotheism*."[54]

Freud's personal physician, Dr. Max Schur, made this pointed observation:

> *Concerning the prosthesis, I must add that while Pichler was a superb surgeon and an excellent physician, his art as a dental technician may not have been quite the equal of his surgical skill. In later years, two other specialists [one of whom was Kazanjian] were asked to try their hand at creating a prosthesis. Perhaps, given an opportunity to be in constant attention, they could have produced a more efficient and less troublesome instrument.*[55]

Paul E. Stepansky, in a recent book, *Freud, Surgery and the Surgeons* (1999), has observed that "Freud realized he was literally waging war with the prosthesis in a fateful struggle for minimally acceptable oral functions . . . but the changing contours of Freud's oral landscape outpaced his surgeons' mechanical ministrations time and again, so that the ego-sustaining, ego-alien device remained refractory, an instigator of oral warfare without truce to the end of his days. Adjustment after adjustment, prosthesis after prosthesis, an end never in sight." He added, "Nor could the surgeons who subsequently tried their hand at an improved prosthesis do any better than Pichler."[56]

"When I left Vienna," Dr. Kazanjian later recalled, "Prof. Freud was content and I did not hear anything more after I left. Freud was a very mild-mannered man, a gentleman, a very cooperative patient. While I was working he recited from Shakespeare, Goethe and went back to the Classics. He was extremely sensitive physically."[57] During his lifetime, Dr. Kazanjian never made a public statement about Freud's illness.

The prosthetic appliances made for Freud by Kazanjian were creatively designed, skillfully fabricated, and technically sound. Kazanjian's treatment modality and accomplishments, given the constraints and limitations under which he was forced to work, merit recognition and commendation. He had to endure the problem that Freud, an inveterate addicted smoker, would not give up his cherished cigars. As a result, his mouth tumor kept reappearing in enlarged form.

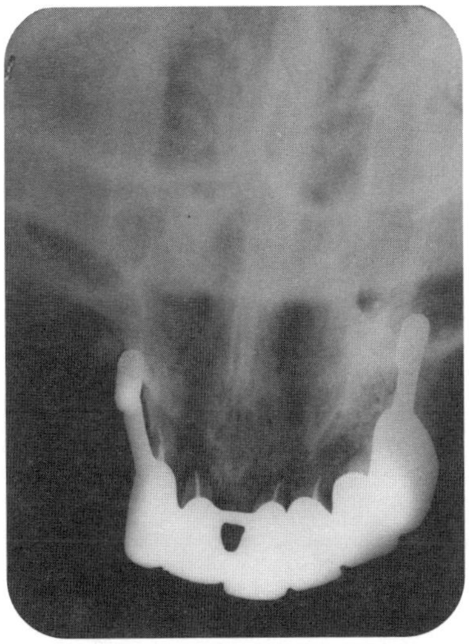

X-ray of Freud's maxillary anterior area: showing the fixed cuspid to cuspid bridgework with the right and left extra-coronal male attachments
Courtesy Freud Museum, London, Michael Molnar, Research Director

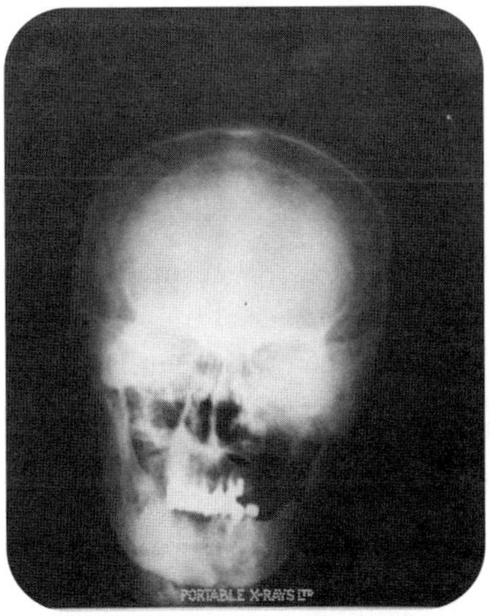

X-ray of Freud skull
Courtesy Freud Museum, London, Michael Molnar, Research Director

NOTES

1 For a synopsis of the progress of aviation during the twentieth century, see Bill Gunston, *Aviation: the First One Hundred Years* (Hauppauge, N.Y.: Barrons, 2002), from which a few sentences are quoted or paraphrased here.

2 "Slide Rule Hawks Speed Demon," *Outlook* 157 (March 25, 1931): 432-433, and "World's Greatest Salesman of Speed," *American Magazine* 111 (June 1931): 42-43.

3 Biographical information on Frank M. Hawks comes mainly from a posthumous biography which appeared in *The National Cyclopaedia of American Biography* 29 (1941): 170-171.

4 "Noted Flier Hits Wall in Take-off," *Worcester Telegram*, Extra edition, April 7, 1932, p. 1, cols 7-8; *The New York Times*, April 8, 1932, p. 1, col. 4.

5 "Six Weeks in Hospital for Famous Flier," *Worcester Telegram*, April 8, 1932, p. 1, col. 8.

6 Walter M. Merkel, "Hawks Badly Battered But He'll Pull Through," *Worcester Telegram,* April 8, 1932, p. 1, col. 5.

7 "Plastic Surgery To Be Used For Hawks," *Worcester Telegram,* April 9, 1932, p. 1, cols. 4-5.

8 "Hawks Face to Be Restored; Noted Harvard Plastic Surgeon to Remove Scars of Crash; Flyer Is Confident of Quick Recovery," *Boston Herald*, April 9, 1932, p. 1, col. 7.

9 "Plastic Surgery for Hawks," *The New York Times*, April 18, 1932, p. 15, col. 1.

10 "Hawks Faces Third Operation," *The New York Times*, May 4, 1932, p. 21, col. 8.

11 "Hawks Leaves Hospital," *The New York Times*, June 6, 1932, p. 17, col. 4.

12 "Hawks Flies to Boston from Floyd Bennett Field," *The New York Times*, June 15, 1932, p. 15, col. 4.

13 "Capt. Hawks Flies to Hospital," *The New York Times*, December 28, 1932, p. 14, col. 5.

14 Peter Gay, ed., *The Freud Reader* (New York: W. W. Norton & Co., 1989), p. 738 and footnote no. 9. "For many, this late essay, in which Freud sums up his long-held theories of culture, is the only Freudian text they ever read" (p. 722). This book first appeared in 1929. The remainder of the paragraph of the text quoted is as follows:

"Nevertheless, he is entitled to console himself with the thought that this development will not come to an end precisely with the year 1930 A.D. Further ages will bring with them new and probably unimaginably great advances in their field of civilization and will increase man's likeness to God still more. But in the interest of our investigation, we will not forget that present-day man does not feel happy in this Godlike character."

15 Sharon Romm, *The Unwelcome Intruder: Freud's Struggles with Cancer* (New York: Praeger, 1983), pp. 17-31, describes the first operation which the dentist Hans Pichler performed on Freud in 1923. Cancers associated with cigar smoking were called the "rich man's cancer," since only rich men could afford to smoke fifteen to twenty cigars a day (p. 38). In a foreword to Romm's book, Dr. Sanford Gifford uses the characterization of "the flamboyant Armenian-American Kazanjian" (p. xi). Later in the text itself (p. 102) Romm writes, "Kazanjian was generally thought of as a kindly practitioner, ready to be of assistance whenever needed." It is this latter characterization that is far more in keeping with the traditional and overwhelming view of Kazanjian.

16 Ernest Jones, *The Life and Work of Sigmund Freud* (New York: Basic Books, 1957), v. 3 p. 89.

17 Letter from Sigmund Freud to his physician, Wilhelm Fliess, dated November 17, 1893, quoted in Max Schur, *Freud: Living and Dying* (New York: International Universities Press, 1972), p. 42. Schur observes, "Nicotine probably helped Freud tolerate pain and frustration and maintain his equilibrium" and "Freud could do no creative work without smoking"(p. 412). Freud's letter to Wilhelm Fliess is in the Arents Collection, New York Public Library.

18 Quoted in Schur, *Living and Dying*, p. 62.

19 Quoted in Hannelore T. Loevy and Aletha Kowitz, "Freud's Oral Problems: The Chicago Connection," *Chicago Dental Society Review* 88 no. 2 (March 1995): 38.

20 Jones, *Life and Work of Sigmund Freud,* v. 3, p. 468. Appendix B, pp. 469-495 contains Pichler's surgical notes of his treatment of Freud which are preserved in the Freud Museum, London. Hans Pichler was a distinguished Viennese oral and maxillofacial surgeon and dean of the Dental School of the University of Vienna. Romm, *Unwelcome Intruder*, p. 59.

21 Jones, *Life and Work of Sigmund Freud,* v. 3, p. 160.

22 Sigmund Freud, *The Diary of Sigmund Freud, 1929-1939*, translated and annotated by Michael Molnar (London: Hogarth Press, 1992), p. 91. "The new suit from Stefan [the tailor] is again perfect," Freud wrote to his wife. "I shall ask him whether he doesn't also make prostheses." Quoted on p. 91, which records the reference as "Freud-Martha Freud 12.4. 1932," correspondence in the Freud Museum, London.

23 Letter from Sigmund Freud to Maria Bonaparte, September 18, 1931, quoted by Schur, *Living and Dying*, p. 430.

24 Schur, *Living and Dying*, p. 364, footnote. Freud's struggle with the "monster" has been described by Jones: "On his birthday [1938], Freud tried till he was quite exhausted to insert the horrible 'monster' into his mouth." (Jones, *Life and Work of Sigmund Freud*, v. 3, p. 196.) "There was constant trouble with the 'monster' which had to be modified every few days . . . Smoking was allowed but to get a cigar between his teeth he had to force the bite open with the help of a clothes peg" (Ibid., p. 101).

25 Jones, *Life and Work of Sigmund Freud*, v. 3, p. 103. One interpreter theorized that "civilization . . . would be very different today if Freud had had a better partial denture, or if he had never smoked cigars!" Dr. E. J. Neiburger, letter to the editor, captioned "Freud's Oral Cancer Changed Psychotherapy," *Journal of the Massachusetts Dental Society* 45, no. 4 (Winter 1997): 8. Since speech was difficult with his prosthesis, "Freud used less hypnosis, because it required 'commanding' speech . . . and Freud gravitated to the invention of free-association psychotherapy in which the patient did all the talking."

26 Jones, *Life and Work of Sigmund Freud*, v. 3, pp. 102, 126.

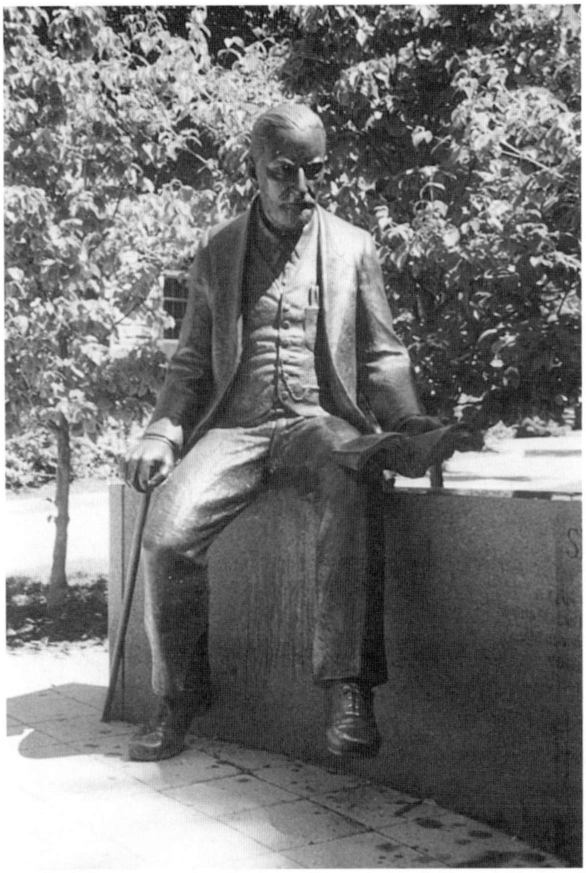

Statue of Freud at Clark University, Worcester, Mass. Robert Shure, sculptor

27 Quoted in Eugene M. Feldman, "Freud's Cancer," *Journal of the History of Dentistry* 47, no. 1 (March 1999): 16. For a comprehensive description of Freud's speech, see Romm, *Unwelcome Intruder*, pp. 69-70. "I do not hear anything on this right side but a constant murmur." (Quoted in Schur, *Living and Dying*, p. 378.)

28 Quoted in Peter Gay, *Freud: A Life for Our Own Time* (New York: W. W. Norton & Co., 1988), p. 539.

29 Romm, *Unwelcome Intruder*, p. 91; Schur, *Living and Dying*, p. 405 (The entire letter in German is quoted on p. 557).

30 Schur, *Living and Dying*, p. 423. "The new Schroeder dentures were a great improvement on

the old ones," (Freud estimated 70 per cent), Davenport wrote. "They were supported by precision attachments that formed part of the bridge that Schroeder had fitted to the upper anterior teeth." See John C. Davenport, "Sigmund Freud's Illness—The Ultimate Team Approach to Head and Neck Cancer?" *Facial Plastic Surgery* 9, no. 2 (April 1993): 129.

31 From obituaries of Princess Marie Bonaparte which appeared in *The New York Times* on September 22, 1962 p. 25, col. 5, and October 13, 1962, p. 24, col. 5.; and the obituary of Ruth Mack Brunswick in *The New York Times* on January 26, 1946, p. 13, col. 3.

32 Jones, *Life and Work of Sigmund Freud*, v. 3, p. 161. Also quoted in Romm, *Unwelcome Intruder*, p. 101.

33 The text mentions Berlin, but in fact Paris was the site of the International Congress of Dentists, August 1-8, 1931.

34 "From 1928 to 1930 Freud's surgeon in Vienna was . . . Dr. Joseph Weinmann . . . a dentist and oral pathologist, not actually a practitioner of oral surgery. He later emigrated to the United States from Vienna, where he devoted his career to research, becoming a professor at the University of Illinois." (Romm, *Unwelcome Intruder*, p. 92.) Also Loevy and Kowitz, "Freud's Oral Problems," p. 39.

35 Transcript of interview of Dr. V. H. Kazanjian conducted in Boston by Dr. Eissler on October 26, 1958, Library of Congress, Washington, D.C., Manuscript Division, Container B55 of the Sigmund Freud collection, pp. 1-2. Appreciation is expressed to Marvin Kranz and the Library of Congress for the use of this material. "Dr. Eissler" is Kurt Eissler, the psychoanalyst and founder of the Sigmund Freud Archives." (Molnar xi)

36 *Diary of Sigmund Freud*, p. 103. The letter to Max Eitingon, July 31, 1931, is in the Freud Museum in London.

37 Ibid.

38 Jones, *Life and Work of Sigmund Freud*, v. 3, appendix B, pp. 482-483. Hans Pichler's notes of Freud's treatment are preserved in the Freud Museum in London.

39 Kazanjian's paper, "Surgical and Prosthetic Treatment of Deformities of the Mandible," International Dental Congress, 8th, Paris, August 2-8, 1931, Section 12, is in the Varaztad H. Kazanjian Archive in The Francis A. Countway Library of Medicine, folder AM-165. Letter from Dr. Robert H. Ivy to Homer S. Samuels, Captain, U.S.N., U.S. Naval Hospital, Philadelphia, February 13, 1968, can be found in the Dr. Samuel D. Harris National Museum of Dentistry, Baltimore. The notion that Kazanjian had been taken by Professor Hans Pichler to Vienna "is at odds with Ernest Jones's" account, which states that Kazanjian was "accompanied by Weinmann." (Jones, *Life and Work of Sigmund Freud*, v. 3, p. 161.) See also *Diary of Sigmund Freud*, entry for August 10, 1931, p. 103. (Ernst-Freud letter 30.8.1931 is in the Freud Archive, Manuscript Division, Library of Congress.)

40 *Diary of Sigmund Freud*, entry for August 10, 1931, p. 103. The Freud-Lamp-de Groot letter 11.8.1931 is in the Freud Museum, London.

41 For further information of the Kazanjian prosthesis, see John C. Davenport, "The Prosthetic Case of Sigmund Freud," *British Dental Journal* 172, no. 5 (March 7, 1995): 205, and "Der Kranke Sigmund Freud und Seine Zahnärzte," *Zm-Zahnärztliche Mitteilungen* 23 (December 1, 1992): 24-28. The author acknowledges his indebtedness to Davenport for the description of Kazanjian's prosthesis. Also Davenport, "The Ultimate Team Approach," pp. 125-131.

42 Vulcanite is a chemical combination of hard rubber, caoutchouc, and sulfur, which have been subjected to vulcanization (steam pressure). It was used as a base of dentures and appliances.

43 The author visited the Freud Museum, 20 Maresfield Gardens, London, on June 12, 2000, and consulted with Michael Molnar, Research Director. The author arranged for a professional photographer to take photographs of the appliance which Dr. Kazanjian fabricated for Freud in 1931, and prints are in the author's possession. Acknowledgment and appreciation are expressed to Michael Molnar and to the Freud Museum for this courtesy.

44 Letter to the author from Professor Dr. Branislav Dimitrijevic, July 24, 1991, Belgrade, Yugoslavia, in the author's possession. "Concerning my opinion, Dr. Kazanjian was sure that Sigmund Freud will refuse to wear any new denture, sooner or later." Sharon Romm,"The Oral Cancer of Sigmund Freud," *Clinics in Plastic Surgery* 10:4

(October 1983): 713, verifies that Kazanjian's "mind was changed by political pressure."

45 Sharon Romm, "The Oral Cancer of Sigmund Freud," *Clinics in Plastic Surgery* 10, no. 4 (October 1983): 713; Transcript of Kazanjian interview conducted in Boston by Dr. Eissler on October 26, 1958, pp. 2-3.

46 *Diary of Sigmund Freud,* entry for August 29, 1931, p. 104. (The Freud-Eitingon 30.8.1931 correspondence is in the Freud Museum in London.)

47 Loevy and Kowitz, "Freud's Oral Problems," p. 39.

48 Transcript of interview of Dr. Kazanjian conducted in Boston by Dr. Eissler on October 26, 1958, p. 2.

49 Romm, *Unwelcome Intruder*, p. 105.

50 Ibid., p. 40.

51 Quoted in Romm, *Unwelcome Intruder*, p. 103. Also, Jones, *Life and Work of Sigmund Freud*, v. 3, pp. 468-495. For many years, the author has been treating post-surgical cancer patients with a clinical diagnosis and situations similar to that of Sigmund Freud. These patients have required the fabrication of maxillofacial prosthetic appliances, some extremely complex. Frequent follow-up appointments are the rule rather than the exception. One such patient required thirty-three appointments one year, thirty-nine the next year, and thirty-five the following year.

52 Sharon Romm and Edward A. Luce, "Hans Pichler: Oral Surgeon to Sigmund Feud," *Oral Surgery, Oral Medicine and Oral Pathology* 47, no. 1 (January 1984): 31-32. John J. Posner, "Dentistry — Vienna to Venice," *Dental Surgery* (April 1934): 41, states that "Professor Hans Pichler is the greatest head surgeon." Schur, *Living and Dying*, p. 362, writes: "Although [Pichler] certainly had no inkling of Freud's place in the history of science, he treated him for 15 years with the utmost respect, tact, and courtesy."

53 Kazanjian offered to be a resource concerning a book that Pichler had written, to determine "whether there would be enough sales in this country to justify the translation." Varaztad H. Kazanjian to Hans Pichler, September 17, 1948, Kazanjian Archive, folder C-335.

54 Romm, *Unwelcome Intruder*, p. 105.

55 Schur, *Living and Dying*, p. 364. Dr. Kazanjian observed that "changes in the device required modification" and said, "I doubt that the physician in Vienna performed those changes adequately." (*Diary of Sigmund Freud,* entry in the section of references for 29 August 1931, p. 283.)

56 Paul E. Stepansky, *Freud, Surgery and Surgeons* (Hillsdale, N.J.: The Analgetic Press, 1999), pp. 143, 146. Dr. Stepansky is a member of the Section on Psychiatric History of the Department of Psychiatry, Cornell Medical College and New York Hospital.

57 Transcript of interview by Dr. Eissler on October 26, 1958, pp. 2-3.

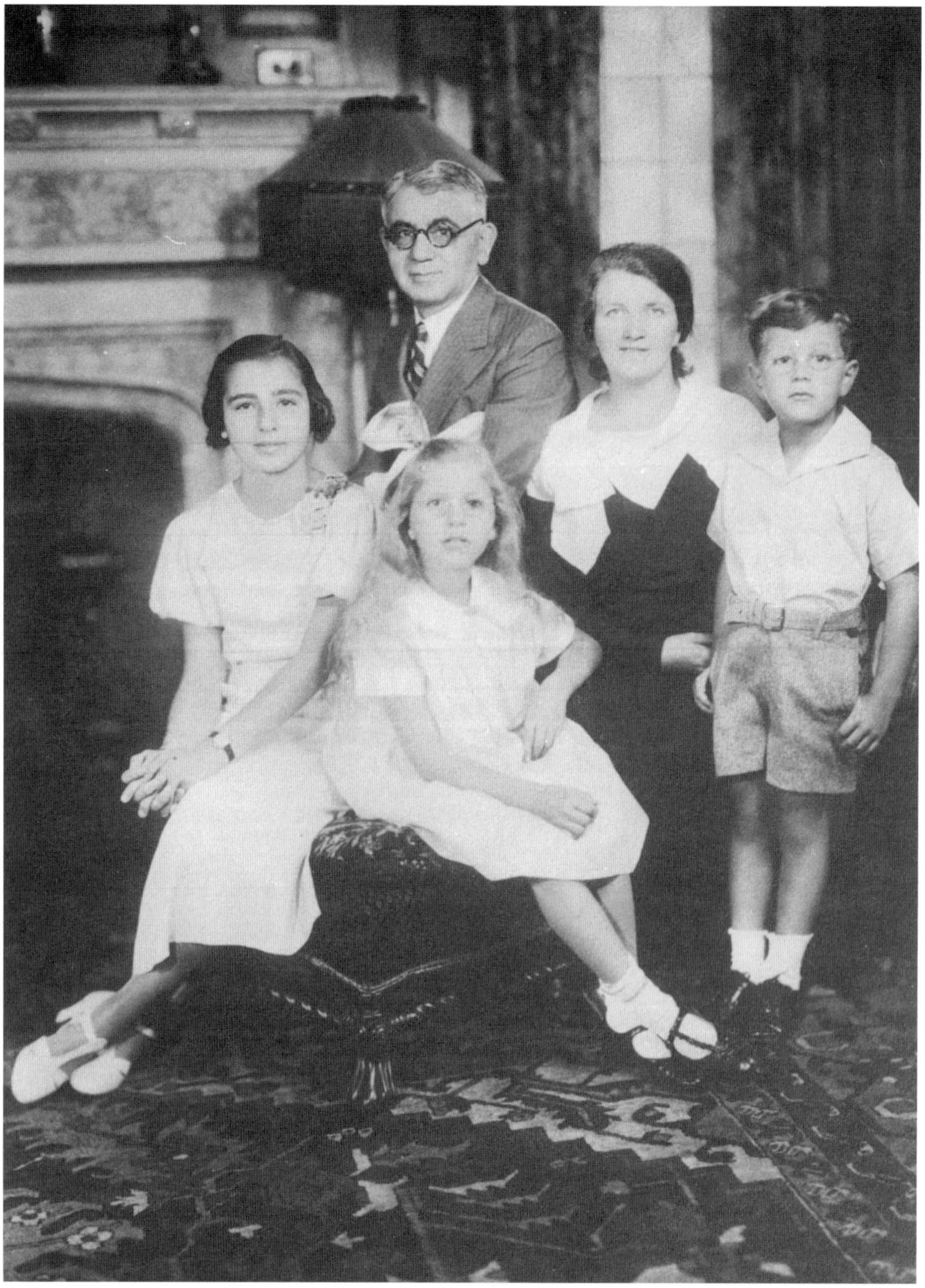

The Kazanjian Family. Seated left, Hélène, Joan and Victor
Courtesy The Rev. Victor H. Kazanjian, Jr.
Photograph by Kaiden-Kazanjian, N.Y.

CHAPTER ELEVEN

World's Most Famous Plastic Surgeon[1]

In 1946 Varaztad H. Kazanjian was sixty-seven years old. In the forty-one years that had passed since his graduation from the Harvard Dental School in 1905 and the twenty-five after he had been awarded the M.D. degree by Harvard in 1921, his career had been marked only with success; and now, in the post World War II world, he continued his activities as he had before—humbly, and in a matter-of-fact manner. Dr. Kazanjian also continued to be a familiar figure at the restructured Harvard School of Dental Medicine, which now contained a greatly diminished student body. Accompanied by Dr. Bradford Cannon, recently returned from service in the U.S. Army, he conducted a clinic there on Fridays and delivered noontime lectures on fractures. "At this clinic," Dr. Walter Guralnick remembered:

> *Methods of preparation of oral and facial prostheses were also developed and appliances constructed for splinting of fractures and post-osteotomy jaw fixation. Operative procedures and consultations were frequently conducted in conjunction with the clinic.*[2]

The ridge extension procedure he devised for improvement of the edentulous ridge (without teeth) was an operation he often did in the School's Surgical Clinic. Patients with jaw deformities were treated there by him, Dr. Henry Carney, and Dr. L. K. Daghlian, prosthetic dentistry instructors whom he had introduced to maxillofacial prosthetics and who became outstanding men in their field. The surgical approach always remained uppermost in Dr. Kazanjian's teaching, but he made expert use of dental appli-

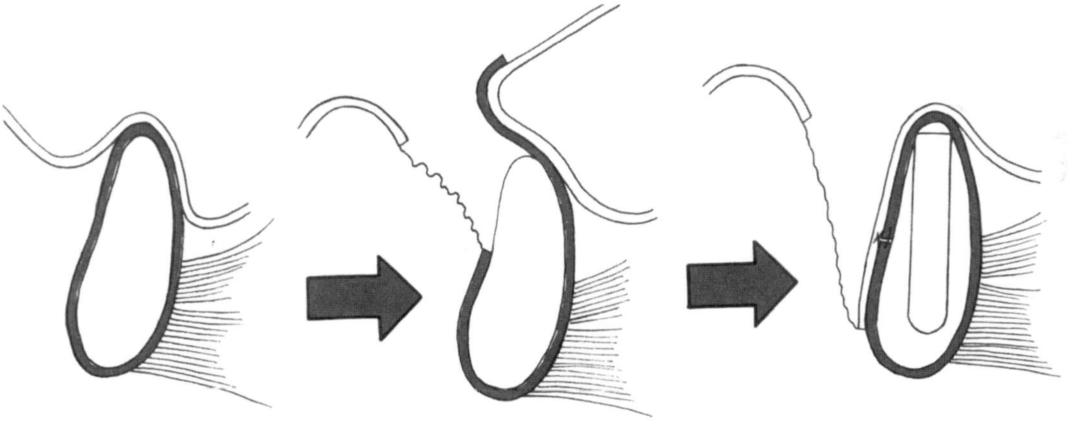

Kazanjian-style vestibuloplasty allows access for implant placement and increased vestibular depth and attached tissue as well. Peterson, Ellis, Hupp, Tucker, Contemporary Oral and Maxillofacial Surgery, *2nd ed. (St. Louis: Mosby, 1993) p. 397. Permission from Elsevier*

ances when indicated. Many of his publications during the decades that followed were based on patient material and experiences originating in this active clinic.[3]

Drs. Kazanjian and Cannon also continued to carry on their Crippled Children's Program at the Mount Auburn Hospital in Cambridge, where they and later their associates "saw large numbers of clefts of the lip and palate, other congenital maladies, varied disfigurements from burns to trauma," and other interesting reconstructive challenges that presented themselves. In his 1990 memoir, Dr. Cannon mentioned that the Mount Auburn Hospital served him in two important ways. "To have done cosmetic surgery at the MGH in the mid 1940s would have been frowned on." The other advantage was the excellence of anesthesia given there; "The chief of anesthesia was willing to listen to the plastic surgeon's special needs, particularly concerning endotracheal intubation, a procedure little understood and seldom used across the river in Boston."[4]

In 1947, Dr. Kazanjian was designated Professor of Plastic Surgery Emeritus at Harvard; and late in 1949, at about the time he reached the age of seventy, the first edition of *The Surgical Treatment of Facial Injuries,* co-authored by him and by Dr. John Converse, was issued by Williams & Wilkins Company in Baltimore.[5] The collaborative work on this book initially began late in 1942 or early 1943 but was interrupted by the war, when Dr. Converse left for army duty in North Africa. For the next ten months, in an Algerian hospital, he treated 375 patients with maxillofacial injuries.[6] It was not until 1946 that the two surgeons resumed their collaboration on the book. The medical secretary at that time who took down the dictation for its text was Virginia Ring. After she worked at the office in the morning, Basil, the chauffeur, would drive her to the Kazanjian residence in Belmont. Following luncheon, Dr. Converse would dictate from the notes that he and Dr. Kazanjian previously had prepared. Traveling from New York, Dr. Converse, accompanied by his wife, would often stay for up to two weeks in the Kazanjian residence and at their summer home in New Hampshire. "Weekends and long evenings of work and discussion resulted in the publication of the book in 1949," Dr. Converse later wrote, "but most of all, resulted in a warm relationship." And, he added, "his [Kazanjian's] interest and enthusiasm never flagged."[7]

The Surgical Treatment of Facial Injuries extended to 574 pages, contained 746 photographs and drawings and other medical illustrations, was dedicated to both of the authors' wives, and sold for ten dollars. Its twenty-five chapters, its authors wrote in their preface, were based upon years of experience in the treatment of many thousands of cases of facial injuries from private practice and institutional clinics, from some of their publications in the surgical literature, and from service in two world wars, Kazanjian's in France in 1914-1918 and Converse's in England, North Africa, Italy and France in the 1940-1946 period. Since the purpose of the book was to stress the viewpoints of the authors regarding the surgical treatment of facial injuries, the text was limited to cases that they had treated personally. They had designed the book to interest not only the specialist in plastic surgery but also the general practitioner in the fields of medicine and dentistry who might be called upon to render emergency treatment in facial injuries; and the otolaryngologist, ophthalmologist, neurosurgeon and oral surgeon would find sections of special interest, since aspects of these specialized fields were intimately related to that of plastic surgery. The authors professed to claim no originality in the operative procedures described, acknowledging that their knowledge and techniques were based on those who had preceded them and on their contemporaries in the field of surgery.

The emphasis in the text was placed on general principles rather than on the details of individual cases, although reference was made to selected illustrations and case histories in order to stress the importance of basic principles employed in treatment. As background for the student and practitioner, the first three chapters dealt with a brief survey of the evolution of the human face, some aspects of anatomy, the healing of wounds, and general principles of operative technique. Subsequent chapters focused on fractures of bones of the face and jaws, with succeeding chapters devoted to general principles of reconstructive surgery and deformities of the upper portion of the face, eyelids, orbital region and nose, and soft tissues and bones of the lower portion of the face. Included also were chapters on the oral cavity and pharynx, temporo-mandibular ankylosis, facial paralysis, deformities of the external ear and burns of the face.

The authors related that they also had attempted to integrate and evaluate the prosthetic and surgical aspects of facial reconstruction. And they added a chapter on anesthetic management on account of the unique requirements of surgery in or near the airway. Facial injury, they believed, was not limited to physical aspects and to disturbance of structure and function alone; psychological and sociological implications of such deformities merited deep concern, because the psychic trauma resulting from facial disfigurement could be of greater consequence than the specific defect. That those suffering from facial disfigurement felt apart from other members of society was demonstrated by the veterans of the first World War in France, who formed an association of mutual assistance of broken faces (*gueules cassées*). But an ever-increasing number of gross facial disfigurements were now being caused by civilian traffic and transportation accidents, industrial mishaps and burns from newly developed physical and chemical agents. They concluded by pointing out that there were three

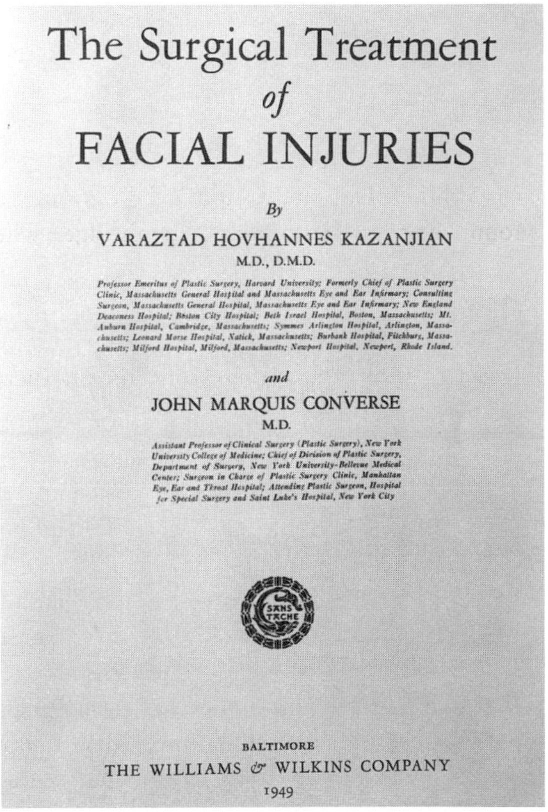
The Surgical Treatment

of

FACIAL INJURIES

By

VARAZTAD HOVHANNES KAZANJIAN

M.D., D.M.D.

Professor Emeritus of Plastic Surgery, Harvard University; Formerly Chief of Plastic Surgery Clinic, Massachusetts General Hospital and Massachusetts Eye and Ear Infirmary; Consulting Surgeon, Massachusetts General Hospital, Massachusetts Eye and Ear Infirmary; New England Deaconess Hospital; Boston City Hospital; Beth Israel Hospital, Boston, Massachusetts; Mt. Auburn Hospital, Cambridge, Massachusetts; Symmes Arlington Hospital, Arlington, Massachusetts; Leonard Morse Hospital, Natick, Massachusetts; Burbank Hospital, Fitchburg, Massachusetts; Milford Hospital, Milford, Massachusetts; Newport Hospital, Newport, Rhode Island.

and

JOHN MARQUIS CONVERSE

M.D.

Assistant Professor of Clinical Surgery (Plastic Surgery), New York University College of Medicine; Chief of Division of Plastic Surgery, Department of Surgery, New York University-Bellevue Medical Center; Surgeon in Charge of Plastic Surgery Clinic, Manhattan Eye, Ear and Throat Hospital; Attending Plastic Surgeon, Hospital for Special Surgery and Saint Luke's Hospital, New York City

SANS TACHE

BALTIMORE

THE WILLIAMS & WILKINS COMPANY

1949

Title page of First Edition, 1949, of Kazanjian and Converse, The Surgical Treatment of Facial Injuries, *(Baltimore: Williams & Wilkins, 1949)*

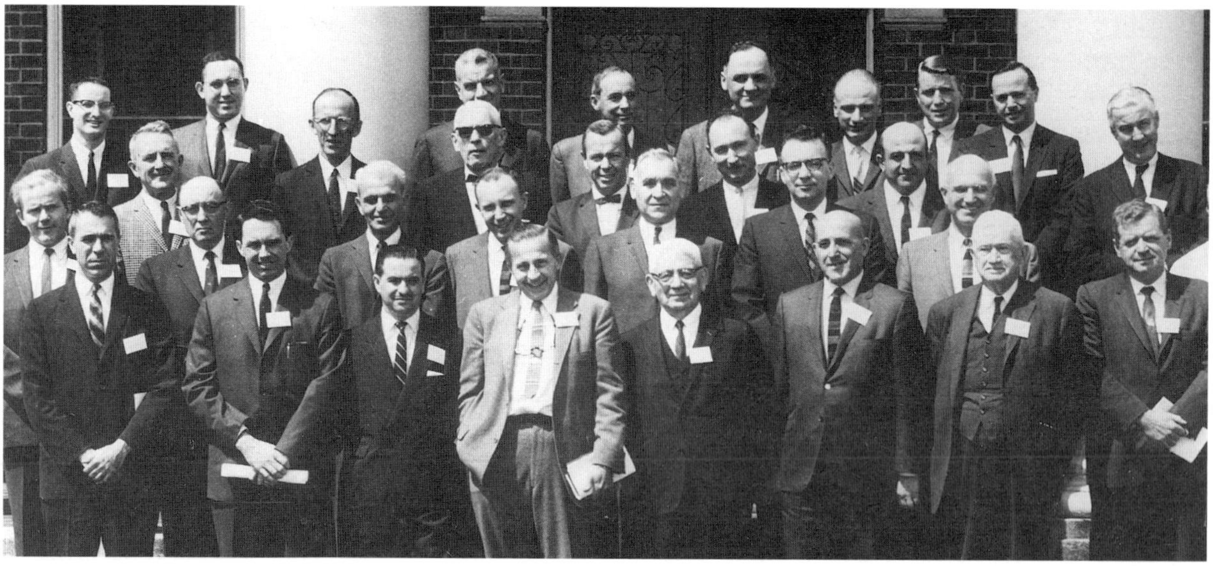

New England Society of Plastic and Reconstructive Surgery, Shriner's Hospital, Boston, Mass., 1964. Dr. Kazanjian, front row, fourth from right. National Archives of Plastic Surgery in the Francis A. Countway Library of Medicine

aspects of the problems associated with the total rehabilitation of the facially disfigured. Highly skillful plastic surgery was an essential requirement; psycho-social rehabilitation was also necessary to insure that the individual could resume his place in society; and the public had to be made aware of its responsibilities in order to avoid exposing the disfigured to attitudes of intolerance when they attempted to follow usual pursuits in society. For Dr. Kazanjian, "the book crowns a brilliant career," Dr. Harris P. Mosher noted. "I happen to know the road was, at times, a hilly one; one which would have stumped all the rest of us."[8]

The Surgical Treatment of Facial Injuries received a number of favorable reviews. One appearing in the *Journal of the American Medical Association* stated that the senior author had originated many new techniques during his service in World War I. "Indeed, in the treatment of wounds he was in advance of his time. Among his contributions were early debridement with delayed primary closure of facial wounds and immediate use of dental prostheses to prevent contracture of soft tissue pending definitive repair." After pointing out that the junior author continued their work in World War II, it related that this magnificent array of case studies formed the basis for their methods, with supplementary materials from a large civilian practice. "Simplicity in design and execution, the use of adjacent tissues rather than free grafts or distant pedicled flaps and the excellent results therefrom attests to the value of this book," which the anonymous reviewer highly recommended.[9]

Another review appearing in *The New England Journal of Medicine* praised the book for many of the same attributes, pointing out that the methods it advocated were developed and applied by its senior author over many years of intensive study in this exacting field.[10]

In the early chapters of the book, particularly those dealing with fractures of the mandible and maxilla, the senior author reproduced photographs of injuries to many of the British soldiers he had treated in France and illustrated some cases with drawings of splints and other devices he had perfected to repair and correct them. One such case, referred to on page 117 and illustrated on page 124, elicited correspondence in 1998 with a descendant of that soldier, more than eighty years after the soldier's wounding and nearly forty years after the initial publication of *The Surgical Treatment of Facial Injuries*. The case had been written up by Major Kazanjian and published in 1918 in the Section of Odontology of the *Proceedings of the British Society of Medicine* under the title, "Splints Combined with Sutures through the Bone for the Immobilization of Extensive Fractures of the Lower Jaw."[11] The article related to a gunshot wound of the face of a "Private C.," who was wounded on February 28, 1917, and admitted to hospital on March 1. The article briefly describes the nature of the wound and the treatment that Dr. Kazanjian provided in the weeks following to stabilize and afterward correct the injury through the application of splints, together with headgear that he devised for immobilizing the patient's lower jaw, both of which devices were illustrated in the article. When describing this type of injury in the 1949 treatise, Dr. Kazanjian provided a brief description of the headgear and a new drawing of both the splint for the jaw and the plaster headcap for maintaining it in position during wound healing.

"Private C" had written Dr. Kazanjian, shortly after his treatment for wounds, after he had been shipped to England for further care.

Weymouth
England
3/10/17

Dear Major Kazanjian:

I am writing to let you know that I am leaving for Australia. Really I do not know how to thank you for all that you have done for me and for the trouble you have taken in sending me photographs, and the medical history. When I look at my photographs when first wounded, I can scarcely imagine I am the same person. The doctors here scarcely credit [i.e., believe] it. In fact, a major here said that you made "too good a job." And now, Sir, I hope you may long enjoy the good name you have justly earned amongst those so badly wounded. Never will I forget all that you did for me. At present, I'm doing really well, and will let you know from time to time of my progress.

Yours faithfully,
E. V. Carroll
Kirkella Stawell
Victoria Aust.[12]

As a footnote, somehow, word got to Australia in the late 1990s that the author was working on a biography of Dr. Kazanjian, and late in 1998 he received an e-mail, out of the blue, from Mrs. Philippa (Pip) Greathead, an Australian speech pathologist, concerning her grandfather — Private Carroll — and the surgical treatment that Dr. Kazanjian had provided to him many decades previously. She related in this letter sent on Sunday, December 13, 1998, that she had become interested in Dr. Kazanjian about fifteen years previously, when she first saw photographs of her grandfather's wounds and surgery. "I was amazed at the quality of the surgery. As a child (my grandfather died of cancer of the jaw when I was 13) I was not aware of any facial deformity at all," she confided in her 1998 e-mail letter. Her interest was renewed, she afterwards related, when she met a plastic surgeon who happened to see her nine-year-old daughter for emergency hand surgery. "I feel a strong connection every time I hear about Dr. K — and I guess that I would not exist! Destiny works in strange ways," she reflected.

Mrs. Greathead related that Ernest Vincent Carroll was twenty-seven years old when he was wounded in February 1917. He had suffered a large gunshot wound on the right side of the jaw. "E. C. spent approximately six months in hospital in France and a further three months in England, where he was under the care of a Dr. MacKay (we think)." He had previously been

Private Ernest Vincent Carroll, wounded February 28, 1917

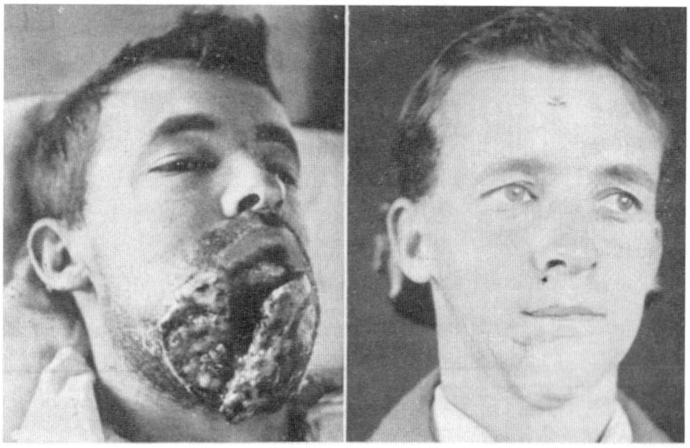

Before and after photos, The Harvard Medical Library in the Francis A. Countway Library of Medicine

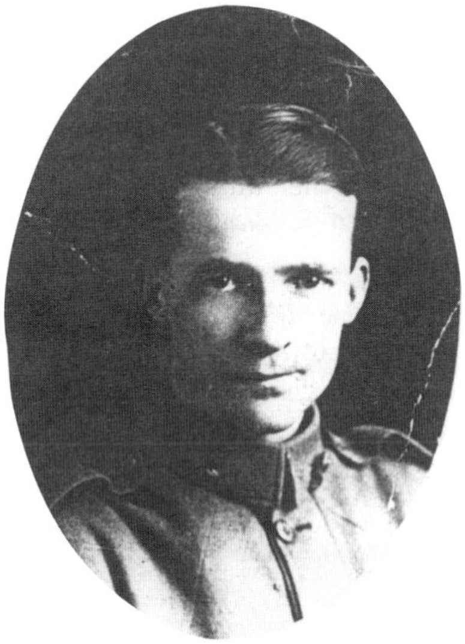

Photograph courtesy of Phillipa Greathead, West Mead, NSW, Australia

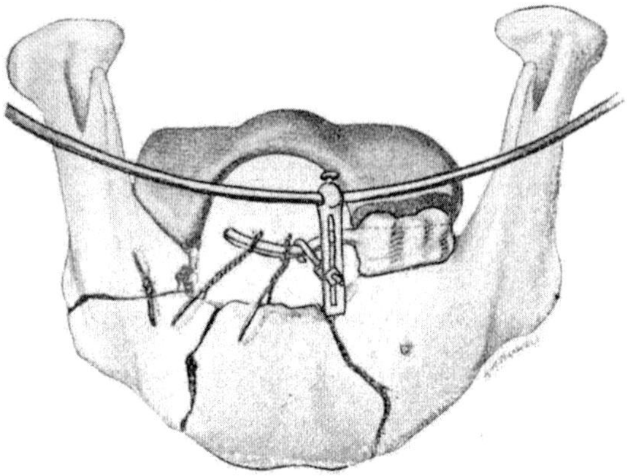

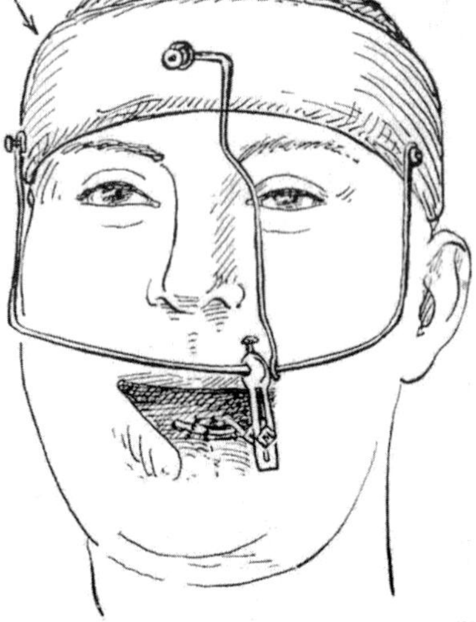

V.H. Kazanjian, "Splints Combined with Sutures through the Bone for the Immobilization of Extensive Fracture of the Lower Jaw." Proceedings of the Royal Society of Medicine, Section on Odontology II (1917-1918): 82-83

reported as missing, but a Red Cross search found him hospitalized in France. She said that her grandmother, Jean, met Ernest Carroll after a "mystic" aunt had told her that she would meet and marry a man who had "a map of the River Darling [an Australian river] on his face." She recalled that her aunt said that when she was a child her grandfather was often in pain and that he had difficulty chewing food. E. C. was apparently often called to the Veteran's Hospital in Sydney during World War II so that the surgeons could examine his jaw repair and use the information to help World War II veterans with similar injuries. Mrs. Greathead said that her grandfather had died of cancer of the jaw in 1967, having survived a previous bout of bowel cancer thirteen years earlier. "I do remember that the doctors wanted to do an autopsy to further examine Dr. K's surgery—but I believe that my grandmother was too upset to allow it to proceed."[13]

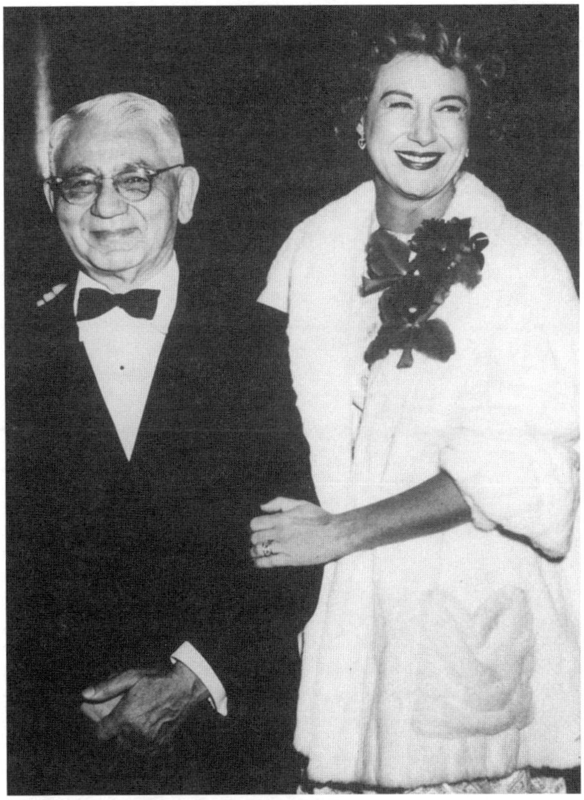

Dr. Kazanjian and Arlene Francis at the event where Dr. Kazanjian received the Notable Achievement Award from Emerson College, 1954
Arber-French & Co., Boston, The Harvard Medical Library in the Francis A. Countway Library of Medicine

Several honors came to Dr. Kazanjian in the early 1950s. In October 1951 he was presented with a metal scroll inscribed with the Special Honorary Citation of the American Society of Plastic and Reconstructive Surgeons.[14] In 1953, Dr. Kazanjian was given the Honor Key Award of the Academy of Ophthalmology and Otolaryngology, and the following year he was granted honorary membership in the Chalmers J. Lyons Academy of the American Society of Oral Surgeons. On this occasion, he delivered a paper, "Advances in Maxillo-facial Surgery during the Past Half Century," in which he challenged "the younger generation of surgeons . . . to surpass the earlier pioneers."[15]

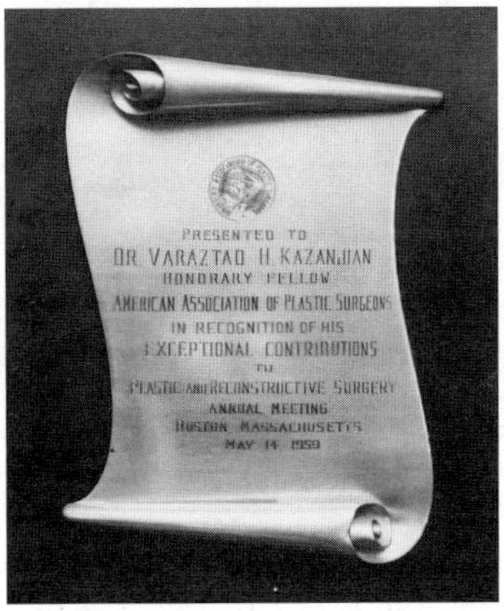
PRESENTED TO
DR VARAZTAD H. KAZANJIAN
HONORARY FELLOW
AMERICAN ASSOCIATION OF PLASTIC SURGEONS
IN RECOGNITION OF HIS
EXCEPTIONAL CONTRIBUTIONS
TO
PLASTIC AND RECONSTRUCTIVE SURGERY
ANNUAL MEETING
BOSTON MASSACHUSETTS
MAY 14 1959

Honorary Fellow American Association of Plastic Surgeons, 1959
The Harvard Medical Library in the Francis A. Countway Library of Medicine
Photograph by Dr. Paul Davis

On December 4, 1954, on the occasion of its seventy-fifth anniversary, Emerson College, in Boston, held a Founder's Day and Diamond Jubilee Banquet, at which an honor citation was presented to Dr. Kazanjian, "whose great ability has been devoted to the rehabilitation of those suffering under the psychological, social and economic handicap of defects in speech and appearance." A

WORLD'S MOST FAMOUS PLASTIC SURGEON

To Dr Kazangian's Office In Boston Come People From Nearly All Parts Of The World

Is Former Worcester Man

By Ivan Sandrof

Next Thursday evening at a formal dinner of the Women's Auxiliary to the Worcester District Dental Society in the Bancroft Hotel, the principal speaker will be Dr. Varaztad H. Kazanjian of Boston.

Despite his white hair, he looks much younger than 78. He is short, with a benign, perceptive look, conservatively dressed in banker's gray. He will speak on "The Rehabilitation of Patients With Facial Deformities."

You may never have heard of him. For when it comes to publicity and there are only two doors from which to leave, Dr. Kazanjian manages to skip out of the window.

Here is a former Worcester boy who rose to become the most famous plastic surgeon in the world. To his office on Commonwealth Avenue, come people from nearly all parts of the world—people with hurt faces and bodies seared by fire, broken in auto crashes, industrial accidents, or deformed from birth. People, it must be added, who have been treated before by other capable surgeons.

"Often they come to you when all hope has been given up, do they not, doctor?" he was asked.

"Do not say that," he suggested quickly. "If you have to say it, state that they come because they are seeking someone who, possibly, has had a little more experience."

So be it!

Dr. Kazanjian's experience has made him a Fellow of the American College of Surgeons and the American College of Dentists. He is also a member of State and National Medical and Dental Societies and a Fellow of the American Academy of Ophthalmology and Otolaryngology. In addition he is a Diplomate of the American Board of Plastic Surgery and holds membership in the American Association of Plastic Surgeons, American Society of Plastic and Reconstructive Surgery, the American Society of Maxillo-facial Surgeons, the American Society of Oral Surgeons, Boston Surgical Society and the International Society of Surgery.

Coming back to Worcester is in a sense, like coming home. For Worcester was Dr. Kazanjian's first American home. He was last here on April 26, 1946 when he spoke in Thayer Hall of City Hospital.

Interviewing the medical man is apt to be somewhat of an experience. Dr. Kazanjian is extremely pleasant, good-natured, sympathetic. But he talks in generalities and he tells you nothing you can take hold of.

But by taking what you do get and adding a bit from someone else, an extract from an honor conferred, some facts from an ancient interview, a talk with a former patient, the opinions of other medical men. . . the story shapes up.

He was born on March 18, 1879 in Verzinga, Armenia, the son of Hovhannes and Anna (Sirounian) Kazanjian, and came to the United States when he was 16. Behind this soft-spoken stripling with the dark complexion and the warm, bright, brown eyes who knew no English to speak of, there was the heritage of the persecuted—a fierce determination to excel.

Kazanjian in Armenian stands for coppersmith. The tradition had been in the family for many generations. Dr. Kazanjian's father was one. The memory of the bright ruddy-orange metal shaped and ball-peened into samovar and bowl is in the family consciousness like the clash of a cymbal.

To save his life, young Varaztad had been smuggled out of Armenia by an uncle. The boy had fought for Armenian freedom by passing forbidden political pamphlets in pre-dawn darkness. Turkish authorities were springing a net around all suspects; the boy had to leave—or lose his life.

Accompanied by two older half-brothers, Varaztad joined an Armenian group of refugees en route to Cherbourg. Here exploiters stuffed them into steerage for America. There were 60 immigrants in one cabin. The vomit-tossed voyage ended at Ellis Island.

The emaciated stripling with the hollow cheeks and the large, smoldering eyes saw the great lady looming high with the torch of liberty, lit only 10 years before. This he could understand; he had fought for liberty and freedom himself. She was also built of copper—and did not Kazanjian mean coppersmith? The lady of liberty loomed like a second mother.

At Ellis Island the boy came very close to not making it, lest he became a public charge. He was held for several days, while his case was considered. All he had was a few cents—the old copper theme—a slip of paper with the name of a family relative in New York and his faith in the future and the lamp beside "the open door."

While he waited he learned from new arrivals of the continuing massacre of Armenians—some 2,000,000 of whom were killed between 1894 and 1915. Kazanjian had no way of knowing then that his family was still alive.

From New York he was sent to a countryman in Worcester, together with his half-brothers. "If I remember correctly," said Dr. Kazanjian, "Worcester then had the largest number of Armenians in the nation—about 900. The first Armenian church in the nation was built there on Laurel Street."

Now began the big push. Kazanjian's first job was in a factory making springs. Piece work. Since he didn't understand English, he didn't know how to handle the procedure. At the end of the week he was handed his first pay: $0.90.

He learned fast. The next week he made $3 and the week after that $6 for a 10-hour, six-day week. Things were looking up. From springs, he sprang into another job at the American Steel and Wire Co., where with frequent overtime he collected $15 a week.

The need for learning English—to project himself into a career now loomed uppermost. He enrolled nights at Dix Street School. "For seven years," he said, "I did not miss a single night."

He read as many books and other matter as he could stuff into his free time. He attended lectures, took correspondence courses and private tutoring in English. Looking back, he remembered some details.

"There was one teacher—I'm ashamed to say I don't remember her name. At the wire mill, I worked 10 to 12½ hours a day, and she used to wait for me to teach me English after work. There are some nice people who want to help others—."

He was trying to do too much

Continued on Next Page

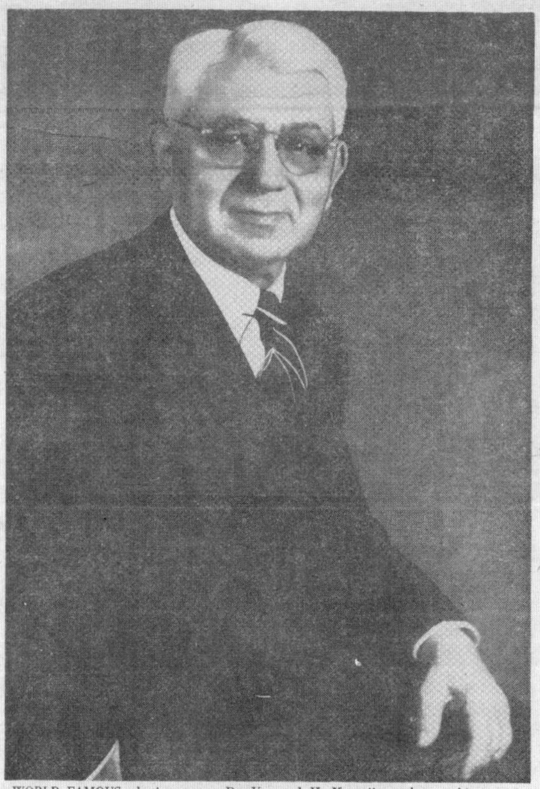

WORLD FAMOUS plastic surgeon, Dr. Varaztad H. Kazanjian, who got his start in Worcester, will talk on his work here next Thursday night.

FEATURE PARADE SECTION WORCESTER SUNDAY TELEGRAM, JAN. 12, 1958 PAGE 3

Ivan Sandrof, "World's Most Famous Plastic Surgeon," Worcester Sunday Telegram, January 12, 1958, Feature Parade, Section F, p. 3
Reprinted with permision of the Worcester Telegram & Gazette

surprise guest at this occasion was Arlene Francis, the noted actress and television personality, who, it was noted earlier, was Dr. Kazanjian's grand niece. Unknown to her uncle, she had flown to Boston between her television commitments to take part in the presentation at her alma mater.[16] (On the day after he received the citation, Dr. Kazanjian performed a facial operation on Capt. W. Peter Cary, an airline pilot who had crashed on a New Hampshire mountain.)

> *Bowdoin College, in Brunswick, Maine, awarded Dr. Kazanjian a Doctor of Science Degree,* honoris causa, *on June 7, 1956: Varaztad Hovhannes Kazanjian, of Boston, plastic and oral surgeon whom hundreds of wounded veterans bless for his discoveries and work in skin grafting and the removal of facial and other scars, decorated by the British Government for his services in World War I, honored today partly because he is the father of a Bowdoin son but chiefly because Bowdoin cherishes those who by scientific research and skill have benefitted the human race.*[17]

In 1959 there was a second edition of *The Surgical Treatment of Facial Injuries*. This revised edition contained over 400 new illustrations and the following six new chapters: 5. Introduction to Fractures of the Facial Bones; 10. Fractures of the Bones of the Frontal-Ethmoidal Region; 12. Facial Injuries in Children; 13. Roentgen Examination of the Frontal Bones; 15. The Transplantation of Tissues; and 16. The Scars of the Face. The book was dedicated posthumously "To the memory of Harry H. Shapiro, D.M.D., anatomist and dental surgeon, poet, and composer of music. His wish was that this book be dedicated to the facially disfigured and to the relief of their suffering." And in their preface the authors expressed "a general debt of gratitude . . . to the inspiring encouragement of Dr. Harry H. Shapiro, Assistant Professor of Anatomy, College of Physicians and Surgeons, Columbia University," who helped edit and condense the manuscript "rendering it more explicit."[18]

There are several references in the correspondence regarding the initial edition to Dr. Shapiro's pivotal role in editing it, such as the letter Kazanjian wrote to Converse on June 29, 1949: "I received a batch of galley proof illustrations from Williams & Wilkins yesterday and mailed them to Dr. Shapiro."[19] Dr. Henry Kaplan, a Harvard dental student from 1944, remembered Dr. Shapiro as an orthodontist who practiced in New York City and was looked upon as a Renaissance man who, in 1947, had published a book entitled *Applied Anatomy of the Head and Neck* that contained photographs of Dr. Kazanjian's treatment of jaw fractures in its Chapter eight. Dr. Shapiro served as Executive Director of the Society of the Rehabilitation of the Facially Disfigured in 1951. Mrs. Lane, who, as previously noted, did much of the secretarial work on the 1949 edition, remembered that on occasion Dr. Shapiro accompanied Dr. Converse to the Kazanjian home to work on the book.[20] A third and final edition, containing 1,400 pages and 1,494 figures in its two volumes, was issued in 1974 under the name of John M. Converse alone and the title *Kazanjian & Converse's Surgical Treatment of Facial Injuries*. It also appeared in Spanish translation.[21]

In 1958, when Dr. Kazanjian was eighty-one years old, Dr. Joseph E. Murray, who was then Chief of Plastic Surgery at the Peter Bent Brigham Hospital, and Dr. Robert M. Goldwyn, then a resident in general surgery, visited him at his office with a patient for consultation. They found him to be "still vigorous and keen," and wearing a head mirror. The qualities that had characterized and endeared him throughout his life remained in place: his modesty, his quiet and courteous manner, his warmth, and his advice given carefully and thoughtfully, his kindness, his maturity, as evidenced when he listened more than he talked.

The two surgeons, together with the patient, realized "that we were in the presence of history."[22]

Dr. Renée Bennett O'Sullivan, a practicing plastic and reconstructive surgeon in Wellesley, Massachusetts, recalled an incident involving Dr. Kazanjian that took place when she was starting her private practice. It also involved Dr. Anthony Zovickian, Chief of Plastic Surgery at Boston City Hospital, who, in her opinion, was an extraordinary plastic surgeon.[23] She felt that Dr. Zovickian was unusual for that time, and even today, because he saw to it that there was an excellent selection of plastic surgery instruments in the hospital operating room. He set a standard of excellence as he sat down and spent hours at the operating table, performing his plastic and reconstructive surgical procedures. She knew him to be respected by the staff and by all who knew him, and she found him to be very welcoming to her as she began her practice. One day, she remembered,

> *he asked if I would assist him for a large surgical procedure he was performing at another hospital. As I was just beginning my practice, I was not very busy. I learned a great deal from working with him, and I was very honored to be asked. After the operation was over, he took me to lunch at the hospital cafeteria. He then asked me how everything was going, and I told him that it was difficult to assess, because I was alone in my practice; I changed in the nurses' changing room and was the only woman surgeon on the staff, and thus I had little interaction with the male surgeons, and the rest of the hospital staff as well, for that matter, particularly in view of the fact that I was the only plastic surgeon on the staff of the hospital at that time and for many years thereafter. He then told me that he was going to give me some advice that had been given to him years ago when he started in practice by his mentor, Dr. Kazanjian, and he would pass it on to me. It was: "Do your own work and mind your own business." Well, I thought to myself, is that all there is? It seemed so simple and not very profound. I waited for more and that was the end of it. So I thanked him for his advice and tucked it into the back of my mind.*

Her story had its ending many years later, she related, when Dr. Kazanjian was beginning to close down his practice. However, he still had his office open, although he was no longer operating. She had inherited one of his complex reconstructive patients who required further surgery, and she needed information regarding the case, previous operating procedures and so forth. She telephoned him to see if she could have copies of his operative notes and possibly see some of the pre- and post-operative photographs that had been taken for each of the stages. Dr. Kazanjian told her that he was very happy to share these with her and invited her to his office to discuss the case. His office was located in one of the old buildings along Commonwealth Avenue, she recalled. Dr. Kazanjian did not hear her approach. He was sitting at a large mahogany desk reading a plastic surgery journal through a magnifying glass.

> *He greeted me, then came around his desk to the front where I was standing. He took me by the arm and walked me over to a grandly upholstered bench that was just inside the door. He invited me to sit down and then sat next to me. He then patted me on the knee and asked how everything was going. I explained the same things that I had to Dr. Zovickian so many years earlier: that I was alone in practice, that it was difficult to tell, but essentially that I was hanging in there. He gave my knee a few more pats and said: "Let me give you a little bit of advice . . . Do your own work and mind your own business." So many years had passed since Dr. Zovickian had said that to me long ago. At last I was able to understand and appreciate these simple words of advice that were so wise and so profound. I remember them to this day and have passed them onto my three physician daughters.*[24]

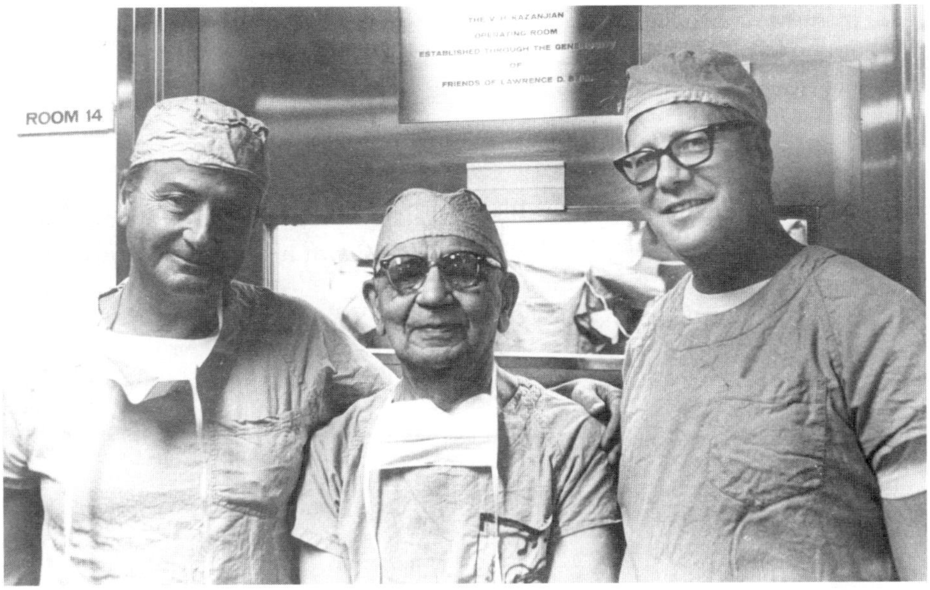

Dr. John M. Converse, Dr. Kazanjian, and Robert E. Bochat, Executive Director of the Society for the Facially Disfigured, standing before the V. H. Kazanjian operating room at the New York University Medical Center, 1970s
The Harvard Medical Library in the Francis A. Countway Library of Medicine

Primarily through Dr. Converse's efforts and with the financial assistance of friends and former patients, the V. H. Kazanjian Visiting Professorship in Plastic Surgery was established at the New York University Medical Center Institute of Reconstructive and Plastic Surgery in 1962. Dr. Kazanjian received the New York University presidential citation and delivered the Inaugural Lecture in 1962, at which he spoke of "Remembrances of Things Past."[25] He was awarded the first certificate issued to honorary membership in the British Association of Plastic Surgeons in 1966, and the following year he was made Honorary Fellow in Dental Surgery of the Royal College of Physicians and Surgeons in Edinburgh.[26]

Dr. Kazanjian continued his surgical practice until 1965, when, at the age of eighty-six, his vision began to decline, and, to a lesser extent, his hearing. He had enjoyed international recognition for over five decades, and for nearly seventy years "he was the outstanding figure in New England plastic surgery" and "the doyen of his specialty in America."[27] He was respected abroad, as Dr. Walter C. Guralnick tells in this warm anecdote:

> *A distinguished Austrian oral surgeon and famous elder statesman in the field was invited to lecture at the Massachusetts General Hospital two years ago. Unknown to him, Dr. Kazanjian was invited to attend and arrived just as the lecturer was about to begin. On seeing Kazanjian, the speaker, Professor Richard Trauner, rushed to embrace him, and was overcome by emotion and joy. When he regained his composure, he said, almost in disbelief, "I never thought I would be so honored as to speak before Dr. Kazanjian. There was nothing that could have give[n] me more joy, in my trip to America, than to see this great and good man again."*[28]

One of the last tributes paid to Dr. Kazanjian took place in 1972, when the American Society of Plastic and Reconstructive Surgeons conferred on him its Neal Owens Award at the Society's forty-first annual meeting. He was in his ninety-third year and unable to attend, but the award was fittingly accepted by Dr. Robert H. Ivy, his warm and intimate friend for over fifty years; both had been trailblazers and had entered their specialty by way of dentistry.[29]

Varaztad Hovhannes Kazanjian died on October 19, 1974, in his ninety-fifth year. (Dr. Ivy had preceded him in death about four months earlier, on June 21.) A simple, dignified service was conducted on October 22, 1974, at the Harvard Memorial Church by the Reverend Samuel W. Hale, Jr., a family friend, of the Grace Episcopal Church in Elmira, New York. He was buried in Mount Auburn Cemetery in Cambridge in a plot beside his first wife, Sophie, his mother, Anna, and his step-brother, Harootiun Siroonian. Marion, his second wife, was interred there following her death on March 9, 1990.[30]

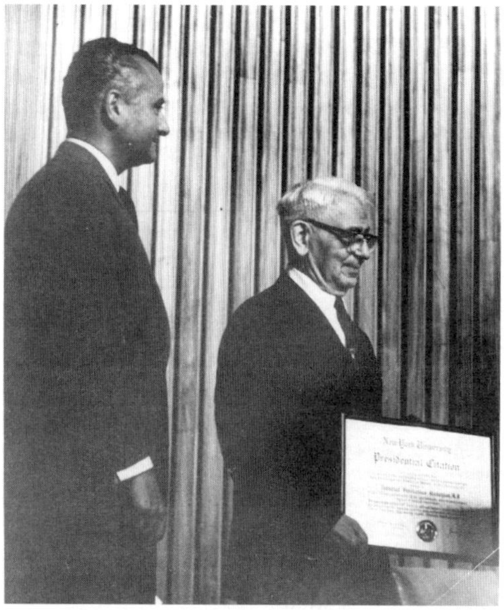

VHK with John Marquis Converse at the inaugural lecture of the V. H. Kazanjian Visiting Professorship in Plastic Surgery at the New York University Institute of Reconstructive Plastic Surgery, 1962
The Harvard Medical Library in the Francis A. Countway Library of Medicine

Tributes were read before professional organizations and appeared in the leading medical, dental and lay publications. Dr. Kazanjian's portrait, painted in oil by Dr. Robert Shaw Wesson, one of his former dental students, was hung over the stairway in the foyer of the Harvard School of Dental Medicine.[31] An exhibit devoted to his life and work was presented at The Francis A. Countway Library of Medicine in September 1976, the same year that the gift shop of the Massachusetts Eye and Ear Infirmary was dedicated to Marion Kazanjian. His life and work were also featured in a program in the "Leaders of American Medicine" series sponsored by the Boston Medical Library and held in the Countway Library on October 11, 1978, at which the speakers were Drs. Bradford Cannon and Walter Guralnick, with a response by his son, Victor Kazanjian. The Massachusetts General Hospital established the Varaztad H. Kazanjian Fellowship in Plastic and Reconstructive Surgery in 1981. An annual Kazanjian visiting professorship in his honor was sponsored by the Plastic Surgical Service of the Massachusetts General Hospital.[32]

A television documentary produced by Station WGBH of Cambridge in its "Nova" series, entitled "A Normal Face: The Wonders of Plastic Surgery," which aired on November 22, 1983, focused on his heroic and pioneering work, particularly in France in 1915. Dr. Joseph E. Murray, who was a participant in the program and who knew him quite well, said in the course of the documentary:

> *It was on his foundations that the successive steps have been built. If you try to put it in sort of a step ladder progression, Dr. Kazanjian worked on the relationship of the jaws, and these were very difficult problems at that time*

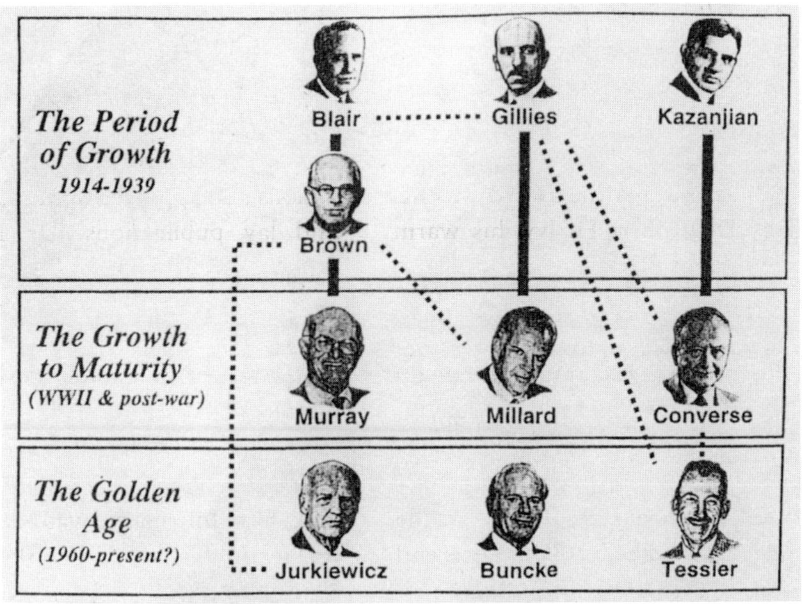

The dominant plastic surgery personalities in each era of the 20th century and their relationships
Geoffrey G. Hallock, Plastic and Reconstructive Surgery, *107:4, April 1, 2001, p. 1023, fig. 11*
Illustrations by Carol Varma.

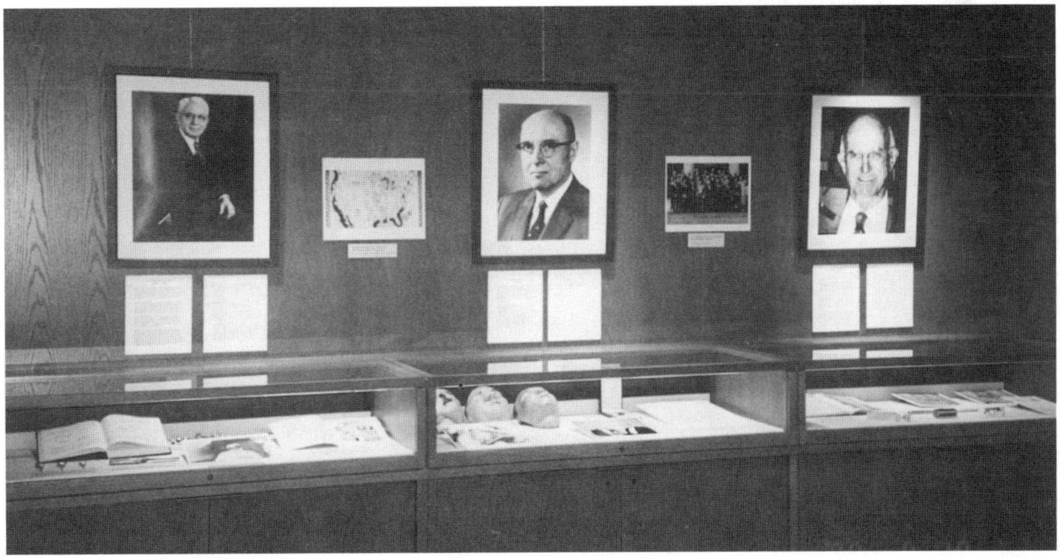

Exhibit at the Francis A. Countway Library, Rare Books
"Plastic Surgery in Boston--Then and Now."
Unveiled April 4, 2001, picturing left to right Drs. Kazanjian, Bradford Cannon and Joseph Murray
Photograph by Dr. Paul Davis

and now Dr. Tessier has combined the orbits and the brain so now we can get at the whole facial structure.[33]

The Nova program pointed out that Dr. Paul Tessier of Paris, who "indisputably founded cranial facial surgery" and who was "one of the most notable mavericks of our time," has been called "the modern Kazanjian." The Nova script related that Dr. Tessier "developed a unique method of cutting across the scalp to rebuild the skull with bone grafts, leaving no scars.[34] Finally, the Massachusetts Eye and Ear Infirmary named the ENT Harvard Teaching Room in Dr. Kazanjian's honor in 1984 in recognition of his role as its first chief of plastic surgery.[35]

On his ninety-fifth birthday, a few months before his death, Dr. Kazanjian received from Dr. Murray a letter that serves as a testament:

It is one of our treasured experiences in life that we have had a chance to know you and share to some degree in your skill and activities on behalf of plastic surgical patients.

Your life is an example for all future generations of plastic surgeons.[36]

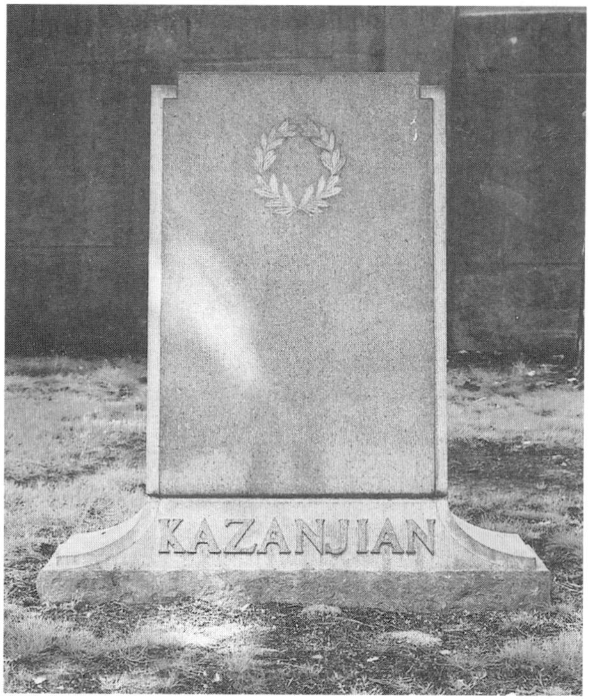

Kazanjian burial site, Mt. Auburn Cemetery, Cambridge, Mass. Photograph by Armen James

As his son Victor pointed out in responding to a tribute to his father that was made on the occasion of the forty-fifth annual convention of the American Society of Plastic and Reconstructive Surgeons in 1976, he had been recognized by "kings, and cardinals, presidents of great universities, noted political leaders, and the press of the world." He would say, "I'm just a technician," and he remained "happy and unruffled." Above all, he confessed, "It does please me when my colleagues . . . think that I have done well."[37]

Varaztad Hovhannes Kazanjian's place of honor in the history of medicine remains secure, whether he be remembered as "The" or "A" Founding Father of Modern Plastic Surgery. What is undeniable is that he was "the last of the great leaders responsible for the stature of plastic surgery as a highly respected and much sought-after medical and surgical specialty" as Dr. Cannon has observed.[38]

If one time and place were to be singled out when the future direction of Dr. Kazanjian's life was determined, as an epiphany, it would be 1900 in Worcester, Massachusetts, when the Reverend K. G. Benneyan convinced him to renounce the idea of returning to Armenia, and someone suggested, "You take dentistry, that's a good profession."[39]

ON THE OCCASION OF DR. KAZANJIAN'S 90TH BIRTHDAY

*A poem written and read by Dr. Claude E. Welch**

The shades of night are falling fast
As in Armenia's wintry blast
A youth was born whose fame would spread
Wherever he would lay his head.
Kazanjian!

For ninety years he's worked and slaved,
A thousand noses he's remade.
Throughout the world, his autograph
Is found on trunk, on head, on calf.
Kazanjian!

And rightly helpers laud his skill,
His mild commands to do his will.
To lift up, flatten, or expand
"Mop, sister, mop" his sole demand.
Kazanjian!

While in the woods he often looks
For Lady slippers, hidden nooks.
And loves to fish in Kolelemook
Though bass refuse to bite his hook.
Kazanjian!

And in his home where'er we look
Are slides and pictures for his book,
Degrees and honors, bale on bale
So, Dean of Plastic Surgeons, Hail.
Kazanjian!

We bring him on these festive days
Our friendship, love and humble praise
For fruitful years, for future things
For Popsy, Katsy, King of kings.
Kazanjian!

The Harvard Medical Library in the Francis A. Countway Library of Medicine

*Dr. Claude E. Welch (1906-1996) was an internationally known authority on abdominal surgery, past president of the American College of Surgeons, the American Surgical Association, and the Massachusetts Medical Society, holder of the highest honor of the American Medical Association (its Distinguished Service Award) and the author of several books, including *Surgery of the Stomach and Duodenum. MGH News 40:4 (May 1981), 8.*

NOTES

1 The title of this chapter comes from the title of Ivan Sandrof's article, "World's Most Famous Plastic Surgeon," *Worcester Sunday Telegram*, January 12, 1958, Feature Parade section.

2 Walter C. Guralnick, et al., "V. H. Kazanjian, A Pioneer in Dentistry and Plastic Surgery," *Harvard University Gazette*, May 2, 1975, p. 9.

3 An obituary of Dr. Henry Carney appeared in the *Boston Globe* on March 16, 1982, p. 23. col. 1. He specialized in facial reconstructive surgery and was also affiliated with Massachusetts General Hospital and the Harvard Dental School. Dr. Carney served overseas in the Army during World War I and World War II, and received the Legion of Merit during World War II. Dr. Levon Krikor Daghlian was born in Aintab, Turkey, and graduated from the Harvard Dental School *cum laude* in 1927. His dental office was at 53 Bay State Road in Boston. His widow, Lucy Daghlian, reported that her husband and his family were often invited to parties at the Kazanjian home. (Personal interview by the author of Lucy Daghlian, August 15, 1996, at Albany, N.Y., in the author's possession.)

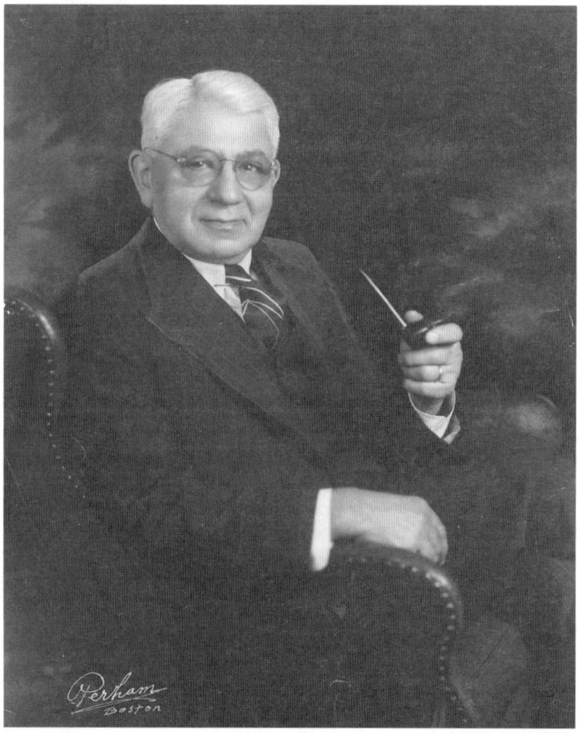

Photograph of Dr. Kazanjian taken in 1952, The Harvard Medical Library in the Francis A. Countway Library of Medicine, Perham Studio, Boston, Mass. MHG staff photograph #34

4 Bradford Cannon, "The Flowering of Plastic Surgery," *Journal of the American Medical Association* 263, no. 6, (February 9, 1990): 863-864.

5 Some idea of the book's date of issue is afforded by the advertisement appearing in the November 1949 issue of the *Journal of Plastic and Reconstructive Surgery* with the notice that it had been published.

6 Blair O. Rogers, "John Marquis Converse (1909-1981), Obituary," *Annals of Plastic Surgery* 8, no. 4 (April 1982): 144, 146

7 Interview by the author of Mrs. Virginia (Ring) Lane, February 15, 1999, Shrewsbury, Mass. Also, John M. Converse, *Kazanjian & Converse's Surgical Treatment of Facial Injuries*, 3rd ed., (Baltimore: Williams & Wilkins, 1974) v. 1, Preface, p. ix.

8 Letter from Dr. Harris P. Mosher to Varaztad H. Kazanjian, December 25, 1949, in the Varaztad H. Kazanjian Archive in The Francis A. Countway Library of Medicine, folder C-300.

9 "The Surgical Treatment of Facial Injuries . . . ," *Journal of the American Medical Association* 144, no. 6 (October 7, 1950): 504.

10 "The Surgical Treatment of Facial Injuries . . .," *The New England Journal of Medicine* 243, no. 21 (November 23, 1950): 840-841.

11 V. H. Kazanjian, "Splints Combined with Sutures Through the Bone for the Immobilization of Extensive Fractures of the Lower Jaw," *Proceedings of the Royal Society of Medicine, Section on Odontology* 11 (1917-1918): 82-83. Also, Kazanjian and Converse, *The Surgical Treatment of Facial Injuries*, (1949), p. 124.

12 Letter from E. V. C. to V. H. Kazanjian, October 30, 1917, can be found in the V. H. Kazanjian Archive in The Francis A. Countway Library of Medicine, Section IV, file on Ernest Carroll.

13 E-mail letter from Philippa Greathead to H. Martin Deranian c/o Brady and Berg, December 13, 1998,

also letter from Greathead to Deranian, February 24, 1999, in author's possession. "My family would not have existed without the brilliance of Varaztad Kazanjian over 80 years ago!" She was also gracious enough to enclose medical records and photographs of her grandfather's treatment during World War I.

14 "Special Awards of the American Society of Plastic and Reconstructive Surgery and the Foundation of the Society of Plastic and Reconstructive Surgery," p. 299. Also Kazanjian Archive, folder PAM-16, for Special Honorary Citation presentation.

15 Section on "Introduction iv," Kazanjian Archive, folder PAM 17. The paper was published in the *Journal of Oral Surgery* 13 (April 1955): 97-102.

16 Emerson College, Boston, Massachusetts, "Press Release," December 5, 1954, Emerson College Archives. Letter to the author from Robert Fleming, Archivist, Emerson College, May 17, 1999, in the author's possession. Kazanjian Archive, folder C-638, contains the program of the evening and correspondence. For more information on Arlene Francis see her book *That Certain Something: The Magic of Charm* (New York: Julian Messner, Inc., 1960). Her obituary appeared in *The New York Times*, June 2, 2001, p. B7, col. 1.

17 *The Bowdoin Orient*, June 7, 1952, p. 2, Kazanjian Archive, folder PAM-47. Also, letter from Sean M. Monahan, Assistant, Special Collections and Archives, Bowdoin College Library, May 25, 1999, in the author's possession. "It seems that Dr. Kazanjian was a great man who greatly deserved the honor Bowdoin bestowed upon him and whose efforts are long deserving of a book!"

18 Varaztad H. Kazanjian and John Marquis Converse, *The Surgical Treatment of Facial Injuries*, 2nd ed. (Baltimore: Williams & Wilkins, 1959).

19 Letter from V. H. Kazanjian to J. M. Converse, June 29, 1949, in the Kazanjian Archive, folder C-89.

20 Harry H. Shapiro, *Applied Anatomy of the Head and Neck: Clinical Application of Anatomy in Dental Practice*, 2nd ed. (Philadelphia: Lippincott, 1947). The Society of Rehabilitation of the Facially Disfigured was founded in New York City through the efforts of Dr. Converse, who obtained support from Lawrence D. Bell, the head of Bell Aviation (See Rogers, "John Marquis Converse"). Also, interview by author of Mrs. Virginia (Ring) Lane, February 15, 1999, Shrewsbury, Mass.

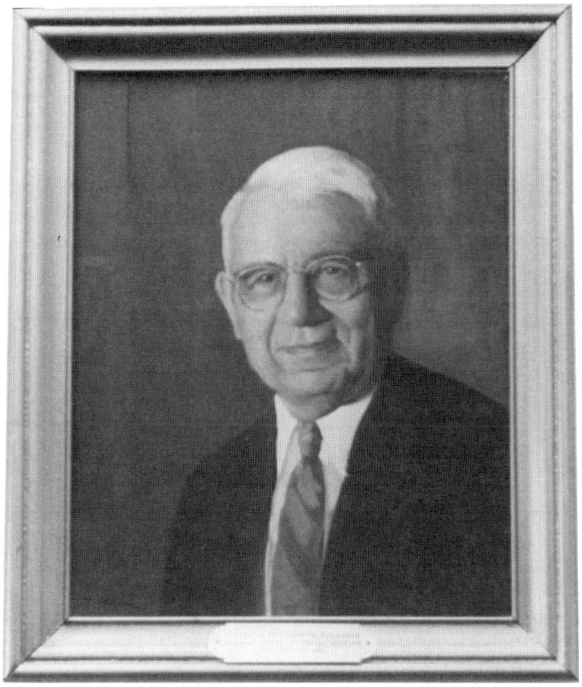

Portrait of Dr. Kazanjian painted by Dr. Robert Shaw Wesson (1879-1974) D.M.D. '28. Courtesy Harvard School of Dental Medicine, and Harvard University Art Museum, Cambridge, Mass., #H-717

21 John M. Converse, *Kazanjian & Converse's Surgical Treatment of Facial Injuries*, 3rd ed., (Baltimore: Williams & Wilkins, 1974), 2 v. Bradford Cannon, "Varaztad H., Kazanjian, 1879-1974. Obituary," *Harvard Medical Alumni Bulletin* 49, no. 3 (January-February 1975): 64. The Kazanjian-Converse book, Spanish-language edition of the *Tratamiento Quirurgico de los Traumatismos de la Cara*, translated by Hector Marino, published at Buenos Aires in 1952, may be found in books from the library of Dr. Varaztad H. Kazanjian given to the National Archives of Plastic Surgery at The Countway Library of Medicine, June 16, 1976.

22 Robert M. Goldwyn, "Dr. Varaztad H. Kazanjian: Relevant or Irrelevant to Our Times?" p. 1, paper delivered to the American Society of Maxillofacial Surgeons, Seattle, Wash., September 24, 1991, in the author's possession.

23 Dr. Anthony Zovickian, F.A.C.S., the son of a physician, was born in Boston in 1918. He received his A.B. degree from Harvard in 1940 and his M.D. from Yale in 1943. He served his residency at Johns Hopkins in plastic surgery and practiced in Boston. *Who's Who in the East,* 12th ed. (Chicago: Marquis Publications, 1969), pp. 1238-1239.

24 Letter to the author from Renée Bennett O'Sullivan, December 20, 1999, in the author's possession.

25 The original typescript of this memoir is in the Kazanjian Archive, folder PAM-18 and AM 198. Published in *Plastic and Reconstructive Surgery,* 35:5, 1965. Robert M. Goldwyn, "The Kazanjian Lecture: What Remains," *Aesthetic Plastic Surgery, 18,* 1994, p. 233. Dr. Goldwyn was chosen to deliver the Kazanjian lecture in 1993. He stated that Dr. Converse "commented, somewhat mournfully, that Dr. Kazanjian, because of his personality and his inclination, never had a residency program, and, in fact, the only person whom he truly trained was Dr. Converse."

26 British Association of Plastic Surgeons, *Newsletter*, October 1, 1966, pp. 3-4.; *British Journal of Plastic Surgery* 20, no. 1 (January 1967): 106; Stephen Plumpton, "Kazanjian," *Dental Magazine and Oral Topics* 84. no. 5 (October 1967): 207.

27 John M. Converse, "The Extraordinary Career of Doctor Varaztad Hovhannes Kazanjian," *Plastic and Reconstructive Surgery* 71, no. 1 (January 1982): 141; Bradford Cannon, "Varaztad H. Kazanjian, 1879-1974," *Harvard Medical Alumni Bulletin*, 49. no. 3 (January-February 1975): 64; Plumpton, "Kazanjian," p. 207.

28 Guralnick, "Pioneer," p. 807. A bond of friendship existed between Dr. Kazanjian and colleagues in many parts of the world. One such colleague was Dr. Alfred Kantorowicz, who had been forced by the Nazi regime into exile in Turkey, where he taught in the dental and medical school of the University of Istanbul between 1934 and 1950.

29 *Newsletter, P.R.S. for Plastic and Reconstructive Surgery* 10:1 (Jan. 1973), in the Kazanjian Archive, folder PAM-20.

30 The Commonwealth of Massachusetts, Division of Vital Statistics, "Standard Certificate of Death, No. 261, October 19, 1974." In a letter to the author, dated December 20, 1974, in author's possession, Marion H. Kazanjian wrote, "Dr. Kazanjian always felt very close to you and spoke of you often." The location of the cemetery plot is 6781, Western Avenue, Mount Auburn Cemetery records.

31 Dr. Robert Shaw Wesson (1879-1974), a former dental student of Dr. Kazanjian's, painted the portrait in the 1960s, according to information in the Harvard School of Dental Medicine archive.

32 MGH [Massachusetts General Hospital] *News,* vol. 40, no. 4 (May 1981): 7.

33 WGBH Educational Foundation, *Nova Booklet n. 1015*, 1983, contains the transcript of "A Normal Face: The Wonders of Plastic Surgery." The quotation comes from p. 5, which contains Dr. Murray's remarks. Also, letter from Kathy White, production assistant, NOVA series, to the author, June 29, 1983, in the author's possession: "Your assistance has been invaluable regarding the understanding of the life and times of Dr. Kazanjian." Also, *Worcester Sunday Telegram,* November 27, 1983, Section A, p. 28A, "Plastic Surgery Pioneer Had Ties Here." "I have no hobbies," Dr. Kazanjian said, "my work is my life."

34 *The Dial* (Chicago) 4, no. 11 (November 1983), contains a review of the Nova Television program, "A Normal Face: The Wonders of Plastic Surgery."

35 Kazanjian Archive, folder C-304.

36 Letter from Joseph E. Murray to Varaztad H. Kazanjian, May 15, 1974, in the Kazanjian Archive, folder C-304.

37 Response of Victor C. Kazanjian to a tribute to his father, Varaztad H. Kazanjian, on the occasion of the forty-fifth annual convention of the American Society of Plastic and Reconstructive Surgeons, its Educational Foundation, and the American Society of Maxillofacial Surgeons at Boston, Mass., on September 28, 1976, Kazanjian Archive, folder PAM-20.

38 Bradford Cannon, "Varaztad H. Kazanjian, 1879-1974," *Harvard Medical Alumni Bulletin* 49, no. 3 (January-February 1975): 63.

39 In a letter that Dr. Kazanjian wrote to J. Jelal on May 26, 1936, he related that "I have the greatest respect and love for Rev. Mr. Benneyan. I have known him for many years and consider him one of the noblest characters in Armenian public life—a great friend and counsellor." (Kazanjian Archive, folder C-218.) Also Carl W. Waldron, "A Testimonial to Varaztad Kazanjian," *Journal of Oral Surgery* 13, no. 2 (April 1955): 94.

The major portion of the research conducted in the preparation of this book was done at the Harvard Medical Library in The Francis A. Countway Library of Medicine. The Varaztad H. Kazanjian papers. (HMS c51) are owned by the National Archives of Plastic Surgery, which is housed in The Francis A. Countway Library of Medicine.

The organization of this archive was supported by the National Archives of Plastic Surgery under the sponsorship of:

American Association of Plastic Surgeons
American Board of Plastic Surgery
American Society for Aesthetic Plastic Surgery, Inc.
American Society of Maxillofacial Surgeons
American Society of Plastic and Reconstructive Surgeons, Inc.
Plastic Surgery Educational Foundation

The Kazanjian Archive was donated by Dr. Kazanjian's family to the National Archives of Plastic Surgery in The Countway Library of Medicine. It spans the years 1905 to 1984 and consists of 204 Paige boxes and 21 card file drawers.

Material from this collection, including Dr. Kazanjian's papers cited herein, can be found in Paige boxes HMS c51.

ACKNOWLEDGMENTS

It is a good thing to give thanks...

— Book of Psalms 92:1

The story of the life and times of Dr. Varaztad Hovhannes Kazanjian has captured my imagination and interest for over half a century. Over this long gestation period, many persons have assisted me, have encouraged me and have shared their remembrances. I publicly acknowledge all these individuals with gratitude; many are no longer alive. My apologies are expressed to anyone whose name I have inadvertently omitted.

Dr. Joseph E. Murray, 1990 Nobel Prize Laureate in Medicine, not only knew Dr. Kazanjian "quite well," but considered him "one of the kindest physicians" he ever knew and one who helped him "get established in Boston." By writing the foreword to this book, Dr. Murray has assured the preservation of the legacy of Dr. Kazanjian. This gracious gesture of remembrance is acknowledged with gratitude.

I conducted much of my research at the Harvard Medical Library in the Francis A. Countway Library of Medicine/Boston Medical Library which houses the Varaztad H. Kazanjian Archive.

Richard J. Wolfe, Curator of Rare Books and Manuscripts of the Harvard Medical Archives, had the uncanny ability of unearthing a lost reference. At a critical time during the later stages of the preparation of my manuscript, he offered his abundant talents in helping revise and edit my work, notwithstanding that he was no longer in Boston, but in Philadelphia.

Madeleine W. Mullen, former Curatorial Associate at the Countway, expertly assisted with research. Dr. Robert M. Goldwyn, Chair of the Archives Committee of the National Archives of Plastic Surgery at the Countway Library, offered me his unwavering encouragement. He granted me permission to use the Archives and to reproduce in my book the photographs in the collection, and he made a critical review of my manuscript. The same may be said for Peter Rawson, Archivist.

Dr. Leonard J. Morse, long-standing friend, was president of the Boston Medical Library at the time I was completing my manuscript. Our convivial lunches provided an opportunity to discuss progress on my book. I am grateful to him and the Boston Medical Library for granting me honorary fellowship.

J. Norma Bedrosian, my faithful secretary-assistant for over twenty years, took my handwritten scribbled notes, deciphered them, and entered them into the computer. She assisted me in many ways, and she took far more than a passing interest in this book, more in the role of collaborator. The book never would have reached the printer without her dedication.

It was Kim Cutler, graphic artist, who designed and laid out this book with a high degree of professionalism and artistry.

Edward D. Simsarian, my friend and lawyer, reviewed my manuscript, providing grammatical and stylistic corrections.

Barbara Merguerian, Ph.D. offered many valuable suggestions as she carefully went over my

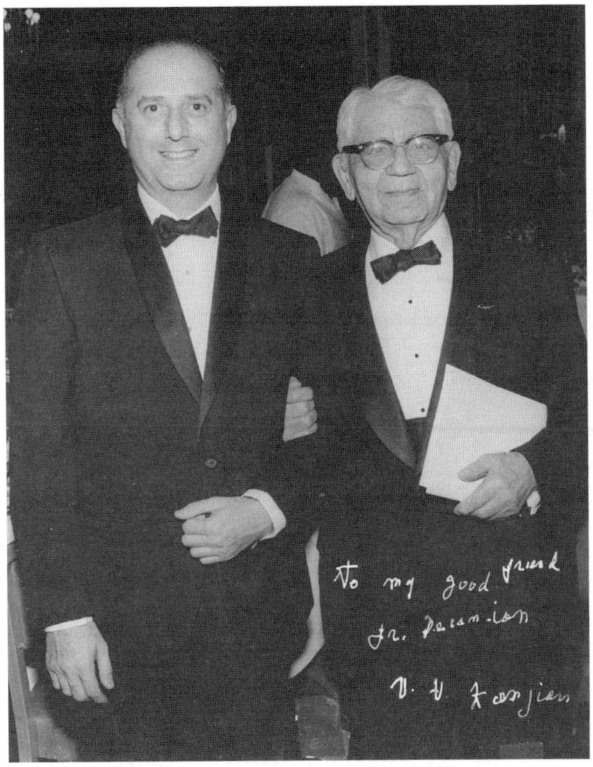

Dr. Kazanjian and Dr. Deranian, October, 1967,
American Academy of Dental Science,
Centennial Meeting, Boston, Mass.

manuscript, particularly in the areas of references and footnotes.

Dr. Adrian F. Bom, retired plastic surgeon, lent me his books on plastic surgery and served as my "sounding board."

Dr. Bradford Cannon, Clinical Professor of Surgery, Emeritus, Harvard Medical School, whom I interviewed, considered Dr. Kazanjian "fast friend, admirer and professional colleague."

Dr. Walter C. Guralnick, Professor of Oral Surgery, Emeritus, at the Massachusetts General Hospital, Harvard School of Dental Medicine, had a knowledge of Dr. Kazanjian as a teacher at Harvard Dental School that was unsurpassed. I interviewed him, and he considered Dr. Kazanjian to be "a genius."

Indirectly, yet omnipresent, has been the influence and memory of Dr. Robert H. Ivy, who lectured to my class in dental school.

Among the other individuals who have assisted me are: Professor James R. Russell, Harvard University Department of Near Eastern Languages and Civilizations, for determining the meaning of the name "Varaztad"; Victoria Stambolian and Florence Chakerian for material on Sivas; Alice Aroian, whose father worked at the wire mill with Dr. Kazanjian; Diana Der Hovanessian, whose grandfather did the same; Dr. Ferdinand Brigham, who served with him in France from 1915 to 1919, and who remained his life-long friend; Dr. Ronald M. King, who was at Hospital No. 5 during World War I and in whose office I served as an associate in Boston from 1947 to 1951; Ann Reardon for providing the diary of her father-in-law, Dr. Daniel Bartholomew Reardon; Dr. Edward Vartan Malcom, whose mother was the sister of Sophie Augusta Kazanjian; Drs. Carnig J. Thomason and Henry Kaplan, who were taught by Dr. Kazanjian as dental students at Harvard, as was Dr. Wallace J. Gardner, whose impassioned remembrance and affection for him will remain as a legacy; Michael Molner, Research Director, Freud Museum, London, for granting permission to professionally photograph the Kazanjian prosthesis and to use the museum archive; Dr. John C. Davenport for identifying and describing the Kazanjian appliance; George Aghjayan for helping pinpoint the date of Dr. Kazanjian's arrival at Ellis Island and the name of the ship; Andrea Pogarian for material on her father, Dr. Kenneth A. Kazanjian; Dr. Richard C. Webster, one of Dr. Kazanjian's earlier protegés; Virginia (Ring) Lane, who was medical secretary in Dr. Kazanjian's office from 1944 to 1948; Mrs. Lucy Daghlian, widow of Dr. Levon K. Daghlian, for recalling her husband's relationships with Dr. Kazanjian; Harry Sogigian, who discovered in the

February 7, 1897 minutes of the Church of Our Saviour a reference to Varaztad Kazanjian delivering a talk in "Readings"; Dr. Renée Bennett O'Sullivan, who provided me with her remembrances of Dr. Kazanjian and of Dr. Anthony Zovickian.

Drs. Malvin E. Ring and Eric Curtis, both eminent dental historians, gave freely of their wealth of knowledge.

Dr. William W. Montgomery, John W. Merriam Professor of Otology and Laryngology at Harvard Medical School, assisted with his personal knowledge of Dr. Kazanjian and Dr. Roopenian at the Massachusetts Eye and Ear Infirmary. Dr. William G. Levelle, Professor and Chairman of the Department of Otolaryngology and Head and Neck Surgery at the University of Massachusetts Medical Center, shared with me the video taken of his interview of Dr. Aram Roopenian, which was most valuable. I also thank Dr. Cliff A. Mergerian, formerly Associate Professor and Director of Otology and Neurotology, University of Massachusetts Medical Center for his strong support and the doors which he opened for me. Gratitude is also expressed to Drs. Adam Moore, Mack L. Cheney, Mark B. Constantian, Raffi Der Sarkissian, Raymond M. Dunn, Joshua C. Brooker, Howard M. Ecker and Sherman Santoian.

Drs. Charles P. Pietrafesa, Gerald Shklar, Andrew Christopher and Robert Babigian, "listened and heard." Dr. John M. Hyson, Jr., of the Harris National Museum of Dentistry, shared with me any information on Dr. Kazanjian that came across his desk. Dr. Pierre Gremeaux of France personally obtained photographs of Drs. Claude Martin, Hyppolyte Morestin and Georges Villain from Paris. Albert Southwick, his daughter, Martha, and her husband, Franz Schwediauer, in Vienna obtained, with great difficulty, a photograph of Dr. Hans Pichler. Jean F. Edmunds, Joan Fouhy, Sandi Bishop and Harold Gregory graciously provided editorial assistance.

Acknowledgment is expressed to the following for the use of photographic material: Project Save, (Armenian Photograph Archives, Inc.) for photographs of Sivas; Melikian Studio, Worcester, Mass., for photographs of early Worcester and the Kazanjian family; Victoria Manoogian for photographs of the Kazanjian family; Rebecca Reynolds of the staff of the Museum of Fine Arts, Boston, for material on Anna Coleman Ladd; The Reverend Manasseh H. Shnorhokian and Dr. Arto Shahrik for assistance in the translation of Armenian sources into English.

In addition to the Countway Library, I have used the facilities of several other libraries, and I wish to thank the librarians at the Boston Public Library and the Worcester Public Library, Imperial War Museum, London, the University of Pennsylvania School of Dental Medicine Library, the University of Massachusetts Medical School Library, and The Webster Collection at the Columbia University School of Medicine.

The unexpected communication from Australia from the granddaughter of one of the facially wounded patients whom Major Kazanjian had treated in France was an omen of success.

There was a patient, who shall remain unnamed, who was treated successively by Drs. Kazanjian, Roopenian and Converse, and who appeared in my office for dental treatment years later and who shared his vivid personal impressions of each of them with me for which I am grateful.

I wish to pay particular homage and appreciation to members of Dr. Kazanjian's family:

I have called upon Dr. Kazanjian's daughter, Hélène Kazanjian Sargeant, who on more than one occasion provided invaluable information and interpretations on her father's life. Before his untimely death, I had the good fortune to talk with Dr. Kazanjian's son, Victor. Later, Victor's son, The Reverend Victor H. Kazanjian, Jr., Dean of Religious Life at Wellesley College, provided rare personal insights into the lives of his grandparents.

Happily, Dr. Kazanjian's grand-nephew, Dr. Roger Ohanesian carries on the family medical tradition as an ophthalmologist in California. His mother, Flora, is the daughter of Dr. Kazanjian's sister, Nouvart. I interviewed both.

Virginia Deranian, my wife, accompanied me on many successful searches and some "wild goose chases" in my search for the Kazanjian legend. Thank you, Virginia.

Over the years, there have been others to whom I am beholden who remain unnamed on these pages but who influenced me more than they could have imagined, some of them dating back to my student days and others to my father's generation.

Above all, it was the invaluable opportunities that Dr. Kazanjian provided for me to meet personally and relate to him on several levels which merit my gratitude and indebtedness. May my work convey to the reader a benevolent yet realistic portrayal of this "gentle genius of plastic surgery."

APPENDIX A

Chronology

1879 Born March 18 in Erzincan, Turkish Armenia, to Hovhannes and Anna (Siroonian) Kazanjian

Attended French Jesuit missionary school in Sivas

1893 Moved to Samsun to live with and work for older half-brother; later worked in a post office in Samsun

1895 Emigrated to United States, entering through Ellis Island in October. Lived in Armenian community in Worcester, took correspondence courses, attended Worcester Evening High School

1900 Became U. S. citizen on October 15

1902 Attended Boston English High School

Admitted to Harvard Dental School, Class of 1905

1905 Awarded D.M.D. from Harvard Dental School on June 28

Established private dental practice in Boston

1906 Appointed Assistant in Mechanical Dentistry, Harvard Dental School

1907 Appointed Assistant in Prosthetic Dentistry, Harvard Dental School

1909 Appointed Demonstrator of Prosthetic Dentistry, Harvard Dental School

1911 Entered second year class (admitted with advanced standing) at Boston University Medical School

1912 Appointed Head of the Prosthetic Dentistry Department, Harvard Dental School. Left Boston University Medical School

Married Sophie Augusta Cuendet in Boston on December 21, (She died in Boston, August 10, 1919)

1913 Appointed Head of the Department of Prosthetic Dentistry, Harvard Dental School

1915 Appointed Chief Dental Officer, Harvard Medical Unit, British Expeditionary Force, with rank of Honorary Lieutenant. Served in Camiers, France, at General Hospitals No. 20 and No. 22

1916 Promoted Honorary Major, Land Forces, Royal Army Medical Corps

1918 Appointed Companion of Saint Michael and Saint George, June 3

Appointed Professor of Military Oral Surgery, Harvard Dental School

1919 Discharged from Royal Army

Invested as Companion of Saint Michael and Saint George by King George V at Buckingham Palace in May

Returned to United States in May and admitted as third year student to Harvard Medical School, Class of 1921

Rejoined faculty at Harvard Dental School as Professor of Military Oral Surgery

1921 Received M.D. degree. Established private practice in Boston in plastic surgery of face, surgical prostheses, and oral surgery

1922 Appointed Professor of Clinical Oral Surgery at Harvard

1923 Married Marion Victorine Hanford in New York City on August 25

1931 Named Surgeon for Plastic Operations at Massachusetts Eye and Ear Infirmary and Special Consultant in Plastic Surgery at Massachusetts General Hospital. (First appointment to M.E.E.I. staff in 1923 and to M.G.H. staff in 1921)

1932 Received Award from Rhode Island State Dental Society

1937 President of American Academy of Dental Science

1940 Served as President of American Association of Plastic Surgeons

1941 Appointed Professor of Plastic Surgery, Harvard Medical School (Appointment created for VHK)

1943 Received Alfred E. Fones Medal, Connecticut State Dental Society

1947 Appointed Professor Emeritus of Plastic Surgery, Harvard Medical School

Appointed Guest Lecturer in Oral Surgery, Graduate School of Medicine, University of Pennsylvania

1949 Publication of first edition of *The Surgical Treatment of Facial Injuries*, co-authored with Dr. John Marquis Converse.

1951 Received Special Honorary Citation of the American Society of Plastic and Reconstructive Surgeons for his leadership in the organization and development of the specialty of plastic surgery

Appointed Visiting Lecturer in Oral Surgery, Graduate School of Medicine, University of Pennsylvania

1952 Awarded honorary degree of Doctor of Science by Bowdoin College

1953 Awarded Honor Key Award of the Academy of Ophthalmology and Otolaryngology

1954 Received Society Award of American Society of Oral Surgeons

Awarded Honorary Membership Chalmers J. Lyons Academy of Oral Surgery, University of Michigan

1956 Received Honorary Award from American Society of Maxillofacial Surgeons

Awarded Leonard Wood Memorial Medal, Boston City Hospital Alumni Association

1956 Made Honorary Member, Massachusetts Dental Society

1957 Became Honorary Member and received Award from New England Society of Oral Surgeons

Awarded Honorary Membership, Worcester Dental Society

1958 Dr. Aram Roopenian joined the practice of V.H.K.

1959 Award from American Association of Plastic Surgeons

Publication of Second Edition of *The Surgical Treatment of Facial Injuries*, co-authored with Dr. John Marquis Converse

1960 Served as first president of New England Society of Plastic Surgeons

1962 Awarded New York University Presidential Citation

V.H. Kazanjian Visiting Professorship in Plastic Surgery established at New York University Medical Center, Institute of Reconstructive Plastic Surgery, by friends and former patients

1964 Retired from private practice

1966 Became Honorary Fellow of British Association of Plastic Surgeons in London

1967 Became Honorary Fellow of Royal College of Physicians and Surgeons in Glasgow

Received Harvard Dental Centennial Award

1972 Received Award of Neal Owens Society for Plastic and Reconstructive Surgery

1974 Died October 19 at his home in Belmont, Massachusetts. Survived by his wife, Marion H. Kazanjian (d. 1980), and three children, Hélène K. Sargeant, Dr. Jean K. Leavitt, Victor H. Kazanjian (d. 1985) and five grandchildren.

APPENDIX B

Professional Appointments

Assistant in Mechanical Dentistry, Harvard Dental School, 1906

Assistant in Prosthetic Dentistry, Harvard Dental School, 1908

Demonstrator of Prosthetic Dentistry, Harvard Dental School, 1909-1916

Lecturer, Harvard-Forsyth Post Graduate School of Orthodontia, 1919-1920

Dental Surgeon, Peter Bent Brigham Hospital, 1920

Visiting Surgeon for Oral and Plastic Surgery, The Boston City Hospital, 1921

Graduate Assistant, Massachusetts General Hospital, Laryngological Clinic of the Out-Patient Department, 1921-1922

Dental Surgeon, Peter Bent Brigham Hospital, 1922

Professor of Clinical Oral Surgery, Harvard Medical School, 1922

Visiting Surgeon for Oral and Plastic Surgery, The Boston City Hospital, 1923

Assistant in the Laryngological Department, Massachusetts General Hospital, 1923

Visiting Surgeon for Oral and Plastic Surgery, The Boston City Hospital, 1924

Assistant Laryngologist, Massachusetts General Hospital, 1924

Visiting Surgeon for Oral and Plastic Surgery, The Boston City Hospital, 1925

Assistant Laryngologist, Massachusetts General Hospital, 1925

Consulting Oral Surgeon, Cambridge Hospital, 1925

Visiting Surgeon for Oral and Plastic Surgery, The Boston City Hospital, 1926

Assistant Surgeon in Oto-Laryngology, Massachusetts Eye and Ear Infirmary, 1926

Assistant Laryngologist, Massachusetts General Hospital, 1926

Consulting Oral Surgeon, Cambridge Hospital, 1926

Visiting Surgeon for Oral and Plastic Surgery, The Boston City Hospital, 1927

Assistant Surgeon in Oto-Laryngology, Massachusetts Eye and Ear Infirmary, 1927

Assistant Laryngologist, Massachusetts General Hospital, 1927

Consulting Oral Surgeon, Cambridge Hospital, 1927

Visiting Surgeon for Oral and Plastic Surgery The Boston City Hospital, 1928

Assistant Surgeon in Oto-Laryngology, Massachusetts Eye and Ear Infirmary, 1928

Consulting Oral Surgeon, Cambridge Hospital, 1928

Assistant Surgeon in Oto-Laryngology, Massachusetts Eye and Ear Infirmary, 1929

Consulting Oral Surgeon, Cambridge Hospital, 1929

Special assignment on plastic surgery of the face, Massachusetts General Hospital, 1929

Visiting Surgeon for Oral and Plastic Surgery, The Boston City Hospital, 1930

Special Consultant in Plastic Surgery, Massachusetts General Hospital, 1930

Assistant Surgeon in Oto-Laryngology, Massachusetts Eye and Ear Infirmary, 1930

Consulting Oral Surgeon, Cambridge Hospital, 1930

Special Assignment on Plastic Surgery Massachusetts General Hospital, 1930

Visiting Surgeon for Oral and Plastic Surgery, The Boston City Hospital, 1931

Surgeon for Plastic Operations, Massachusetts Eye and Ear Infirmary, 1931

Special Consultant in Plastic Surgery, Massachusetts General Hospital, 1931

Consulting Oral Surgeon, Cambridge Hospital, 1931

Special Assignment of General Plastic Surgery, Massachusetts General Hospital, 1931

Visiting Surgeon for Oral and Plastic Surgery, The Boston City Hospital, 1932

Surgeon for Plastic Operations, Massachusetts Eye and Ear Infirmary, 1932

Special Consultant in Plastic Surgery and Honorary Surgeon, Massachusetts General Hospital, 1932

Consulting Oral Surgeon, Cambridge Hospital, 1932

Visiting Surgeon for Oral and Plastic Surgery, The Boston City Hospital, 1933

Surgeon for Plastic Operations, Massachusetts Eye and Ear Infirmary, 1933

Special Consultant in Plastic Surgery, Massachusetts General Hospital, 1933

Consulting Oral Surgeon, Cambridge Hospital, 1933

Visiting Surgeon for Oral and Plastic Surgery, The Boston City Hospital, 1934

Surgeon for Plastic Operations, Massachusetts Eye and Ear Infirmary, 1934

Special Consultant in Plastic Surgery, Massachusetts General Hospital, 1934.

Consulting Oral Surgeon, Cambridge Hospital, 1934

Visiting Surgeon for Oral and Plastic Surgery, The Boston City Hospital, 1935

Surgeon for Plastic Operations, Massachusetts Eye and Ear Infirmary, 1935

Visiting Surgeon, Massachusetts General Hospital, 1935

Consulting Oral Surgeon, Cambridge Hospital, 1935

Surgeon for Plastic Operations, Consulting Surgeon, Massachusetts Eye and Ear Infirmary, 1936

Visiting Surgeon, Massachusetts General Hospital, 1936

Consulting Oral Surgeon, Cambridge Hospital, 1936

Visiting Surgeon for Oral and Plastic Surgery, The Boston City Hospital, 1936

Visiting Surgeon for Oral and Plastic Surgery, The Boston City Hospital, 1937

Surgeon for Plastic Operations, Consulting Surgeon, Massachusetts Eye and Ear Infirmary, 1937

Visiting Surgeon, Massachusetts General Hospital, 1937

Consulting Oral Surgeon, Cambridge Hospital, 1937

Visiting Surgeon for Oral and Plastic Surgery, The Boston City Hospital, 1938

Surgeon for Plastic Operations, Consulting Surgeon, Massachusetts Eye and Ear Infirmary, 1938

Visiting Surgeon, Massachusetts General Hospital, 1938

Surgeon for Plastic Operations, Massachusetts General Hospital, 1938

Consulting Oral Surgeon, Cambridge Hospital, 1938

Visiting Surgeon for Oral and Plastic Surgery, The Boston City Hospital, 1939

Consultant in Maxillo-Facial Surgery, Beth Israel Hospital, Boston,1939

Consulting Staff, The Jordan Hospital, Plymouth, Massachusetts, 1939

Surgeon for Plastic Operations, Massachusetts Eye and Ear Infirmary, 1939

Consulting Oral Surgeon, Cambridge Hospital, 1939

Surgeon, Cambridge Hospital, 1939

Consulting Oral and Plastic Surgeon, The Burbank Hospital, Fitchburg, Massachusetts, 1940

Visiting Surgeon for Oral and Plastic Surgery, The Boston City Hospital, 1940

Surgeon, Cambridge Hospital, 1940

Professor of Plastic Surgery, Harvard Medical School, 1941

Visiting Surgeon for Oral and Plastic Surgery, The Boston City Hospital, 1941

Surgeon in Department of General Surgery Cambridge Hospital, 1941

Visiting Surgeon for Oral and Plastic Surgery, The Boston City Hospital, 1942

Surgeon, Cambridge Hospital, 1942

Visiting Surgeon for Oral and Plastic Surgery, The Boston City Hospital, 1943

Surgeon in the Department of Surgery, Cambridge Hospital, 1943

Visiting Surgeon for Oral and Plastic Surgery, The Boston City Hospital, 1944

Lecturer in Otolaryngology, Tufts College Medical School, 1944

Surgeon, Cambridge Hospital, 1944

Visiting Surgeon for Oral and Plastic Surgery, The Boston City Hospital, 1945

Surgeon, Cambridge Hospital, 1945

Visiting Surgeon for Oral and Plastic Surgery, The Boston City Hospital, 1946

Surgeon, Cambridge Hospital, 1946

Consulting Oral and Plastic Surgeon, Henry Heywood Memorial Hospital, Gardner, Massachusetts, 1946

Visiting Surgeon for Oral and Plastic Surgery, The Boston City Hospital, 1947

Member of the Consulting Medical Staff, Cambridge Hospital, 1947

Professor of Plastic Surgery, Emeritus, Harvard Medical School, 1947

Consulting Surgeon for Oral and Plastic Surgery, The Boston City Hospital, 1948

Member of the Consulting Staff, Glover Memorial Hospital, Needham, Massachusetts, 1948

Consulting Medical Staff in Plastic Surgery, Mount Auburn Hospital, Cambridge, 1948

Consulting Surgeon for Oral and Plastic Surgery, The Boston City Hospital, 1949

Consultant in Plastic Surgery, Mount Auburn Hospital, 1949

Consulting Surgeon for Oral and Plastic Surgery, The Boston City Hospital, 1950

Consultant in Plastic Surgery, Mount Auburn Hospital, 1950

Consulting Surgeon for Oral and Plastic Surgery, The Boston City Hospital, 1951

Consultant in Plastic Surgery, Mount Auburn Hospital, 1951

Consulting Surgeon for Oral and Plastic Surgery, The Boston City Hospital, 1952

Courtesy Staff, Sancta Maria Hospital, Cambridge, 1952

Consultant in Plastic Surgery, Mount Auburn Hospital, 1952

Consulting Staff, Mount Auburn Hospital, 1953-1954

Consulting Surgeon for Oral and Plastic Surgery, The Boston City Hospital, 1953-1957

Consulting Staff in Plastic Surgery, Mount Auburn Hospital, 1957

Consultant in Oral and Plastic Surgery, The Boston City Hospital, 1958

Consulting Staff in Plastic Surgery, Mount Auburn Hospital, 1958

Consultant in Surgery, Beth Israel Hospital, 1959

Consultant in Plastic Surgery at Tufts University School of Dental Medicine, Cleft Palate Institute, 1960

Consultant in Oral and Plastic Surgery, The Boston City Hospital, 1959-1961, 1963-1965

Honorary Surgeon, Massachusetts General Hospital, 1965

Plastic Surgeon, Active Staff, New England Deaconess Hospital, Boston, 1967

Honorary Medical Staff in Surgery-Plastic and Reconstructive, Symmes Hospital, Arlington, Massachusetts, 1967

Consultant in Surgery (Plastic), Beth Israel Hospital, Boston, 1967

Honorary Surgeon, Massachusetts General Hospital, 1967

Senior Consulting Surgeon for Plastic Operations, Massachusetts Eye and Ear Infirmary, 1968

Consultant in Surgery (Plastic), Beth Israel Hospital, 1968

Honorary Staff, New England Deaconess Hospital, 1968

Honorary Medical Staff in Surgery - Plastic and Reconstructive, Symmes Hospital, Arlington, 1968

Honorary Surgeon, Massachusetts General Hospital, 1968

Senior Consulting Surgeon for Plastic Operations, Massachusetts Eye and Ear Infirmary, 1969

Consultant in Surgery (Plastic), Beth Israel Hospital, 1969

Honorary Staff, New England Deaconess Hospital, 1969

Honorary Medical Staff in Plastic and Reconstructive Surgery, Symmes Hospital, 1969

Honorary Surgeon, Massachusetts General Hospital, 1969

Consultant in Surgery (Plastic), Beth Israel Hospital, 1970

Honorary Staff, New England Deaconess Hospital, 1970

Honorary Medical Staff in Surgery (Plastic and Reconstructive), Symmes Hospital, 1970

Honorary Surgeon, Massachusetts General Hospital, 1970

Senior Consulting Surgeon for Plastic Operations, Massachusetts Eye and Ear Infirmary, 1971

Honorary Staff, New England Deaconess Hospital, 1971

Honorary Medical Staff in Plastic and Reconstructive Surgery, Symmes Hospital, 1971

Senior Consulting Surgeon for Plastic Operations, Massachusetts Eye and Ear Infirmary, 1972

Honorary Staff, New England Deaconess Hospital, 1972

Honorary Medical Staff in Plastic and Reconstructive Surgery, Symmes Hospital, 1972

Board of Consultation, Massachusetts General Hospital, 1972

Senior Consulting Surgeon in Otolaryngology (Plastic Surgery), Massachusetts Eye and Ear Infirmary, 1973

Honorary Staff, New England Deaconess Hospital, 1973

Honorary Medical Staff in Plastic and Reconstructive Surgery, Symmes Hospital, 1973

Board of Consultation, Massachusetts General Hospital, 1973

Senior Consulting Surgeon in Otolaryngology (Plastic Surgery), Massachusetts Eye and Ear Infirmary, 1974

Honorary Staff, New England Deaconess Hospital, 1974

Board of Consultation, Massachusetts General Hospital, 1974

APPENDIX C

Bibliography

1911 "The Retention of Artificial Dentures," *Journal of the Allied Dental Societies*, 6:95.

1915 "Prosthetic Restoration of Acquired Deformities of the Superior Maxilla," *Journal of Allied Dental Societies*, 10:14.

1916 "Immediate Treatment of Gunshot Fracture of Jaws," *British Dental Journal*, War Supplement, 37:297 and *Journal of the Allied Dental Societies*, 12:29

"Treatment of Maxillary Fractures," *British Medical Journal*, 1:266 and *British Dental Journal*, War Supplement, 37:50.

1917 "The Dentist and the Army," *The Mirror* (Yearbook of the Senior Class) of the Harvard University Dental School, p. 45.

"The Department of Oral Surgery of the Harvard Surgical Unit," *British Medical Journal* 2:3 and *British Journal of Dental Science*, 60:454

Five articles in Comunications et Présentations au Congrès Dentaire Interallié, Paris 10-13 November 1916. Compte Rendu, Tomes 1 and 2, Paris. "Traitement Précoce des Blessures de la Face et de la Machoire," p. 116. "Quelques Problèmes de Prosthèse Rélatifs à la Destruction des Os Maxillaires Supérieurs," p. 557. "Pont Nasal Artificiel," p. 606. "Appareil Destiné à Prévenir la Contraction Cicatricielle des Joues," p. 741. "Appareil Universel Externe de Soutien de la Face, du Nez et du Maxillaire," p. 963.

"Suture des Esquilles Osseuses pour L"Immobilsation des Fractures Étendues du Maxillaire Inférieur," *La Restauration Maxillo-Faciale*, 1:168.

(With Harold Burrows) "The Treatment of Haemorrhage Caused by Gunshot Wounds of the Face and Jaws," *British Journal of Surgery*, War Supplement, 5:126.

1918 "Some Problems of Prosthesis as a Result of Destruction of the Superior Maxilla," *British Dental Journal*, 39:26.

"Splints Combined with Sutures through the Bone for the Immobilization of Extensive Fractures of the Lower Jaw," *Proceedings of the Royal Society of Medicine* (Section of Odontology), 11:67.

(With Harold Burrows) "The Treatment of Gunshot Wounds of the Face Accompanied by Extensive Destructions of the Lower Lip and Mandible," *British Journal of Surgery*, 6:74.

"Sutures of Osseous Splinters for Fixing Extensive Fractures of the Mandible," *Ash's Monthly*, (Jul-Aug) 241.

"The Use of Appliances in the Treatment of Injuries of Soft Parts of the Face and Mouth," *La Restauration Maxillo-Faciale*, 2:427 and same article in French on p. 345.

1919 "Early Suturing of Wounds of the Face," *Journal of the American Medical Association* 72:626

"Prosthetic Appliances in Surgical Treatment of Wounds of the Face and Jaws," *Journal of the American Medical Association*, 73:1265.

"Wounds of the Face and Jaws," Chapter 10 in *A Manual of War Surgery* by Seymour Barling and John T. Morrison. London: Oxford University Press.

1920 "An Analysis of Gunshot Injuries to the Face," *International Journal of Orthodontia and Oral Surgery*, 6:96.

"Observation on War Surgery of the Face and Jaws," *Dental Cosmos*, 62:283.

1921 "Plastic Surgery of the Lip," *Journal of the American Medical Association*, 77:1959.

1922 "Problems of Prosthetic Restoration Following Injuries of the Face and Jaws," *Military Dental Journal*, 5:69.

1924 "Surgical Operations as Related to Satisfactory Dentures," *Dental Cosmos*, 66:387.

1925 "Treatment of Nasal Deformities," *Journal of the American Medical Association*, 84:177.

1926 "Immediate Care and Treatment of Traumatic Injuries of the Mandible and Maxilla," *The Apollonian*, 1:16.

Two articles in Transactions of the Seventh International Dental Congress, Philadelphia, August 23-27, 1926. "Unilateral Deformity of the Mandible," p. 1549. "Treatment of Injuries of the Upper Part of the Face," p. 2133.

"Urgent Treatment of Face and Jaw Injuries," *Journal of the American Dental Association*, 13:712.

1927 "Treatment of Injuries of the Upper Part of the Face," *Journal of the American Dental Association*, 14:1607.

1928 "The Treatment of Postoperative Complications Following the Extraction of Teeth," *Dental Cosmos*, 70:135.

"Unilateral Deformity of the Mandible," *Journal of the American Dental Association*, 15:105.

1929 "A Method of Locating Broken Dental Needles," *The Apollonian*, 4:79.

"Surgery in Relation to Orthodontia," *Dental Cosmos*, 70:141

"Tumors of Jaws and Mouth," *New England Journal of Medicine*, 201:1200.

1930 "Prosthetic Restoration of Deformities of Face and Jaw," Chapter 28 in *Prosthetic Dentistry,* by Ira G. Nichols, St. Louis, C.V. Mosby

1931 "Surgical and Prosthetic Treatment of Deformities of the Mandible," International Dental Congress, 8th Paris, 2-8 August, 1931, Section 12.

"Treatment of Acute Infections of the Mouth," *The Apollian*, 6:24

1932 "Modern Accomplishments in Dental and Facial Prosthesis," *Journal of Dental Research*, 12:651.

(With A.T. Rowe and H.A. Young) "Prosthesis of the Mouth and Face," *Journal of Dental Research*, 12:651.

"Surgical Treatment of Mandibular Prognathism," *International Journal of Orthodontia, Oral Surgery and Radiography*, 18:1224

1933 "Injuries to the Face and Jaws Resulting from Automobile Accidents," *Transactions of the American Academy of Ophthalmology and Otolaryngology*, 38:275

"Nasal Deformities and Their Repair," *Laryngoscope*, 43:955.

"The Treatment of Automobile Injuries of the Face and Jaws," *Journal of the American Dental Association*, 20:757.

1934 "Dental Prosthesis in Relation to Facial Reparative Surgery," *Surgery, Gynecology and Obstetrics*, 59:70.

"Traumatism of the Face and Jaws with Special Reference to Complications," *Journal of American Dental Association*, 21:1138.

1935 "Benign Giant Cell Tumor of the Mandible," *The Apollonian*, 10:152.

"Dental Restoration for an Edentulous Patient with Perforation of the Palate," *The Apollonian*, 10:11

Discussion of "The Value of Speech Training in Cleft Palate and Other Mouth Conditions," *Otolaryngology*, 22:594

"Surgery as an Aid to More Efficient Service with Prosthetic Dentures," *Journal of the American Dental Association*, 22:566.

"Surgical Treatment of Dental Root Cysts at the Anterior Part of the Maxilla," *The Apollonian*, 10:227.

1936 "Consideration of Abnormalities, Deformities and Pathological Conditions of Edentulous Mouths," *International Journal of Orthodontia and Oral Surgery*, 22:735.

"Dentigerous Cysts Involving the Maxillary Sinus," *The Apollonian*, 11:26.

"Plastic Surgery of the Face," American Academy of Ophthalmology and Otolaryngology Graduate Lecture Conference no. 322.

"The Repair of Contractures Resulting from Burns," *New England Journal of Medicine*, 215:1104.

"Surgical Correction of Deformities of the Jaws and Its Relation to Orthodontia," *International Journal of Orthodontia* and Oral Surgery, 22:259.

"Surgical Preparation of the Mouth for Artificial Dentures," Chapter 13 in *Essentials of Oral Surgery* by Vilray P. Blair, Robert H. Ivy and James B. Brown St. Louis, C.V. Mosby.

"Surgical Treatment of Deformities of the Mandible," *The Apollonian*, 11:226.

"Surgical Treatment of Dental Cysts Involving the Mandible," *The Apollonian*, 11:154.

1937 "Book Review: *Oral Diagnosis and Treatment Planning* by Samuel C. Miller," *Harvard Dental Record*, 11:7.

"Deformities of Mandible Following Fracture," *The Apollonian*, 12:85.

"Fractures of the Edentulous Mandible," *The Apollonian*, 12:146.

"Fractures of the Nasal and Malar Bones," Chapter 35 in Volume 11, *Practitioners Library of Medicine and Surgery*. New York, D. Appleton Century.

"Plastic Repair of Deformities about the Lower Part of the Nose Resulting from Loss of Tissue," *Transactions of the American Academy of Ophthalmology and Otolaryngology*, 42:338.

"Prosthetic Restoration for Large Palatal Defect," *The Apollonian*, 12:242.

"The Surgical Treatment of Deformities of the Mandible Resulting from Osteomyelitis," *The Apollonian*, 12:9.

1938 "Ankylosis of the Temporomandibular Joint," *Surgery, Gynecology and Obstetrics*, 67:333.

"Fractures of the Facial Bones," Chapter 17 in *Experience in the Management of Fractures and Dislocations* edited by Philip D. Wilson. Philadelphia, J.B Lippincott.

(With Kurt Thoma) "Fractures of the Facial Bones Including Nasal, Malar and Mandibular Bones," Chapter 21 in *The Treatment of Fractures*, 11th ed., rev. by Charles L. Scudder, Philadelphia, W.B. Saunders.

"Large Odontoma of the Mandible with Impacted Lower Third Molar and Alveolar Abscess," *The Apollonian*, 13:87.

"Lateral Pressure Splint for the Nose," *Archives of Otolaryngology*, 27:474.

"Molar Root in Antrum -Twelve Years' Duration," *The Apollonian*, 13:25.

1939 "Book Review: *Fractures of the Jaws*, 2nd ed. by Robert H. Ivy and Lawrence Curtis," *Harvard Dental Record*, 13:11.

"Congenital Absence of the Ramus of the Mandible," *Journal of Bone and Joint Surgery*, 21:761.

"Jaw Reconstruction," *American Journal of Surgery*, 43:249.

"Secondary Deformities in Cleft Palate Patients," *Annals of Surgery*, 109:442.

1940 "The Interrelation of Dentistry and Surgery in the Treatment of Deformities of the Face and Jaws," *Proceedings of the Dental Centenary Celebration*, Baltimore, MArch 18-20, 1940

(With John M. Converse) "Reconstruction after Radical Operation for Osteomyelitis of the Frontal Bone," *Archives of Otolaryngology*, 31:94.

"The Surgical Treatment of Abnormalities of the Edentulous Alveolar Processes and the Palate," *American Journal of Orthodontics and Oral Surgery*, 26:263

(With Somers H. Sturgis) "Surgical Treatment of Hemiatrophy of the Face," *Journal of the American Medical Association*, 115:348.

"Tumors of the Jaws," a chapter in *Cancer: A Manual for Practitioners* by The Committee on Publication of the Massachusetts Medical Society and the American Society for the Control of Cancer. Boston, Rumford Press.

1941 "Dental Autonomy: A Policy of Isolation," *Journal of the American Dental Association*, 28:1671.

"Interrelation of Dentistry and Surgery in Treatment of the Harelip," *American Journal of Orthodontics* (Oral Surgery section), 27:10.

"Primary Care of Facial Wounds," *American Journal or Orthodontics* (Oral Surgery Section), 27:448.

"Primary Care of Injuries of the Face and Jaws," *Surgery, Gynecology, and Obstetrics*, 72:431.

"Synopsis of Treatment of War Time Injuries of the Face and Jaws," *The Apollonian*, 15:57.

"Treatment of Benign Tumors of the Jaws," *Journal of the American Dental Association*, 28:208.

1942 (With Moses S. Strock) "Early Treatment of Fractures of the Mandible," *Journal of the American Dental Association*, 29:76.

"Immobilization of Wartime, Compound, Comminuted Fractures of the Mandible," *American Journal of Orthodontics and Oral Surgery*, 28:551

"An Outline of the Treatment of Extensive Comminuted Fractures of the Mandible," *American Journal of Orthodontics and Oral Surgery*, 28:265.

"Primary Treatment of Gunshot Wounds of the Face," Chapter 1 in *Ophthalmology and Otolaryngology by the National Research Council.* Philadelphia, W.B. Saunders.

"The Treatment of Congenital Atresia of the Choanae," *Annals of Otology, Rhinology and Laryngology*, 51:704.

1943 "Jaw Reconstruction," a chapter in *Rehabilitation of the War Injured* by William B. Doherty and Dagobert D. Runes. New York, Philosophical Library.

"Plastic Surgery," *Bulletin of the American College of Surgeons*, 28:140.

"Reconstruction of Deformities of the Forehead and the Frontal Bone," Transactions of the Twelfth Annual Meeting of the American Society of Plastic and Reconstructive Surgery, New York City, October 9, 1943.

(With Carl W. Waldron and Douglas B. Parker) "Skeletal Fixation in the Treatment of Fractures of the Mandible," *Journal of Oral Surgery*, 1:59.

"Synopsis of Treatment of War Time Injuries of the Face and Jaws." American Academy of Ophthalmology and Otolaryngology Graduate Lecture Continuous Course No. 54.

"Treatment of Extensive Loss of the Mandible and Its Surrounding Tissues," *Journal of Oral Surgery*, 1:30.

1944 Discussion of "Problems in Reconstructive Treatment of Gunshot Wounds of the Face," by Michael Lewin, *Transactions of the American Academy of Ophthalmology and Otolaryngology*, 49:281.

"Early Treatment of Gunshot Wounds of the Face and Jaws," *Surgery*, 15:22.

(With Edgar M. Holmes) "Reconstruction after Radical Operation for Osteomyelitis of the Frontal Bone," *Surgery, Gynecology and Obstetrics*, 79:397.

"Treatment of Deformity from Burns," *Connecticut State Medical Journal*, 8:661.

1945 "Stenosis of the Oropharynx," *Journal of Oral Surgery*, 3:164.

1946 "The Repair of Nasal Defects with the Median Forehead Flap," *Surgery, Gynecology and Obstetrics*, 83:37.

"Spontaneous Regeneration of Bone Following Excision of Section of the Mandible," *American Journal of Orthodontics and Oral Surgery*, 32:242.

(With Edgar M. Holmes) "Stenosis of the Nasopharynx and Its Correction," *Archives of Otolaryngology*, 44:261.

"Surgical Treatment of Ichthyosis Hystrix," *Plastic and Reconstructive Surgery*, 1:91.

(With Richard C. Webster) "The Treatment of Extensive Losses of the Scalp," *Plastic and Reconstructive Surgery*, 1:360.

1947 "Estlander-Abbe Operation in Treating Secondary Harelip Deformities and Defects of the Upper Lip Resulting from Cancer," *Plastic and Reconstructive Surgery*, 2:307.

(With Edgar M. Holmes) "New Rongeur for Removing a Nasal

Hump," *Archives of Otolaryngology*, 45:361.

"Prosthetic Restoration of Congenital and Acquired Deformities of Hard and Soft Palate," *Journal of Oral Surgery*, 5:181.

"Restoration of the Nose, Lip and Maxilla by Surgery and Prosthesis," *Plastic and Reconstructive Surgery*, 2:531

1948 "The Inter-relation of Dentistry and Surgery of the Face and Jaws," *Australian Journal of Dentistry*, 52:336.

"Nasal Deformities of Syphilitic Origin," *Plastic and Reconstructive Surgery*, 3:517.

1950 (With Alfred T. Joseph) "Beryllium Granuloma of the Nose," *Plastic and Reconstructive Surgery*, 6:156.

(With Aram Roopenian) "Total Avulsion of the Scalp," *New England Journal of Medicine*, 242:539.

"The use of Skin Flaps in the Repair of Facial Deformities," *Plastic and Reconstructive Surgery*, 5:337.

1951 "Book Review: *Breast Deformities and Their Repair* by Jacques W. Maliniac," *New England Journal of Medicine*, 245:956.

"Book Review: *Plastic and Reconstructive Surgery* by Ferris Smith," *New England Journal of Medicine*, 245:196.

"Congenital Deformity of the Maxilla and Mandible," *Plastic and Reconstructive Surgery*, 7:396.

"Resection of Tumor of the Mandible and Repair of the Deformity," *Journal of Oral Surgery*, 9:59.

"Secondary Deformities of Cleft Palates," *Plastic and Reconstructive Surgery*, 8:477.

"The Treatment of Mandibular Prognathism with Special Reference to Edentulous Patients," *Oral Surgery, Oral Medicine and Oral Pathology*, 4:680.

1952 "Bone Transplanting to the Mandible," *American Journal of Surgery*, 83:633.

Discussion of "Plastic Surgery Methods Used in the Treatment of Korean Casualties," by Bernard N. Soderberg, Transactions at Symposium on Military Medicine, Murphy Army Hospital, Waltham, Massachusetts, June 23-23, 1952, p. 277.

"Fractures of the Nasal Bones," *Transactions of the American Academy of Ophthalmology and Otolaryngology*, 56:565

1953 "Book Review: *Ophthalmic Plastic Surgery* by Sidney A. Fox," *New England Journal of Medicine*, 249:826.

"Damage to Bones and Soft Tissues," *Transactions of the American Academy of Ophthalmology and Otolaryngology*, 57:873.

"Repair of Partial Losses of the Scalp," *Plastic and Reconstructive Surgery*, 12:325.

1954 (With Aram Roopenian) "Clinical Experience in the Treatment of Hemangiomata," *Plastic and Reconstructive Surgery*, 13:325.

"The Surgical Treatment of Prognathism," *American Journal of Surgery*, 87:691.

(With Aram Roopenian) "The Treatment of Lip Deformities Resulting from Electric Burns," *American Journal of Surgery*, 88:884.

1955 "Book Review: *Surgery of Hare-Lip and Cleft-Palate* by Frantisek Burian," *New England Journal of Medicine*, 253:623.

"Advances in Maxillofacial Surgery During the Past Half Century," *Journal of Oral Surgery*, 13:97.

"Open-Bite Deformities of the Jaws Surgical Treatment," *Fortschritte der Kiefer- und Gesichts-Chirurgie*, 2:195.

"Temporomandibular Joint Ankylosis with Mandibular Retrusion," *American Journal of Surgery*, 90:905.

1956 "Bilateral Absence of the Ascending Rami of the Mandible," *British Journal of Plastic Surgery*, 9:77.

"Book Review: *Fractures of the Facial Skeleton* by N.L. Rowe and H.C. Killey," *New England Journal of Medicine*, 255:725.

"Mandibular Retrusion with Ankylosis of the Temporomandibular Joint," *Plastic and Reconstructive Surgery*, 17:91.

(With Aram Roopenian) "Median Forehead Flaps in the Repair of Defects of the Nose and Surrounding Areas," *Transactions of the American Academy of Ophthalmology and Otolaryngology*, 60:557.

1957 "Book Review: *The Principles and Art of Plastic Surgery* by Harold Gillies and D. Ralph Millard, Jr.," *New England Journal of Medicine*, 257:432.

1958 "Observations in the Treatment of Deformities and Injuries of the Facial Bones During the Last Fifty Years," *Massachusetts Dental Society Journal*, 7:9.

"Surgical Treatment of Congenital Deformities of the Ears," *American Journal of Surgery*, 95:185.

(With Edgar M. Holmes) "The Surgical Treatment of Edentulous Prognathic Patients," *American Journal of Surgery*, 96:833.

"Treatment of Dermoid Cysts of Nose," *Plastic and Reconstructive Surgery*, 21:169.

1959 (With Aram Roopenian) "The Repair of Full Thickness Eyelid Defects with Special Reference to Malignant Lesions," *Plastic and Reconstructive Surgery*, 24:262.

(With Edger M. Holmes) "Treatment of Median Cleft Lip Associated with Bifid Nose and Hypertelorism," *Plastic and Reconstructive Surgery*, 24:582.

1962 (With John M. Converse and Edgar M. Holmes) "Traumatic Injuries of the Face," American Academy of Ophthalmology and Otolaryngology Instruction Section Course 317.

"El Tratamiento Quirurgico de los Grandes Quistes Benignos del Maxilar Superior," *Revista de la Asociacion Odontologica, Argentina*, 50:420.

1963 (With Aram Roopenian) "The Surgical Treatment of Basal Cell Carcinoma of the External Nose."' *Transactions of the American Academy of Ophthalmology and Otolaryngology*, 67:37.

1964 "Foreword," in *Reconstructive Plastic Surgery* by John M. Converse. Philadelphia W.B. Saunders.

1965 "Remembrance of Things Past," *Plastic and Reconstructive Surgery*, 35:5.

"Tratamiento de las Deformidades Consecutivas a Resecciones en la Cara y la Mandibula," *Revista Latino-Americana de Cirurgia Plastica*, 9:89.

"Treatment of Deformities resulting from Resections of Face and Mandible," *Revista Latino-Americana de Cirurgia Plastica*, 9:98

1966 (With John M. Converse) "Comminuted Nasal Fractures," *Oral Surgery*, 4th ed,. by W. Harry Archer. Philadelphia, W.B. Saunders, p. 890.

1968 "Repair of Congenital Defects of the Mandible," Chapter 32 in *Cranofacial Anomalies* by J.J. Longacre. Philadelphia, J.B. Lippincott.

1975 (With John M. Converse) "Comminuted Nasal Fractures," *Oral and Maxillofacial Surgery*, 5th ed., by W. Harry Archer. Philadelphia, W.B. Saunders, p. 1319.

SOURCES

PRIMARY SOURCES

Archival Material

American Steel & Wire Collection, Baker Library, Harvard Business School, Cambridge, Mass.

Aharonian, A. Grace. "Early Armenians in Worcester." April 5, 1937, Industrial Museum Case 7, Folder VCB-987

Archive du Val-de-Grace, Paris.

Baillaud, Hélène, "Mémoires d'une Infirmière du Val-de-Grace."

Arents Collection, New York Public Library.

Freud, Sigmund. Letter to Wilhelm Fliess, November 17, 1893.

Dr. Samuel D. Harris National Museum of Dentistry, Baltimore. Ivy, Dr. Robert H. Letter to Homer S. Samuels, February 13, 1968.

Massachusetts Eye and Ear Infirmary Archives, Boston. Aram Roopenian, M.D. Interview conducted by Dr. William G. Lavelle. January 28, 1989.

National Archives of Plastic Surgery, Francis A. Countway Library of Medicine, Harvard Medical School, Boston.

Varaztad H. Kazanjian (1879-1974): An Inventory of His Records and Papers. 1989.

Anderson, Robin. Taped interview with V. H. Kazanjian, 1971.

New York City, Borough of Manhattan. Municipal Archives. 1923.

Official Documents

Commonwealth of Massachusetts. *Registry of Vital Records and Statistics*, 1909, 1912, 1918, 1919, 1974.

Commonwealth of Massachusetts. *Worcester Superior Court #2003,* April 27, 1900, Worcester County Mass.

Harvard University, Cambridge, Mass. *Alumni Bulletin*, 1915, 1916, and 1921.

——, *Catalogue,* 1902-03, 1904-05, 1906-97.

——, *Reports of the President and Treasurer, 1914-15.*

U. S. Congressional Record. 1920.

U. S. Department of Commerce, Bureau of Census. Thirtieth Census, 1910, and Fortieth Census, 1920.

U. S. Department of State. Dispatches, 1895.

Worcester City Documents. 1900.

Worcester Directory, 1895, 1896, 1898, 1899, 1900, 1901, 1902, 1905, 1912, 1918.

Worcester House Directory. 1908.

Unpublished Reports

Anderson, Major W. D. Report, March 29 to April 11, 1916.

Catheron, Robert S. "The Work of the Dental Section of the Harvard Surgical Unit." Paper delivered to the Harvard Dental Alumni between May 1916 and Aug. 1917.

——, "Remembrances of Kazanjian." Unpublished and undated manuscript.

Deranian, H. Martin. "The First Honor Society for Dentists." Paper delivered at the American Academy of Dental Science, April 14, 1987.

Eresian, John G. "A History of the Tomajian and Eresian Families." Chevy Chase, MD., Jan. 30, 1993.

Fickling, B. W. Address at memorial service for William Warick James, the Middlesex Hospital Chapel, Nov. 11, 1965.

Goldwyn, Dr. Robert M. "Dr. Varaztad H. Kazanjian: Relevant or Irrelevant to Our Times?" Paper delivered at American Society of Maxillo-facial Surgery, Seattle, Wash., September 24, 1991.

Leatherman, G. H. "The American Dental Society of London, An Historical Record (1908-1958)." Paper read at the American Dental Society of London, Oct. 14, 1958.

Macalister, A. D. "The Queen's Hospital, Sidcup." Manuscript, unpaged, 1987.

Minutes of Ladies Visiting Committee, *Archivist*, Massachusetts Eye and Ear Infirmary, June 19, 1976

Interviews and Letters (in author's possession)

Aroian, Ruth. Interview, April 19, 2001.

Bom, Adrian. Interview, May 23, 1996.

Booker, Dr. Joshua Charles. Interview, January 13, 2003.

Brigham, Dr. Ferdinand. Interview, October 19, 1967.

Cannon, Dr. Bradford. Interview, January 5, 1979, June 3, 1996 and November 11, 2002

Chakerian, Florence. Letter of June 4, 2001 and October 9, 2002

Cherken, Harry S., Jr. Interview, July 11, 1996.

Chiofaro, Diane. Interview, November 25, 1999.

Cohen, R.A. Letter, March 14, 1996.

Constantian, Dr. Mark B. Letter, February 17, 2000.

Daghlian, Lucy. Interview, August 15, 1996.

Deradoorian, Grace. Interview, September 10, 1989.

Der-Hovanessian, Diana. Letter, November 7, 1988.

Der Kazarian, Marion H. Letter, December 20, 1974.

Desteian, Sylvie (Tahmizian). Personal communication, December 12, 1994.

Dimitrijevic, Dr. Branislav. Letter, July 24, 1991.

Ecker, Dr. Howard M. Interview, November 3, 1999 and Jan. 13, 2003.

Eissler, Kurt. Interview of V. H. Kazanjian, October 26, 1958, Library of Congress, Washington D.C.

Fleming, Robert, Archivist, Emerson College. Letter, May 17, 1999.

Fouey, Joan. Letter, November 19, 2001.

Gardner, Dr. Wallace J. Letter, October 29, 2001.

Goldwyn, Dr. Robert M., and Mullen, Madeleine W. Taped interview of Louise Roopenian, November 22, 1991.

Goldwyn, Dr. Robert M. Letter, Apr. 24, 2002; Interview, April 22, 2002.

Greathead, Philippa. E-mail letters, December 13, 1998 and February 24, 1999.

Guralnick, Dr. Walter C. Interview, June 24, 1996.

Heller, Pat, Librarian, University of Pennsylvania School of Dental Medicine. Letter, March 6, 1998.

Holmes, Martha. Interview, February 4, 2002.

Horrocks, Thomas A. Letter, November 2003 and May 20, 2004.

Kaplan, Dr. Henry. Interview, May 25, 1998.

Kassabian, John. Interview, December 22, 1993.

Kazanjian, Victor C. Interview, September 28, 1976. Letter, March 15, 1982.

Kazanjian, Reverend Victor H., Jr. Interview, February 4, 2002.

Kazanjian, V. H. Letter, April 14, 1945, February 27, 1958 and December 30, 1960. Interview, January 17, 1961, October 19, 1967 and unrecorded dates.

Lane, Virginia (Ring). Interview, February 15, 1999.

Lavelle, Dr. William G. Interview, July 8, 1999.

Malcom, Dr. Edward. Letters, November 28, 1994 and February 27, 1996. Interview, August 5, 1995

Mergerian, Dr. Cliff A, Interview, April 20 and July 8, 1999.

Molnar, Michael. Letter, September 2, 1997 and August 8, 2000.

Monahan, Sean M., Assistant, Special Collections and Archives, Bowdoin College Library. Letter, May 25, 1999.

Montgomery, Dr. William W., John W. Merriam Professor of Otology and Laryngology, Harvard Medical School. Interview, April 20, 1999.

Morse, Dr. leonard J. Letter, November 18 2000 to Janet Sloven and Janice B. Yost.

Murray, Dr. Joseph. Interview, January 23, 1996.

Ogasapian, Marion. Interview, April 6, 1990.

Ohanian, Dr. Roger, and his mother, Flora. Interview, May 5, 1997.

O'Sullivan, Renée Bennett. Letter, December 20, 1999.

Pogarian, Andrea. Letter, August 5, 1999.

Roopenian, Louise. Letter to Virginia Ring Lane, August 11, 1972.

Rustigian, Edward. Interview, April 6, 1990.

Russell, James, Harvard University. Letter, March 2, 1995.

Santoian, Dr. Sherman. Interview, July 15, 1987.

Sargeant, Hélène K. Letter, May 1, 1997 and November 20, 2000. Interview, July 15, 2002, July 29, 2002 and August 16, 2002.

——, Letter to Dr. Robert M. Goldwyn, November 7, 1991.

Stomboulian, Victoria. Interview, March 6, 1995 and Novmber 4, 1992.

Thomason, Dr. Carnig. Interview, July 19, 1995.

Topjian, Betty. Interview, March 1, 1991. Letter, April 1, 1991.

Tenuta, Robert J. Letter. June 6, 1999.

Vickery, Bess P. Letter, December 20, 1998.

Webster, Dr. Richard C. Interview, unrecorded date.

——, Letter to Robert M. Goldwyn, June 4, 1975.

——, Letter to author, August 9, 1948.

Wolfe, Richard J. Letter, September 26, 1969, June 6, Auguat 22, and October 13, 2002.

SECONDARY SOURCES

Books

Aftandilian, Gregory. *Armenia: Vision of a Republic, The Independence Lobby in America*. Boston: Charles River, 1981.

American Guide Series. The Armenians in Massachusetts. American Historical Society, written and compiled by the Federal Writers Project of the Works Progress Administration. Boston, 1937.

Aroian, John H. *Mountains Stand Firm*. New York: Green Hill Publishing, 1977.

Asbell, Milton B. *Dentistry: A Historical Perspective*. Bryn Mawr, Penn.: Dorrance, 1988.

——, *A Century of Dentistry: A History of the University of Pennsylvania School of Dental Medicine*, 1878-1978. University of Pennsylvania, 1977.

Avakian, Linda L. *Armenian Immigrants, Boston 1891-1901, New York 1880-1897*. Camden, Me.: Pictron, 1996.

Bainbridge, William S. *Report on Medical and Surgical Developments of the War*. United States Naval Medical Bulletin. Washington, D.C.: Government Printing Office, 1919.

Barling, Seymour, and Morrison, John T. *A Manual of War Surgery*. London: Oxford University Press, 1919.

Bedoukian, Kerop. *Some of Us Survived: the Story of an Armenian Boy*. New York: Farrar, Straus, Giroux, 1978.

Blair, Vilray P. *Surgery and Diseases of the Mouth and Jaws*. St. Louis: Mosby, 1912.

——, *Surgery and Diseases of the Mouth and Jaws, a Practical Treatise on the Surgery of the Diseases of the Mouth and Allied Structures...3rd ed Revised So As To Incorporate the Latest War Data Concerning Gunshot Injuries of the Face and Jaws*. St. Louis: Mosby, 1917.

Bliss, Edwin M. *Turkey and the Armenian Atrocities*. New York: M. J. Cohlan, 1896.

Boardman, W. E. *Biographies of the Founders of the Masssachusetts Dental Society*. Boston: Frank Brown, 1914.

British Documents on Ottoman Armenians, vol. 2. Ankara: Publication of the Turkish Historical Society, 1983.

Brown, Percy. *American Martyrs to Science Through the Roentgen Rays*. Springfield, Il: Charles Thomas, 1936.

Buck, Gordon. *Contributions to Repairative Surgery*. New York: Appleton, 1876.

Carson, Gerald. *The Dentist and The Empress*. Boston: Houghton Mifflin, 1983.

Castleman, Benjamin; Crockett, David C.; and Sutton, S. B.; eds., *The Massachusetts General Hospital*, 1955-1980. Boston: Little Brown, 1983,

Cheney, Mack L. *Facial Surgery Plastic and Reconstructive*. Baltimore: Williams & Wilkins, 1997.

Converse, John M. *Reconstructive Plastic Surgery.* Philadelphia: Saunders, 1964 vol. 1; also, 2nd ed. Philadeiphia: Saunders, 1977.

——, *Kazanjian & Converse's Surgical Treatment of Facial Injuries*, 3rd. ed. 2 vols. Baltimore: Williams & Wilkins, 1974.

Cushing, Harvey. *The Life of Sir William Osler*. Oxford, England: Clarendon Press, 1925. 2 vols.

——, *From a Surgeon's Journal 1915-1918*. Boston: Little Brown, 1936.

Davis, John S. *Plastic Surgery - Its Principle and Practice*. Philadelphia: Blackiston, 1919.

Dawson, Coningsby. *Carry On, Letters in War-Time*. New York: John Lane, 1917.

de Morgan, Jacques. *History of the Armenian People*, trans. Ernest F. Barry. Boston: Hairenik Press, 1918.

Der Manuelian, Lucy. *Weavers, Merchants and Kings: The Inscribed Rugs of Armenia*. Fort Worth, Tex.: Kimball Art Museum, 1984.

Deranian, Hagop Martin. *Worcester Is America*. Worcester, Mass: Mercantile Press, 1998.

Deranian, Marderos. *Hussenig*. Belmont, Mass.: Armenian Heritage Press, 1994.

Dorland, W. A. Newman. *The American Illulstrated Medical Dictionary*. Philadelphia: Saunders, 1932.

Dunning, James M. *The Harvard School of Dental Medicine: Phase Two in the Development of a University Dental School.* Cambridge, Mass.: The Harvard School of Dental Medicine, 1981.

Filian, George H. *Armenia and Her People.* Hartford: American Publishing Co., 1896.

Foure, Jacques. *American Dental Club, Paris: The First Hundred Years.* Paris Club, 1990.

Francis, Arlene. *That Certain Something: The Magic of Charm.* New York: Julian Messner, Inc., 1960.

——, *Contemporary Theater, Film and Television.* Detroit: Gale Research, 1988.

——, (with Florence Rome) *Arlene Francis, A Memoir.* New York: Simon and Shuster, 1978.

Freud, Sigmund. *Civilization and Its Discontents.* London: Hogath Press, 1955.

Fulton, John F. *Harvey Cushing, a Biography.* Springfield, Il.: Thomas, 1941.

Gaidzakian, Ohan. *Illustrated Armenia and the Armenians.* Boston:

published by author and B. H. Aznive, 1898.

Garretson, James E. *A System of Oral Surgery.* Philadelphia: Lippencott, 1873.

Garsoian, Nina G. *The Epic Histories Attributed to Pawstos Buzand.* Cambridge, Mass: Harvard University Press, 1989.

Gay, Peter, ed. *The Freud Reader.* New York: W. W. Norton & Co., 1989.

——, *Freud A Life for Our Times.* New York: Morton, 1988.

Gillies, H. D. *Plastic Surgery of the Face.* London: Oxford University Press, 1920.

——, and Millard, Ralph, Jr. *Plastic and Reconstructive Surgery.* Boston: Little Brown, 1957.

——, and Millard, Ralph, Jr. *Principles and Art of Plastic Surgery.* Baltimore: Williams & Wilkins, 1971.

Glubb, John. *Into Battle: A Soldier's Diary of the Great War.* London: Book Club Associates, 1978.

Golden, Richard L., and Roland, Charles G., eds. *Sir William Osler, An Annotated Bibliography with Illlustrations.* Norman Bibliography Series, no. 1. San Francisco: Norman

Publishing, 1988.

Graber, G. S. *Caravans to Oblivion, The Armenian Genocide, 1915.* New York: John Wiley, 1996.

Grabill, Joseph L. *Protestant Diplomacy and the Near East.* Minneapolis: University of Minnesota Press, 1971.

Grey, Vincent Edward of Fallodon. *Twenty-five Years, 1892-1916.*New York: Frederick A. Stokes, 1925.

Gunston, Bill. *Aviation: The First One Hundred Years.* Hauppauge, N.Y.: Barrons, 2002.

Haiken, Elizabeth. *Venus Envy: A History of Cosmetic Surgery.* Baltimore: Johns Hopkins Press, 1997.

Handlin, Oscar. *The Uprooted.* New York: Gosset and Dunlap, 1951.

Hapgood, Richard Locke. *History of the Harvard Dental School.* Peterboro, N.H.: Transcript Printing Co., 1930.

Hemingway, Ernest. *A Movable Feast, Sketches of the Author's Life in Paris in the Twenties.* New York: Scribners, 1964.

——, *A Farewell to Arms.* New York: Scribners, 1929.

Holmes, Oliver Wendell. *The Claims of Dentistry.* Boston: Rand, Avery, 1872.

Hopkins, J. Castell. *The Sword of Islam or Suffering Armenia.* Toronto, Canada: Bradley-Garretson, Ltd., 1896.

Hopkins, Samuel A. *The Care of the Teeth.* New York: Appleton, 1902.

Hovannisian, Richard G. *The Republic of Armenia.* Berkley: University of California Press, 1971.

Howe, M. A. DeWolfe, ed. *The Harvard Volunteers in Europe.* Cambridge, Mass.: Harvard University Press, 1916.

Impert, L., and Regal, P. *Fracture of the Lower Jaw.* J. F. Colyer, ed. London: University of London Press, 1918.

Ivy, Robert Henry. *A Link With the Past.* Baltimore: Williams & Wilkins, 1962.

——, and Eby, Joseph D. "Maxillofacial Surgery." *Medical Department of the United States Army in the World War*, vol. 2, Surgery, Part 2. Washington: Government Printing Office, 1924.

James, W. Warwick, and Fickling, B. W. *Injuries of the Jaws and Face with Special Reference to War Casualties.* London: John Bale and Staples, 1940.

Jones, Ernest. *International Psycho-analytical Library, No. 17*. London: Hograth Press, 1930.

——, *The Life and Work of Sigmund Freud*. New York: Basic Books, 1957, vol. 3.

Keegan, John. *The First World War*. New York: Alfred A. Knopf, 1999.

Keep, N. C. *The Aims and Duties of the Dental Profession*. Boston: T. R. Marvin, 1865.

Kévorkian, Raymond H., and Paboudjian, Paul B. *Les Arméniens dans l'Empire Ottoman a la Veille du Génocide*. Paris: Les Éditions d'Art et d'Historie, 1992.

Khorenatsi, Moses. *History of the Armenians*. Robert W. Thomson,trans. Cambridge, Mass: Harvard University Press, 1978.

Kingsley, Norman W. *A Treatise on Oral Deformities as a Branch of Mechanical Surgery*. New York: Appleton, 1880.

Koch, Charles R. E., ed. *Biographies of Pioneer American Dentists and Their Successors*. Chicago: National Art Publishing Co., 1910.

Kolle, Frederick S. *Plastic and Cosmetic Surgery*. New York: Appleton, 1911.

Krikorian, Rebecca K. *Jerusalem*. Kansas City, Missouri: General Foreign Missionary Board Pentecostal Church, 1919.

Kronenberger, Louis, ed. *Alexander Pope, Selected Works*. New York: Random, 1951.

Kurkjian, Vahan M. *A History of Armenia*. New York: Armenian General Benevolent Union of America, 1964.

Lamb, Helen J. *World War I, An American Nurse with the British Troops in France Nov. 1916-Feb. 1919*. Provo, Utah: Stevenson Genealogical Center, 1981.

Lang, David Marshall. *Armenia, Cradle of Civilization*. London: Allen and Unwin, 1970.

Lash, Joseph P. *Eleanor and Franklin: The Story of Their Relationship*. New York: W. W. Norton, 1971.

Latham, Ronald, trans. *The Travels of Marco Polo*. Hammondsworth, N.Y.: 1982.

Lee, Roger I. *Letters from Roger I. Lee, Lt. Col., U. S. Army Medical Corps, 1917-1918*. Brookline, Mass.: Privately printed, 1962.

Lewis, C. Day, ed. *Collected Poems of Wilfred Owen*. Norfolk, Conn.: New Directions, 1963

Luftkin, Arthur W. *A History of Dentistry*. Philadelphia: Lea and Febiger, 1948.

Macdonald, Lyn. *The Roses of No Man's Land*. London: Penguin, 1993.

MacTherson, W. G. *Medical Services General History*, vol. 2. London: His Majesty's Stationery Office, 1923.

Malcom, M. Vartan (Malcom Vartan Malconian). *The Armenians in America*. Boston: Pilgrim Press, 1919.

March, Francis A. *History of the World War*. Philadelphia: United Publishers, 1919.

Martin, Edwin W. *The Hubbards of Sivas, A Chronicle of Love and Faith*. Santa Barbara, Calif.: Fithian Press, 1991.

Marshall, John S. *A Manual of Injuries and Surgical Diseases of the Face, Mouth, and Jaws*. 2nd ed. Philadelphia: S.S. White Company, 1902.

Marshall, S. L. A. *World War I*. Boston: Houghton Mifflin, 1964.

Martin, Claude. *De la Prosthèse Immédiate, Appliqué a la Résection des Maxillaries*. Paris: G. Masson, 1889.

Mason, Francis. *On the Surgey of the Face*. London: Churchill, 1878.

Massachusetts General Hospital, Memorial and Historical Volume. Boston: 1921.

McDowell, Frank. *The Source Book of Plastic Surgery*. Baltimore: Williams & Wilkins, 1977.

Millard, D. Ralph, Jr. *Cleft Craft, The Evolution of Its Surgery*. Boston: Little Brown, 1980.

Miner, Leroy, M. S. *The New Dentistry*. Cambridge, Mass.: Harvard University Press, 1933.

Mitchell, Claudine. *Work and the Image*. London: Ashgate, 2001.

Molnar, Michael. *The Diary of Sigmund Freud, 1929-1939*. London: Hograth Press, 1992.

Mooney, James E. *Worcester Celebration 1722-1972*. Worcester: Commonwealth Press, 1972, section on Armenians by Sadie Takvorian.

Morganthau, Henry. *Ambassador Morgenthau's Story*. Garden City, N.Y.: Doubleday Page, 1919.

Murray, Joseph E. *Surgery of the Soul*. Canton, Mass.: Science History Publications, 2001.

Nalbandian, Louise. *The Armenian Revolutionary Movement*. Berkeley: University of California Press, 1963.

Neary, Michael T. "Industrial Development of the American Steel and Wire Co." M. A. thesis, Clark University, 1933.

Papazian, Bertha S. *The Tragedy of Armenia*. Boston: Pilgrim Press, 1918.

Paletta, Francis X. *History of the American Society of Plastic and Reconstructive Surgery*. Baltimore: Waverly, 1963.

Peter Bent Brigham Hospital Eighth Annual Report for the Year 1921. Cambridge, Mass.: University Press, 1922.

Pound, Reginald. *Harley Street*. London: Michael Joseph, 1967.

——, *Gillies, Surgeon Extraordinary*. London: Michael Joseph, 1964.

Power, D'Arcy, and Lefany, W. R. *Plarr's Lives of the Fellows of the Royal College of Surgeons of England, 1930-1951*. London: The Royal College, 1951. Supplement 1930-1951.

Poynter, F. N. L. *Introduction to Exhibitions [of the Wellcome Institute of the History of Medicine]: Medicine and Surgery in the Great War, 1914-1918*. London: 1968.

Prinz, Herman. *Dental Chronology*. Philadelphia: Lea & Gebiger, 1945.

Reardon, Daniel Bartholomew. *A Brief Biography*. Undated, privately published.

Reynolds, Francis J., and Churchill, Allen L., eds. *World's War Events*, vol. 1. New York: Collier, 1919.

Rice, Franklin P. *Dictionary of Worcester and Its Vicinity.* Worcester: F. S. Blanchard, 1893.

——, ed. *The Worcester of Eighteen Hundred and Ninety-eight*. Worcester: F. S. Blanchard, 1899.

Roberts, John B. *Surgery of Deformities of the Face Including Cleft Palate.* New York: William Wood, 1912.

Romm, Sharon. *The Unwelcome Intruder: Freud's Struggle With Cancer*. New York: Praeger, 1983.

Rosenweig, Roy. *Eight Hours For What We Will: Work and Leisure in an Industrial City, 1870-1920*. Cambridge: Cambridge University Press, 1983.

Schur, Max. *Freud: Living and Dying*. New York: International Universities Press, 1972.

Service With Fighting Men, An Account of the Work of the American Young Men's Christian Association in the World War. New York: Association Press, 1924.

Shapiro, Harry H. *Applied Anatomy of the Head and Neck: Clinical Application of Anatomy in Dental Practice*. 2nd ed. Philadelphia: Lippincott, 1947.

Stepansky, Paul E. *Freud, Surgery and Surgeons.* Hillsdale, N.J.: The Analgetic Press, 1999.

Stevens, Charles E. *Worcester Churches 1719-1889.* Worcester: Lucius Paulinus Goddard, 1890.

Stone, Frank A. *Academies For Anatolia*. Lanham, N.Y.: University Press of America, 1984.

Stone, Orreal L. *History of Massachusetts Industries.* Boston: S. J. Clarke, 1930.

Story of U. S. Army Base Hospital No. 5. Cambridge, Mass.: Harvard University Press, 1919.

Taylor, A. J. P. *Illustrated History of the First World War*. New York: Putnam, 1964.

Taylor, J. A. *History of Dentistry*. Philadelphia: Lea and Febiger, 1922.

The Story of U. S. Army Base Hospital No. 5. Cambridge: University Press, 1919.

Thornton, Jessie May. "Character, Composition, and Distribution of the Southeastern Europeans in Worcester." M.A. thesis, Clark University, 1934.

Thorpe, Burton Lee. "History of Dental Surgery," in Charles E. Koch, ed. *Biographies of Pioneer American Dentists and Their Successors*. vol. 3. Chicago: National Art Publlishing Co., 1910.

Thoumin, Richard, ed. *The First World War*. New York: Putnam, 1963.

Transactions of the New Hampshire Medical Society, May 16, 1916. Manchester, N.H.: John B. Clarke Co., 1916.

Tuchman, Barbara W. *The Guns of August*. New York: Ballantine, 1962.

Villard, Henry S., and Negal, James. *Hemingway in Love and War*. Boston: Northeastern Univ. Press, 1989.

Walker, Christopher J. *Armenia, the Survival of a Nation*. London: Croom Helm, 1980,

Wallace Anthony R. *The Progress of Plastic Surgery: An Introductory History*. Oxford: William H. Meeuws, 1982.

Washburn, Charles G. *Industrial Worcester*. Worcester: Davis Press, 1917.

Wolfe, Richard J., and Menczer, Leonard F., eds. *I Awaken to Glory*. Boston Medical Library, 1994.

Wolfe, S. Anthony, and Berkowitz, Samuel. *Plastic Surgery of the Facial Skeleton*. Boston: Little Brown, 1989.

Work of Anna Coleman Ladd. Boston: Seaver-Howland Press, 1920.

Zeller, Rose. "Changes in the Ethnic Composition and Character of Worcester's Population." PhD. diss., Clark University, 1940.

Books

Armenian

Armenian Encyclopedic Almanac 1925. Boston: Hairenik Press, 1925.

Church of Our Saviour, Minutes.

Dzotsikian, S. M. *The Western Armenian World*. New York: 1947.

Everyone's Yearbook, 1921. Istanbul: H. Hovagimian.

Jizmejian, Manug K. *Kharpert and Her Children*. Fresno: 1955.

Najarian, Hagop T. *The Story of the Armenian Communities in the Diaspora*. New York: Tankian Publishing, Undated.

Patrik, Arakel, ed. *History of the Armenians of Sebastia and Neighboring Villages*. Beirut: Mesrob Press, 1974.

Seropian, Bishop Mushegh. *The American-Armenian Annual Yearbook*. Boston: Cilicia Press, 1913.

Soviet Armenian Encyclopedia, vol. 3. Erevan, Armenia: 1977.

Surmenian, K. *Erzican*. Cairo: Sahag Mesrob Press, 1947.

Tarbassian, Hratch A. *Erzurum [Garin]:Its Armenian History and Traditions*. Garin Compatriotic Union of the U.S., 1975.

Articles and Pamphlets

American Medical Association. *Program of the Scientific Assembly of the Seventy-second Annual Session*. Boston, June 7-10, 1921.

Bainbridge, William S. "Report on Medical and Surgical Developments of the War. *United States Naval Medical Bulletin* (1919).

Battersby, H. F. Prevost. "Surgery's Miracle at the Western Front." *Daily Graphic* (April 22, 1916) and *British Dental Journal* 37 (January-June 1916).

Battle, Richard. "Plastic Surgery in the Two World Wars and the Years Between." *Journal of the Royal Society of Medicine* 71 (November 1978).

Benison, Saul; Barger, A. Clifford; and Wolfe, Elin L. "Walter B. Cannon and the Mystery of Shock: A Study of Anglo-American Co-operation in World War I." *Medical History* 35 (1919).

Blair, Vilray P. "The Aims of the Sub-section of Plastic and Oral Surgery." *Gynecology and Obstetrics* 25 (July to December 1917).

——, "The Maxillofacial Services of the American Army in the War." *Journal of the American Medical Association* 73:5 (August 3, 1919).

——, "The Role of the Plastic Surgeon in the Care of War Injuries." *Annals of Surgery* (May 1941).

——, discussion of paper: V. H. Kazanjian, "Prosthetic Appliances in Surgical Treatment of Wounds of Face and Jaws." *The Dental Summary* (December 1919).

"Princess Marie Bonaparte." Obituary. *New York Times* (September 22 and October 13, 1962).

Brigham, Ferdinand. "Harvard Goes to War." *Harvard Dental Alumni Bulletin* 24:4 (1964).

——, "Dentistry in the Harvard Surgical Unit." *The Mirror (1919)*, Harvard Dental School.

Brophy, Truman W. in Thomas L. Gilmer, "Fifty Years Observation of Oral Surgery." *Journal of the National Dental Association* 9:7 (July 1922).

"Ruth Mack Brunswick." Obituary. *New York Times* (January 26, 1946).

Cabot, Hugh. "Harvard Surgical Unit with the British Expeditionary Force in France." *The Harvard Graduate Magazine* 25:9 (1916-1917).

——, "The Harvard Unit R.A.M.C." *The Harvard Graduates' Magazine* (1919-1920).

Cannon, Bradford. "The Flowering of Plastic Surgery." *Journal of American Medical Association* 263:6 (February 9, 1990).

——, "Varaztad H. Kazanjian 1879-1974," Obituary. *Harvard Medical Alumni Bulletin* (January-February 1975).

——, and Murray, Joseph E. "The Influence of the St. Louis Quadrumvirate of Plastic Surgery." *Plastic and Reconstructive Surgery* 94:4 (April 1995).

"Dr. Henry Carney." Obituary. *Boston Globe* (March 16, 1982).

Cheever, David. "The Work of the Harvard Unit in France." *Harvard Alumni Bulletin* 18:27 (April 5, 1916).

——, "Experiences of the Harvard Unit with the British Expeditionary Force." *Transactions of the New Hampshire Medical Society* (May 16, 1916).

Chiavaro, Angelo. "Organizzazione Metodi Di Cura." *Odontologia* (Rome, 1920).

Cohen, Morris H. "Worcester Ethnics." *Holy Cross Quarterly* 5:3-4 (1973).

Colyer, J. F. "Injuries of the Mandible in Military Practice." *British Dental Journal* 38:1 (January - June 1917).

Converse, John M. "Plastic Surgery: The Twentieth Century, the Period of Growth (1914-1939)." *Surgical Clinics of North America* 47:2 (April 1967).

——, "Robert H. Ivy, M.D., D.D.S." *Plastic and Reconstructive Surgery*, 51:4 (April 1973).

——,"The Extraordinary Career of Doctor Varaztad Hovhannes Kazanjian." *Plastic and Reconstructive Surgery* 71:1 (January 1982).

Cooke, John W. "Kazanjian and Harvard." *Harvard Dental Alumni Bulletin* 3:2 (January 1943).

Cope, Zachary. "In Memoriam: William Warick James." *Annals of the Royal College of Surgeons of England* 37:5 (November 1965).

Cruse, William P. "Auguste Charles Valadier: A Pioneer in Maxillofacial Surgery." *Military Medicine* 152:7 (July 1987).

Currier, Isabell. "The Gentle Genius of Plastic Surgery." *Worcester Sunday Telegram* (May 3, 1932).

Curtis, E. C. "Harvard Men in Hospital Work." *Harvard Graduates Magazine* 24 (September 1915).

Cushing, H. C. "The American Ambulance." *Military Surgeon* 38:605 (1916).

——, "Concerning Operations for the Cranio-Cerebral Wounds of Modern Warfare." *The Military Surgeon* (June 1916).

Cutler Elliott C. "The Organization, Function and Operation of an Evacuation Hospital." *Military Surgeon* (January 1920).

Davenport, John C. "The Prosthetic Case of Sigmund Freud." *British Dental Journal* 172:5 (March 7, 1992).

——, "Der Kranke Sigmund Freud und Seine Zahnarzte." *Zim-Zahnarztliche Mitteilungen* (December 1, 1992).

——, "Sigmund Freud's Illness—The Ultimate Team Approach to Head and Neck Cancer?" *Facial Plastic Surgery* 9:2 (April 1993).

Davenport, W. S. "The Pioneer American Dentists in France and Their Successors." *Revue d'Histoire de l'Art Dentaire* (October 1965).

"William Slocum Davenport." Obituary. *Annals of Dentistry*. (March 1938).

"Dr. William Slocum Davenport, Senr." Obituary. *The Dental Magazine and Oral Topics* (May 1938).

——,. "Multiple Fracture of the Mandible and Lost Substance Restored by Bone-Graft." *Dental Cosmos* 58:10 (October1916).

Davis, John S. "Plastic Surgery in World War I and World War II." *Annals of Surgery* 123:4 (April 1948).

Dawson, Coningsby. "The Glory of the Trenches, the Road to Blighty." *Good Housekeeping* (January 1918).

Deranian, Hagop Martin. "With a Passion for Humanity." *Harvard Dental Alumni Bulletin* 38:2, (1978). Also, *Ararat Quarterly* 76:4 (1978).

Der Kazarian, Marion. "My Recollections of the Laurel Street Church." *The Messenger,* Church of Our Saviour, Worcester, Mass, (May 1987).

Derounian, Avedis. "The Noted Surgeon Prescribes Industry." *The Armenian Spectator* (February 7, 1935).

Desfosses, P. "Nos Amis Les Americains." *Presse Médicale* 30 (May 30, 1919).

Dolamore, W. H. "The Treatment of Injuries of the Face and Jaws at Düsseldorf." War Supplement to the *British Dental Journal* 38:1 (January-June 1917).

Faggart, Harold I. "Dr. James E. Garetson and the First Hospital of Oral Surgery." *Bulletin of the History of Medicine* 17.

Feldman, Eugene M. "Freud's Cancer." *Journal of the History of Dentistry* 47:1 (March 1999).

Fickling, B. W., and Boyes, J. "No End to Talk About: Personal Recollections of the Late William Warwick James." *British Dental Journal* 13:5 (March 4, 1975).

Fickling, Ben W. (B. W. F.). "William Warwick James." Obituary *British Dental Journal* 119:7 (October 5, 1965).

——, " V. H. Kazanjian." Obituary. *British Dental Journal* 138:2 (January 21, 1975).

Field, Robinson. "A Few Remarks on the Role of the American Dentist in Paris During the Great War." *Dental Items of Interest* (March 1923).

Fitzgibbon, G. M. "The Commandments of Gillies." *British Journal of Plastic Surgery* 21:3 (July 1968).

Foure, J. L. "Hippolyte Morestin." Obituaty. *La Presse Médicale* (February 20, 1915).

Foure, Jacques. "The First Hundred Years." (Section on William Davenport) *American Dental Club* (Paris, 1990).

"Arlene Francis." Obituary. *Boston Globe* (June 2, 2001) and *New York Times* (June 2, 2001).

Gillies, Harold. "Experiences With Tubes Pedicle Flaps." *Surgery, Gynecology and Obstetrics* 60:2 (February 15, 1935).

Gilmer, Thomas L. "A Case of Fracture of the Lower Jaw With Remarks on the Treatment." *Archives of Dentistry* (1887).

Gilmour, W. H. "Notes on a Visit to the Military Hospitals at the Base in France and Some Hospitals in Paris." *British*

Dental Journal 37:51 (August 1, 1916).

——, "Immediate Treatment of Gunshot Fracture of the Jaws." *British Dental Journal* 37:15 (1916).

Goldwyn, Robert M. "The Kazanjian Lecture: What Remains." *Aestheic Plastic Surgery* 18 (1994).

Gordon, Noah. "Dr. Varaztad Kazanjian of Belmont Still Active at 80: Immigrant Boy Became `A Miracle Man' of Plastic Surgery in World War." *Boston Sunday Herald* (September 20, 1959).

Guralnick, Walter G. "Varaztad H. Kazanjian, M.D." *New England Journal of Medicine* (April 10, 1975).

——, et al. "V. H. Kazanjian, A Pioneer in Dentistry and Plastic Surgery." *Harvard University Gazette* (May 2, 1975).

——, and Cannon, Bradford. "V. H. Kazanjian, A Pioneer in Dentistry and Plastic Surgery." *Harvard Gazette* (May 2, 1975).

——, "Varaztad H. Kazanjian," Obituary. *Harvard Dental Alumni Bulletin* 35:1 (February 1975).

Haiken, Beth. "Plastic Surgery and American Beauty at 1921." *Bulletin of the History of Medicine* 68:42 (1994).

Hait, Pam. "History of the American Society of Plastic and Reconstructive Surgeons, Inc. 1931-1994." *Journal of Plastic and Reconstructive Surgery* 94:4 (September 1994).

Harding, Robert L. "Robert Henry Ivy, 1881-1974." Obituary. *Plastic and Reconstrucitve Surgery* 55:1 (January 1975).

Harper, Grace S. "New Faces for Mutilated Soldiers." *Red Cross Magazine* 13 (November 1918).

"Dr. George Hayes." Obituary. *San Diego Union* (December 27, 1957).

Hayes, George B. "War Dental Surgery; Some Cases of Maxillo Facial Injuries Treated in the Dental Section of American Ambulance at Neuilly (Paris) France." *Dental Cosmos* 58:3 (March 1916).

Helmi, E. "Le Docteur Claude Martin, de Lyon: Un Technicien de Genie." *La Presse Médical* 925:95 (November 27, 1909).

Holbrook, C. Henry. "Impressions of Sivas 1912." *Journal of Armenian Studies* 5:1 (Winter/Spring 1990-91).

Hughes, John. "Special Report—The Eyes of Armenia, Missions of Mercy." *The Armenian Reporter* (January 11, 1997).

Hyson, John M., Jr., and Foley, Gardner P. H. "James Baxter Bean: The First Military Maxillofacial Hospital." *Maryland State Dental Association Journal* 40:2 (Spring, 1997).

——, "Thomas Brian Gunning and His Splint For Jaw Fractures." *Maryland State Dental Association Journal* 40:1 (Winter 1997).

Ivy, Robert H. "The Mysterious Dr. Valadier." *Plastic and Reconstructive Surgery* 74:4 (April 1971).

——, "Personal Recollections of the Organization and Founders of the American Association of Plastic Surgeons." *Plastic and Reconstructive Surgery* 47:5 (May 1971).

——, "Vilray Papin Blair." *British Journal of Plastic Surgery* 5:4 (January 1953).

——, "Some Circumstances Leading to Organization of the American Board of Plastic Surgery." *Plastic and Reconstructive Surgery* (August 1955).

Jenkins, N. S. "The Influence of American Dentists Upon Europe." *Dental Cosmos* 59 (1917).

K., T. P. "The Late Sir Harold Gillies." *British Journal of Plastic Surgery* 21:3 (1960-1961).

—-, "Vilray Papin Blair. "British Journal of Plastic Surgery." (January 1953).

"Dr. Kenneth A. Kazanjian." Obituary, *Boston Globe* (September 26, 1977).

Leceme, P. and Mondor, H. L. "L'Oeuvre Chirurgicale de H. Morestin." *Journal de Chirargie* 16 (1920).

Lindsay, Lillian. "Sir Frank Colyer." Obituary. *British Dental Journal* 96:8 (April 20, 1954).

Loevy, Hannelor, and Kowitz, Aletha A. "Alfred Kantorowicz, Pediatric Dentistry Innovator." *Journal of Dentistry for Children* (October 1993).

——, "Freud's Oral Problems: The Chicago Connection." *Chicago Dental Society Review* 88:2 (March 1995).

Makins, George H. "The Development of British Surgery in the Hospitals of the Lines of Communication in France." *British Medical Journal* (June 16, 1917).

Mangubar, E. Antonio; Hopping, Steve B.; and Smith, Richard. "Leaders in Cosmetic Surgery: Richard Curtis Webster." *International Journal of Esthetic Surgery* 5:1 (November 1, 1997).

"John Sayre Marshall." Obituary, *San Francisco Examiner* (November 22, 1922).

"Claude Martin." Obituary. *Dental Cosmos* 53 (1911): 497-498.

McAuley, J. E. "Charles Valadier: A Forgotten Pioneer in the Treatment of Jaw Injuries." *Proceedings of Royal Society of Medicine, Section of the History of Medicine* 67 (August 1974).

McDowell, Frank. "History of the American Association of Plastic Surgeons to 1963." *Plastic and Reconstructive Surgery* 32 (1963).

Memorial addressed to the President of the United States and to Congress by the Union of American Veterans of Armenian Birth, April 14, 1920.

Mix, Eldridge. "The Armenians of Worcester." *The Worcester Magazine* 9 (August 1902).

Mouchate, "Hippolyte Morestin." Obituaty. *Paris Médical* 32. no.1010 (1919).

Neiburger, Dr. E. J. Letter to editor, "Freud's Oral Cancer Changed Psychotherapy." *Journal of the Massachusetts Dental Society* 45:4 (Winter, 1997).

O'Brien, Mary Murray. "Boston's Famous Plastic Surgeon Once Worked for Ninety Cents a Week." *Boston Sunday Globe* (March 16, 1952).

Peer, Lydon A. "Robert H. Ivy, D.D.S., M.D., F.A.C.S., Sc.D." *Plastic and Reconstructive Surgery* 4:30 (September 1954).

Pickerell, H. P. "The Queen's Hospital Sidcup." *British Journal of Plastic Surgery* 6 (April 1953-January 1954).

Plumpton, Stephen. "Kazanjian." *Dental Magazine and Oral Topics* 84:5 (October 1967).

Posner, John J. "Dentistry—Vienna to Venice." *Dental Surgery,* (April 1934).

R., M. A. "Sir William Kelsey Fry." Obituary. *British Dental Journal* 115:1 (November 19, 1963).

Richards, David. "Dentistry in England in the 1840s: the First Indications of a Movement Toward Professionalization." *Medical History* (1968).

Ring, Malvin E. "The History of Maxillofacial Prosthetics." *Plastic and Reconstructive Surgery* 87:1.

——, "The Life and World of Dr. George Byron Hayes, Pioneer Maxillofacial Surgeon." *Journal of the History of Dentistry* 4:3 (November 1999).

Robinson, Field. "A Few Remarks on the Role of the American Dentists in Paris During the Great War." *Dental Items of Interest* (March 1923).

Rogers, Blair O. "John Marquis Converse, 1909-1981." Obituary. *Annals of Plastic Surgery* (April 1982).

——, "Hippolyte Morestin (1869-1919)." *Aesthetic Plastic Surgery* (1982).

Romm, Sharon. "The Oral Cancer of Sigmund Freud." *Clinics in Plastic Surgery* 10:4 (October 1983).

Romm, Sharon, and Luce Edward A. "Hans Pichler: Oral Surgeon to Sigmund Freud." *Oral Surgery, Oral Medicine and Oral Pathology* (January 1984).

Romm, Sharon, and Zacher, Judith. "Anna Coleman Ladd: Maker of Masks for the Facially Mutilated." *Plastic and Reconstructive Surgery* 70:1 (July 1982).

"Aram Roopenian." Obituary, *Boston Globe* (June 4, 1975).

Rosenthal, James M. Letter to the Editor. *Boston Herald* (July 1, 1930).

Sandrof, Ivan. "World's Most Famous Plastic Surgeon." *Worcester Sunday Telegram* (January 12, 1958).

Seventy-fifth Anniversary Memorial Booklet. Worcester: Church of the Martyrs, 1892-1967.

"Lt. Gen. Sir Arthur Sloggett." Obituary: *Journal of the Royal Army Medical Corps* 54:1.

Smith, Eugene H. "The Harvard Dental School." *The Harvard Graduates' Magazine* 28 (Sepember 1919).

"Special Awards of the American Society of Plastic and Recontructive Surgery, and of the Foundation of the Society of Plastic and Reconstructive Surgery." *Plastic and Reconstructive Surgery* 9:4 (April 1952).

Steinicki, Eric J.; Young, V. Leroy; Francel, Tom; and Randall, Peter. "Vilray P. Blair, His Surgical Descendants and Their Roles in Plastic Surgical Development." *Plastic and Reconstructive Surgery* 103:7 (June 1999).

Swan, Gary E. "Ichabod Washburn Made Worcester World Center of the Wire Industry." *Worcester Sunday Telegram* (July 16, 1972).

Tashjian, James A. *A Bicentennial History of the Armenian Community of America.* Watertown, Mass:, 1976.

——, "Dr. Varaztad H. Kazanjian, A Profile." *Armenian Review* 1:1 (Winter, 1948).

Thorp, Lee. "History of Dental Surgery." in *Biographies of Pioneer American Dentists and Their Successors.* Chicago: National Art Publishing Co., 1910.

Valadier, A. C., and King, L. A. B. "A Few Appliances of Probable Interest to the Dental Surgeon." *La Restauration Maxillo-Faciale* (January 1918).

——, and Whale, H. Lawson. "A Report on Oral and Plastic Surgery and on Prosthetic Appliances." *British Journal of Surgery* 5:17-20 (July 1917 to April 1918).

Villain, G. "The Physiological Treatment of Fractures and Dislocations." *The Lancet* 1 (June 24, 1916).

"M. Georges Villain." Obituary. *The Dental Magazine and Oral Topics* 55 (May 1938).

"Dr. Georges Villain." Obituary. *Journal of the American Dental Association* 25:7 (July 1938).

Villard, Henry S. "A Prize Specimen of Wounded Hero," in "The World Wars Remembered." *Yankee Magazine* (1979).

Verazin, M. "Professor Varaztad Kazanjian: His Surgery During the Great War." *Hairenik Monthly* 8:2/95 (September 1930). [in Armenian]

——, "A Famous Oral and Plastic Surgeon." *Hairenik Daily* (May 8, 1930). [in Armenian]

WGBH Educational Foundation. *Nova Booklet* #1015. 1983.

W., T. G. "Great Teachers of Surgery in the Past: Sir William Kelsey Fry (1889-1963)." *British Journal of Surgery* 53:4 (April 1966).

Waldron, Carl W. "A Testimonial to Varaztad Kazanjian." *Journal of Oral Surgery* 13:2 (April 1955).

Webster, Jerome P. "Vilray P. Blair 1871-1915," in Frank McDowell. *The Source Book of Plastic Surgery.*

——, "In Memoriam: Sir Harold Delf Gillies 1887-1960." *Plastic and Reconstructive Surgery* 27:1 (January 1961).

Webster, Richard C. "Cosmetic Surgery: Its Past, Present and Future." *The American Journal of Cosmetic Surgery* 1 (1984).

"Dr. Richard C. Webster." Obituary. *Boston Globe* (September 28, 1994).

Whale, H. Lawson. "A Report on Oral and Plastic Surgery and on Prosthetic Appliances." *The British Journal of Surgery* (July 1917).

Whitlock, Brad. "The Tragedy of Edith Cavell," in Francis J. Reynolds and Allen L. Churchill, *World's War Events.* New York: Collier, 1919.

Wood, Francis D. "Masks for Facial Wounds." *The Lancet* 1 (June 23, 1917).

INDEX

C

N

O

P

Q

R

S

T

U